T0354051

Praise for *The Modern Herbal Dispensatory*

"*The Modern Herbal Dispensatory* relies on the solid foundation that comes from direct interaction with living, breathing botanicals. To this it adds a specificity gleaned from twenty-first century science: clear guidelines rooted in chemistry and physiology provide definitive answers to questions of extraction method, solvent, timing, and formulation. If you've ever wondered which extraction method to use for a given plant, or felt reluctant to try advanced techniques like percolation, this clear and concise reference guide will become a trusted companion. A must-have for herbal educators, clinicians, and manufacturers alike!"

—Guido Masé, cofounder and codirector, Vermont Center for Integrative Herbalism

"Thomas Easley and Steven Horne have done it once again. In the *Modern Herbal Dispensatory*, historic traditions of medicine making have been captured and shared in a way that empowers the modern lay herbalist to capture the benefits of botanical medicine in the most accessible and potent form. Weaving together folk teachings and scientific perspectives, this book bridges the spectrum of herbal medicine to provide an inspiring, detailed, and practical handbook for herbalists at all levels of experience. This guide should be on the bookshelves of every herbal school, home apothecary, and herbal production facility."

—Emily Ruff, executive director, Florida School of Holistic Living

THE
MODERN HERBAL DISPENSATORY

A MEDICINE-MAKING GUIDE

THOMAS EASLEY

STEVEN HORNE

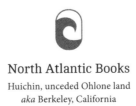

North Atlantic Books
Huichin, unceded Ohlone land
aka Berkeley, California

Published by
North Atlantic Books
Huichin, unceded Ohlone land
Berkeley, California

Cover and book design by Howie Severson/Diana Rosinus
All photos by Terrie Easley unless otherwise noted
Printed in the United States of America

Cover art credits (clockwise from upper-left): (1) "Eupatorium perfoliatum. (bone-set. thoroughwort)." New York Public Library Digital Collections. http://digitalcollections.nypl.org/items/510d47dc-4fde-a3d9-e040-e00a18064a99; (2) "Common Yarrow (Achillea Millefolium)." Public domain. www.briar-gate.org; (3) www.flickr.com/photos/biodivlibrary/10575241163; (4) "Smilacina racemosa" New York Public Library Digital Collections. http://digitalcollections.nypl.org/items/510d47dd-ef5a-a3d9-e040-e00a18064a99; (5) iStockphoto.com/Craig McCausland; (6) Mentha Piperita by J.H. Colen, taken from Illustrations of Medical Botony by Joseph Carson, M.D.; (7) iStockphoto.com/Craig McCausland; (8) "Poppy, California" New York Public Library Digital Collections. Accessed. http://digitalcollections.nypl.org/items/510d47d9-9c7f-a3d9-e040-e00a18064a99; (9) Anicula Europaea, plate 357 by Otto Wilhelm Thomé, Flora von Deutschland, Österreich u.d. Schweiz, Gera (1885).

MEDICAL DISCLAIMER: The following information is intended for general information purposes only. Individuals should always see their health care provider before administering any suggestions made in this book. Any application of the material set forth in the following pages is at the reader's discretion and is their sole responsibility.

The Modern Herbal Dispensatory: A Medicine-Making Guide is sponsored and published by North Atlantic Books, an educational nonprofit based in the unceded Ohlone land Huichin (Berkeley, CA) that collaborates with partners to develop cross-cultural perspectives; nurture holistic views of art, science, the humanities, and healing; and seed personal and global transformation by publishing work on the relationship of body, spirit, and nature.

North Atlantic Books's publications are distributed to the US trade and internationally by Penguin Random House Publisher Services. For further information, visit our website at www.northatlanticbooks.com.

Library of Congress Cataloging-in-Publication Data
Names: Easley, Thomas, 1982– , author. | Horne, Steven H., author.
Title: The modern herbal dispensatory : a medicine-making guide /
    Thomas Easley and Steven Horne.
Description: Berkeley, California : North Atlantic Books, [2016] |
    Includes bibliographical references and index.
Identifiers: LCCN 2016013141 (print) | LCCN 2016013649 (ebook) |
    ISBN 9781623170790 (print) | ISBN 9781623170806 (ebook)
Subjects: | MESH: Plants, Medicinal | Plant Preparations |
    Phytotherapy--methods | Formularies
Classification: LCC RM666.H33 (print) | LCC RM666.H33 (ebook) |
    NLM QV 740.1 | DDC 615.3/21—dc23
LC record available at http://lccn.loc.gov/2016013141

16 17 18 VERSA 27 26 25 24

North Atlantic Books is committed to the protection of our environment. We print on recycled paper whenever possible and partner with printers who strive to use environmentally responsible practices.

To my wife, Terrie. Two books in three years of marriage isn't easy, and I couldn't have done it, or anything for that matter, without you.

—THOMAS

I dedicate this book to the Utah midwives who taught the first class I attended on herbal medicine making and got me started in the wonderful world of making herbal products.

—STEVEN

Acknowledgments

Thomas would like to thank his wife for the incredible photography. It really ties the whole book together. He would also like to thank his former intern and editor Esther Mack for making his contributions to the book more concise and understandable.

Steven wishes to acknowledge the help of his staff at the School of Modern Herbal Medicine, including David Horne, Garret Pittario, and Kenneth Hepworth, for helping to compile and edit some of the material in this book.

Contents

On Herbal Medicine

Herbal medicine is one of the most ancient of the healing arts. It is, and always will be, the medicine of the people. No matter which political party is in power, no matter what is deemed legal versus illegal, not even the FDA in all of its regulatory glory can prevent someone from stepping out their door and using nature's free medicine. Herbal medicine exists, and always has, because we live in symbiosis with plants. As herbalist Sam Coffman says, with every breath we take we perform mouth-to-mouth resuscitation with nature. Plants have been here longer than we have. They have learned their lessons and adapted to their environment, and they have produced a beautiful language to communicate those lessons with other plants, animals, and fungi. The chemical compounds that plants produce, their biochemical language, is so complicated that we haven't even scratched the surface in the thousand or so plants that have been researched, let alone the remaining tens of thousands of plants around the world that are used as medicine.

Although we may not understand how plants act chemically in our body, we have a long and well-documented history of their use as food and medicine. As we move toward a more sustainable world with clean energy production, locally grown organic foods, and nature conservation, we must look at our current model of medicine through the same filter of sustainability. A world that remains totally dependent on high-cost chemical medicines, controlled by multinational pharmaceutical companies whose main purpose is profit, is dependent upon the very institutions that created the environmental problems that are poisoning this world.

Modern medicine and the judicious use of pharmaceuticals are essential for treating many serious illnesses. But although it is a great disease-care system, modern medical care is not a health care system. Any system of medicine that is separated from the greater whole of health, including food production, ecological health, social health, and emotional health, can only put a bandage on a bullet wound, conveniently masking the real issues that are slowly bleeding us to death. Rising costs for disease care and lack of access to care are taking a toll on everyone, and minorities and underprivileged groups bear the brunt of that burden. In America, disease care is the primary cause of financial ruin: Nearly two million people file bankruptcy every year because of medical bills.

USING HERBS AS MEDICINE

Medicinal plants grow everywhere and are easily available for harvest or purchase for a fraction of the cost of modern pharmaceuticals. Learning how to make your own herbal medicines is as easy as learning how to cook. The goal of this book is to empower you to use herbs to help yourself, your family, and others.

Mastering herbalism involves a lot of work. Different herbs with entirely different medicinal actions can have the same common name. Conversely, the same herb can be called many different names depending on what book you are looking at. Learning the Latin (botanical) name of a plant is a good place to start to identify the correct herb, but identifying the right plant is just the first step.

Different parts of a single plant can have different actions on the body. The root of dandelion is a wonderful digestive tonic and gently stimulates phase one liver detoxification. Dandelion leaves, on the other hand, are a strong diuretic; and the flowers, prepared as a flower essence or a wine, are specific for helping overachievers who are tense and stressed to learn to go with the flow.

How you use an herb makes a difference in how it affects the body. Different constituents are soluble in different mediums. Some constituents of plants are exclusively alcohol soluble, whereas others only come out in water. Yarrow is a great herb for fevers when it is prepared as a hot infusion (tea) of the flowers. A hot infusion draws out the aromatic qualities of yarrow that stimulate circulation and promote perspiration, whereas a decoction extracts more of the bitter and astringent principles. Many Native Americans used a cooled decoction of the whole herb (flowers and leaves) as a digestive tonic for weak digestion. The dried leaves make an excellent styptic for cuts and wounds, and encapsulated yarrow clears the lymphatics, stimulates innate immunity, and helps relieve urinary tract infections. Yarrow essential oil is anti-inflammatory, but most of this oil is lost when the herb is dried. Yarrow flower essence is used to help sensitive individuals who overidentify with other people's problems (a characteristic that comes naturally to many herbalists).

Some books list yarrow as being good for toothache; the Diné (Navajo) and other Native Americans use yarrow for this purpose. But swallowing a capsule or tincture won't do anything for a toothache, nor will chewing on dried mature leaves. The part of the plant that is used for toothache is the purplish part of the young leaves, which contain a topical analgesic. The fresh young leaves are chewed to relieve tooth pain. As you can see, knowing how a plant is prepared and how that changes its usage is an important part of effective herbalism.

Much of the information about how to properly prepare and administer herbs is being lost as people increasingly rely on commercial herbal preparations. Traditional herbalists keep the knowledge of how to make and use herbs alive. This book aims to present different methods for preparing and administering herbs to help you choose not only the appropriate remedy but the preparation method that brings forth the actions you want. We hope it will help you learn to use herbs in new and creative ways.

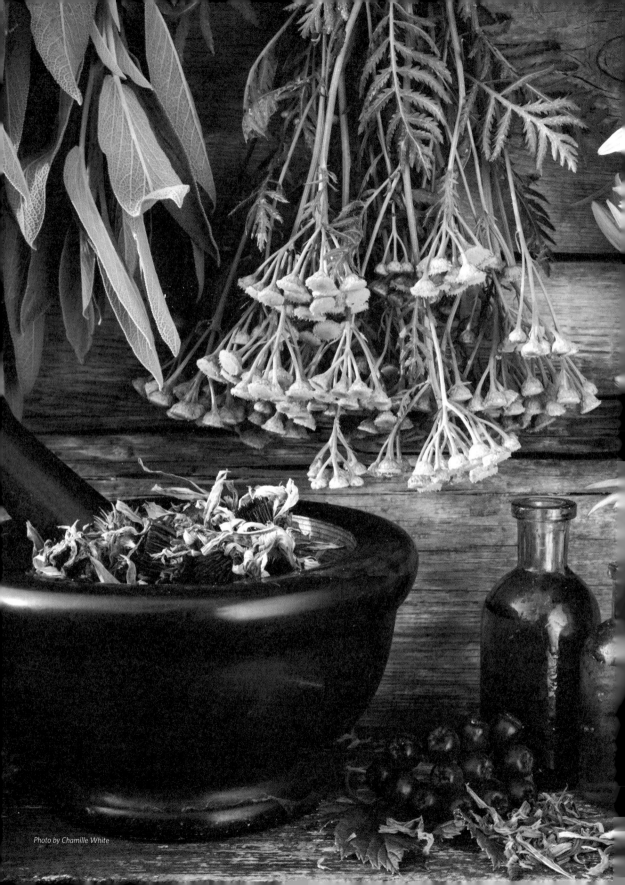

CHAPTER ONE

Getting Started

BASIC CONCEPTS IN HERBAL MEDICINE

This book is about making herbal medicines, and if you're going to make effective herbal medicines, you need to be familiar with some basic concepts.

HERBAL ENERGETICS

The major constituents that give herbs their various actions can be detected using human senses. The effects of these basic constituents can be felt and observed in one's own body. This observation and detection are what modern Western herbalists call energetics.

Herbs can be divided into broad energetic categories based on their taste, constituents, and basic effects on the body. Learning these basic categories is like learning the alphabet or musical notes: They form the basis for understanding the language of herbalism. Just as musical notes are arranged together to create an infinite array of music, the energetic properties of herbs blend together to create thousands of unique herbal profiles.

The twelve basic categories of herbs we're about to introduce you to have some basic qualities in common. We refer to these in energetic terms, using three sets of qualities.

HOW HERBS AFFECT ENERGY PRODUCTION

- **Warming** refers to herbs that stimulate or speed up metabolism, increase energy production and warmth, and bring blood flow and vitality to tissues that are pale and cool.
- **Cooling** refers to herbs that sedate or slow down metabolism to decrease energy production while cooling or soothing irritation and redness.
- **Neutral** describes herbs that are neither warm nor cool. Neutral herbs do not have a strong effect on circulation or cellular metabolism.

HOW HERBS AFFECT THE DENSITY OF TISSUES

- **Moistening** refers to herbs that increase the moisture content of tissues, which means they lubricate and soften dry, brittle, or hardened tissues.
- **Drying** refers to herbs that remove excess fluid from tissue, causing it to become more firm and dense, relieving conditions of dampness and swelling.
- **Balancing** is the term we use for herbs that normalize tissues that are either damp or dry, helping to balance the amount of moisture and solids (minerals) within the tissues.

HOW HERBS AFFECT MUSCLE TONE, FLOW, AND SECRETION

- **Constricting** refers to herbs that increase the tone or tension within muscles and other tissues, which stops excess flow and secretion. These herbs tone up tissues that have become overly relaxed or weak and that are leaking or secreting fluids such as blood or mucus.
- **Relaxing** refers to herbs that relax muscle cramps and spasms, relieving excess tension in the tissues. This promotes easier flow and movement and can help to increase deficient secretion.
- **Nourishing** is the term we use for herbs that provide essential nutrients that aid tissue healing, improving tissue structure and function.

THE TWELVE CATEGORIES OF HERBS

With this basic understanding of energetic terms, let's look at the twelve categories of herbs referred to in this book. Keep in mind that any individual herb may fit into more than one category.

PUNGENT HERBS

Pungent herbs have a spicy or hot taste and typically have a very sharp aroma. These are plants that are used to add spiciness to dishes, such as capsicum (cayenne pepper), ginger, mustard, and onions. The pungent flavor of these herbs is due to the presence of resins, alkamides, allyl sulfides, or monoterpene essential oils.

Herbs with a pungent taste are warming and drying. They move blood and energy upward toward the head and outward from the interior of the body to the skin and mucous membranes. This means they help to dispel stagnation, induce perspiration, and stimulate blood circulation. They stimulate production of digestive secretions, which enhances appetite, expels gas, and increases intestinal peristalsis.

Overuse of pungent herbs depletes the body's energy reserves and cools the body. Some people find these herbs irritating to their digestive tract. Pungent herbs are contraindicated for people who tend to be hot, flushed, and irritable and who have a reddish complexion.

AROMATIC HERBS

Aromatic herbs contain volatile oils (also called essential oils). Volatile oils evaporate when they are exposed to heat and light. Like pungent herbs, many aromatics are used as seasonings in food. The mint and carrot families contain many aromatic herbs, including dill, peppermint, and lemon balm.

Aromatic herbs are also normally warming and drying, but they have a milder action than pungent herbs. They tend to have strong effects on the nervous system, either calming or stimulating. Many essential oils are antimicrobial, which makes aromatic herbs helpful in fighting infections. Aromatics can induce perspiration when taken as hot tea, and they stimulate blood circulation and expel intestinal gas.

Aromatic herbs are very safe. However, pure essential oils should be used almost exclusively in topical applications; even then, they need to be well diluted. Essential oils are highly concentrated extracts, and they are far more likely than whole herbs to create bad reactions.

SIMPLE (NONALKALOIDAL) BITTERS

Simple bitters are herbs that are bitter due to what old herbal textbooks called bitter principles. Today we know these compounds as diterpenes and various glycosides. Anthraquinone glycosides are responsible for the action of stimulant laxatives, which are a subcategory of simple bitters. Nonalkaloidal bitters include artichoke leaf, gentian, wild lettuce, kale, and hops. Stimulant laxatives include cascara sagrada, Turkey rhubarb, buckthorn, butternut bark, and aloe leaf (not the gel).

Most nonalkaloidal bitters are cooling and drying. A few contain aromatic compounds that make them warming and drying, including dong quai and turmeric.

Bitters cause energy to move downward (toward the eliminative organs) and inward (toward the digestive organs). Nonalkaloidal bitters tend to be detoxifying. Some have sedative or calming effects and a few are anodynes, which means they help to relieve pain. One of their primary uses is to stimulate the production of hydrochloric acid, bile, and pancreatic enzymes. This happens only when the bitters are tasted; bitter herbs that are sweetened or swallowed in capsules do not stimulate digestive secretions.

Cooling bitters can deplete digestion over time. Traditional digestive tonics include warming bitters, aromatic or pungent herbs to modulate the depleting effects of cooling bitters. Bitters should be avoided by thin, weak, emaciated, and dry people.

ALKALOIDAL BITTERS

Alkaloidal bitters taste bitter due to the presence of alkaloids. These compounds have names ending in -ine, such as caffeine, nicotine, and berberine.

Coffee and chocolate are alkaloidal bitters. Herbs that contain alkaloids include goldenseal, Oregon grape, and California poppy.

Like nonalkaloidal bitters, alkaloidal bitters tend to be cooling and drying. Many are detoxifying and used to stimulate the digestive system and liver. Alkaloidal bitters that contain berberine, such as goldenseal and Oregon grape, are used to fight infections. Alkaloids have very specific effects on the nervous and glandular systems and can mimic hormones and neurotransmitters, stimulating or sedating specific body processes.

Alkaloidal bitters have the same general contraindications that nonalkaloidal bitters do. They should be avoided by thin, weak, emaciated, and dry people, and can be drying and depleting when excessively used. Pay attention to the specific indications and contraindications for each herb in this category.

FRAGRANT BITTERS

Fragrant bitters are a cross between simple bitters and aromatics. Their primary constituents are sesquiterpene lactones and triterpenes. Examples of fragrant bitters include elecampane, black walnut hulls, wormwood, tansy, and wormseed.

Fragrant bitters are warming and drying. They are used in small amounts to stimulate appetite and digestion. Many are used to expel parasites. Most fragrant bitters are contraindicated in pregnancy, and many are not suitable for long-term use. They also have the same general contraindications as the other two classes of bitters.

ACRID HERBS

Acrid herbs are characterized by a bitter, nasty, burning taste that is much like the taste of throwing up bile. These herbs contain resins (like pungent herbs) and alkaloids (like alkaloidal bitters). The best examples of this taste are lobelia and kava-kava, but this characteristic is found to a lesser degree in black cohosh, skunk cabbage, and blue vervain.

Acrid herbs tend to be relaxing, which means they are diffusive, opening up the flow of blood, lymph, and energy. They may also be cooling and drying. Their primary action tends to be antispasmodic, which means they relax cramps. They are used to relieve what are known as wind disorders in some traditional systems of medicine. These are disorders that involve alternating symptoms like fever and chills or diarrhea and constipation. Pains that migrate from one part of the body to another are also part of the pattern of wind disorders. Acrid herbs will often induce vomiting in large doses, and large doses or long-term use may adversely affect the nerves.

ASTRINGENT HERBS

Astringent herbs are herbs that contain tannins. Tannic acid gives plants a slightly bitter taste and produces a drying, slightly puckering sensation in the mouth. Green tea is astringent. Other astringent herbs include white oak bark, uva ursi, and sage.

Astringent herbs constrict and dry tissues. They are used to arrest excessive secretions, tighten loose tissue, reduce swelling, and help blood coagulate. They are antivenomous when applied topically to bites and stings. Internally, they slow intestinal peristalsis (counteracting loose, watery stool) and tone up intestinal membranes.

Because they tend to inhibit digestive secretions, and may interfere with mineral absorption, astringents are best taken between meals. Large doses can cause constipation, and long-term use can be irritating to the skin and mucous membranes.

SOUR HERBS

Many berries and fruits have a sour taste due to the presence of various fruit acids (citric, malic, and ascorbic acid), which are accompanied by flavonoids. Flavonoids are antioxidant and fever reducing.

Sour herbs are cooling and nourishing. They may be balancing, slightly moistening, or slightly drying. They are used to reduce tissue inflammation and irritation and reduce free radical damage (thought to cause aging and degenerative disease). They can strengthen capillary integrity and tone weak tissues. Sour herbs are considered good for the liver and eyes, two organs that use more antioxidants than any other organs. They are safe foods and have no contraindications.

SALTY HERBS

The salty taste in plants isn't like the taste of table salt. It's a more subtle flavor that is sort of a grassy or green taste. Think of the flavor of celery or spinach. The subtle salty flavor in these foods is due to the presence of mineral salts: Magnesium, potassium, sodium, and calcium. Salty herbs are green herbs like alfalfa, mullein, and seaweeds.

Salty herbs are balancing and nourishing. They can moisten dry tissues and can dry damp tissues. They are nutritive because they supply minerals that help to tone and heal tissues. They clear the lymphatics, promote lymph flow, loosen mucus, and soften swollen lymph nodes. Many salty herbs are nonirritating diuretics that nourish and support kidney function. They are generally mild in action and have no contraindications.

SWEET HERBS

Sweet herbs aren't sweet in the same way that sugar or honey is sweet. It's more like the sweetness of a bar of dark chocolate. This sweetness is due to the presence of polysaccharides or saponins. Obvious examples of sweet herbs include licorice and stevia, and many tonic and adaptogenic remedies such as American or Korean ginseng, codonopsis, and astragalus are sweet as well.

Sweet herbs tend to be moistening and neutral, but they may be slightly warming or cooling. Sweet herbs are used to build up weakened conditions, counteract wasting, strengthen glands, and replenish energy reserves. They counteract dryness and aging in tissues and often act as immune tonics to either stimulate or balance immune functions.

Most sweet herbs are very benign and suitable for long-term use in small doses. Larger doses can overstimulate the body and are abused in the same way as stimulants like coffee, especially when used by younger people. They often work better as part of a formula than taken as single remedies.

MUCILANT HERBS

Most books call these herbs mucilaginous or demulcent herbs, but we use the word "mucilant." Mucilants have a bland or slightly sweet taste, but their most important distinguishing feature is their texture. When moistened, they have a slippery, slimy texture. This is due to water-loving polysaccharides or mucopolysaccharides, such as gums, mucilage, or pectin. They may also contain glycosaminoglycans.

Okra is a mucilant. Herbal examples include aloe vera, slippery elm, and kelp.

Mucilants are moistening, cooling, and nourishing. They are used to soothe tissues that are hot, red, dry, and irritated. Taken internally, they add water-soluble fiber to the stool; they are bulk laxatives when they are taken with plenty of water. They can help to arrest diarrhea, too. Mucilants feed and support friendly gut bacteria and promote general intestinal health. They absorb bile from the gallbladder and liver to help reduce cholesterol and remove toxins from the body. Mucilants protect mucous membranes and are applied topically as poultices to soothe irritated or damaged skin and promote healing.

Because they are absorbent, mucilants should be taken apart from nutrients and medications. Excessive use can slow down and cool gastrointestinal function, but this can easily be counteracted by adding a small amount of an aromatic or pungent herb. Mucilants must be taken with plenty of water in order to work properly.

OILY HERBS

Oily herbs, mostly seeds, have an oily taste and texture due to the presence of fatty acids. Oily herbs include flaxseed, evening primrose seed, and coconut.

Oily herbs are nourishing and cooling. They provide the body with fatty acids that are used for energy production and immune, nerve and glandular function. (Borage and evening primrose oils are marketed as remedies to influence prostaglandin function.) Oily herbs moisten dry tissues and promote tissue flexibility Some are mild laxatives, lubricating the stool for easier elimination. Oily herbs have no real contraindications.

THE SIX TISSUE STATES

The six tissue states model originated with clinical herbalist Matthew Wood. The six tissue terrains refer to the tissues of the body and complement the basic energetics of herbs we introduced in the beginning of this chapter. Tissue terrain imbalances may be systemic or tissue- or organ-specific. Identifying terrain states and using remedies that restore balance to the tissues will achieve far better results than trying to match herbs with diseases.

The tissue states include three basic tissue qualities that are divided into opposing imbalances. The first of these tissue factors is the metabolic rate, which is how fast or slow the tissues generate energy. Tissues can be overactive (hyperactive or hyperfunctioning) or they can be underactive (hypoactive or hypofunctioning). These correspond to the qualities of heat (overactive) and cold (underactive). We call the hyperactive state *irritation,* and the hypoactive state *depression.*

The second tissue quality is density, which relates to the ratio of solid (mineral) elements to fluid elements (water and fats). When fluids exceed solids, the tissues are in a state of *stagnation,* as in a swamp. When solids outbalance fluids, the tissues get hard and dry, a state that is referred to as *atrophy.* These two tissue states are also called dampness (stagnation) and dryness (atrophy).

The third tissue quality is tension. This has to do with the tone of the tissues in general, and specifically with muscle tone. Excess tone results in *constriction,* and a lack of tone results in an atonic state of excess *relaxation.*

These six basic imbalances—irritation (heat), depression (cold), stagnation (dampness), atrophy (dryness), constriction (tension), and relaxation (atony)—can occur in isolation or in combination (such as irritation and constriction or dampness and depression). Start with the basic imbalances and eventually you will be able to identify the more complex mixtures of imbalance.

ENERGY PRODUCTION

Irritation and *depression* have to do with metabolism and energy generation. In irritation energy production is excessive; in depression it is deficient.

Irritation has a strong correlation to oxidation, inflammation, and fever, which is why it is often referred to as "heat" in traditional herbalism. Tissues that are irritated are red and warm to the touch. Irritation is often accompanied by sharp pains. A red tongue, a rapid pulse, a ruddy (or reddish) complexion, and hyperactivity are also signs of heat or irritation.

Irritation can be caused by chemical, infectious, or metabolic irritants. Tissues in the body increase their production of energy to try to overpower the irritant. Irritation is the mechanism by which cells initiate the healing process through inflammation. Part of the job of the inflammatory response is to destroy damaged cells and draw immune and stem cells to the area for tissue repair. Acute irritation isn't a bad thing; it's when that irritation becomes chronic that problems arise.

Irritation is balanced with cooling and moistening herbs. Sour herbs are the primary remedy for reducing irritation, but mucilants, oily herbs, sweet tonics, and some bitters are also cooling to irritated tissues.

Depression is the opposite of irritation. Tissues that are depressed are cool to the touch and pale, which is why depression is often referred to in traditional herbalism as "cold." If pain is present, it tends to be dull and achy. Other signs of tissue depression are hypoactive function, a pale complexion, a pale tongue, and a slow pulse rate.

Tissue depression is tricky to treat because it can be mimicked by false cold caused by low thyroid function and anemia. Infection in depressed tissues can also give rise to false heat. True tissue depression presents with a general feeling of fatigue, a pale or dark-purple tongue, and a slow pulse rate.

Tissue depression is balanced herbally with warming remedies. Aromatic and pungent herbs are the primary category used here, but warming fragrant bitters may also be helpful.

Pay attention to the energetics of the condition and use remedies with the appropriate properties. Treating hot (irritated) conditions with warming herbs, or cold (depressed) conditions with cooling herbs, will not balance the body.

MINERALS AND FLUIDS

Stagnation and *atrophy* have to do with the balance between the solid (mineral) components of the body and the fluid (water and fat) components in the body. In stagnation, there is too much fluid with insufficient minerals to move it. In atrophy, the mineral content is too high and there is not enough fluid to keep it in solution.

In **stagnation,** fluid accumulates in tissues. This can take the form of edema, swollen lymph nodes, and sluggish flow of body fluids. In traditional herbalism, stagnation is often called "dampness." Tissues that have stagnation are soft and spongy or hard and swollen to the touch. The tongue is pale and damp and the pulse feels congested or slippery.

Stagnation was called *torpor* by the Eclectic physicians of the mid-1800s and early 1900s. Herbs that relieved torpor were called alteratives or blood puri-fiers. Alteratives alter the extracellular fluid around the cells by stimulating immunity or improving blood and lymph flow. Bitter herbs break up stagna-tion. Aromatic, pungent, and astringent herbs help to dry up the dampness of stagnation.

Atrophy is seen when tissues become hard and brittle. When tissues are deficient in good fats and water, they become hard and inflexible or brittle. Traditional herbalism refers to this tissue state as "dryness." Many of the dis-eases of aging are dry, including bone spurs, arterial plaque, the stiffness of arthritis, and the loss of elasticity in the lungs in emphysema. Dry, wrinkled skin associated with aging and the brittle bones of osteoporosis are examples of atrophy. The tongue tends to be dry and withered, and the pulse becomes thin and weak.

Herbs used to treat conditions of atrophy are sometimes called tonics, and they help to revitalize people when they become weak or sickly. Sweet, muci-lant, and oily herbs help to balance atrophy.

Drying herbs will not help atrophy, and moistening herbs will not help stag-nation. There are neutral remedies that can be used in atrophy or stagnation to balance the solids and liquids within the body. We refer to them as *balancing*.

TISSUE TONE

The final pair of opposing imbalances has to do with muscle tension or tone. Muscles control the flow of energy and fluids in the body. When muscles tense, flow is reduced or obstructed. When muscle tone becomes too relaxed or tis-sues are damaged, fluids can drain or leak from tissues. In constriction, muscles are tight, and relaxation occurs when muscles are relaxed or tissues are dam-aged and leaking.

Constriction typically happens because muscles get tired from overuse. Muscles expend energy when they contract, and rebuild energy when they relax. When muscles fatigue, either due to excessive use or to nutritional deficiencies, they spasm. This can cause sharp pain and constricted movement. Constriction occurs in some cases of high blood pressure, tension headaches, asthma attacks, and a spastic colon.

Constriction can periodically relax, causing the dam to break and excessive flow or secretion to occur. Alternating diarrhea and constipation, alternating fever and chills, and migrating pains are examples of this. These are called wind disorders in some traditional systems of medicine.

Antispasmodic herbs are used in conditions of constriction. Antispasmodics are primarily acrid in nature, but some are aromatic, relaxing nervines.

Relaxation occurs when tissues are unable to hold fluids due to damage or loss of muscle tone. Relaxation occurs in diarrhea, leaky gut, excessive mucus production, bleeding, urinary incontinence, and excessive sweating. Astringent herbs counteract relaxation.

You can learn more about the tissue states in Matthew Wood's *The Practice of Traditional Western Herbalism* and in his two-volume work *The Earthwise Herbal.*

GETTING THE RESULTS YOU WANT

To get good results with any health care, you need a correct diagnosis or assessment, and you need to select the right remedy, which includes administering it in the correct way and at an effective dose.

STEP ONE: GET A CORRECT ASSESSMENT

The rising interest in holistic health has led to a huge increase in the number of people using herbal medicine. This use is divorced from traditional systems of diagnosis. Western medical diagnosis is useful, but it is often centered around symptomatic relief rather than addressing the root cause for true healing.

People who use herbs as symptom-relieving remedies will often find themselves disappointed with the results. Herbs are not isolated chemical compounds or magic bullets, and most herbs don't target specific biochemical reactions to create rapid changes in symptoms like pharmaceuticals do. Herbs, like foods, contain thousands of chemical compounds that interact with the body in extremely complex ways. There are herbs that do act in the body in strong ways, including some toxic botanicals, but even these remedies have more complex actions than the singular chemical compounds used in modern medicine.

The good news is that this makes them relatively free of side effects. The bad news is that herbs aren't very good at relieving symptoms, which actually isn't so bad when you think about it. Herbs bring about balance in the body, as we've just explained in our discussion of basic herbal categories and biological terrain. Herbs are best used in conjunction with diet and lifestyle changes that address underlying causes of disease.

This leads us to more good news. All traditional systems of medicine, such as traditional Chinese medicine (TCM), Ayurvedic medicine from India, indigenous traditions of medicine, and even traditional Western herbalism, have assessment systems that were designed to identify broad, underlying patterns of imbalance. This means that their diagnostic systems were matched to the way herbs work. A well-trained herbalist will understand these concepts and can help you figure out what herbal remedies will work best for your situation.

The primary goal of an herbalist (or any other well-trained natural healer) is to look at each person's health problems through a wide lens. Herbalists usually spend more than an hour talking with each client, looking at their overall health and health history, and examining their diet and lifestyle and their mental and emotional state. Identifying the underlying imbalances that are causing a person's health problems is a complicated and time-consuming process, but it is essential to getting good results.

There is no specific herbal remedy for chronic fatigue. This is because fatigue has many causes, which could include problems like stress, emotional depression, nutrient deficiencies, or mitochondrial dysfunction. The same principle applies to all complex health problems, including depression, anxiety, and autoimmune disorders. In order to provide anything other than symptomatic relief, the underlying causes must be determined.

Many people learn to use herbs as first aid remedies or to speed recovery from ordinary self-limiting diseases. If you have a serious health issue, we recommend you consult with a professional herbalist for assistance. One way to find a good herbalist is to look for a professional member of the American Herbalists Guild (AHG). Herbalists who are registered with the AHG have passed a peer-review process to ensure their competency and character. Go to www.americanherbalistsguild.com to learn more. Findanherbalist.com lists herbalists who are registered with the AHG in addition to competent herbalists who are not registered. You can also find herbalists listed at herbrally.com.

Find an herbalist you trust. The relationship between healer and patient is an important part of the healing process. Herbalists don't have to worry about huge overheads or how many clients they see in an hour, and they devote a lot of time to developing a relationship with each client.

All of this is not to suggest that you avoid medical doctors. We work with, not against, modern medicine. Although the medical system forces most doctors into a model of practice that doesn't give them enough time to explore the root causes of a person's health problems, medical doctors have advanced diagnostic tools and other equipment at their disposal. Serious health problems should be monitored by a competent medical practitioner.

STEP TWO: SELECT THE PROPER REMEDY

Once you have a correct assessment, it's time to select the appropriate remedy. The right remedy may not be an herb. Herbs aren't going to make up for a lack of sleep, dehydration, or a diet filled with processed and refined foods. Blue vervain isn't the right remedy for anxiety caused by a deficiency of magnesium.

Find the gentlest approach that will get the results you desire. Modern medicine is focused on strong, fast-acting remedies. These produce rapid changes in symptoms, but negatively impact health in the long term. People who are used to rapid results may choose a strong herb over a mild one, or may think that if a little is good, more will be better.

This is not the way traditional herbalism works. Physicians in ancient Baghdad had their market license revoked if they used a strong medicine when a gentle one would suffice, a gentle medicine when food would suffice, or food when simple advice about lifestyle would suffice.

The correct remedy must be administered in the right way. Many books about herbs do not provide information about dosage forms or methods of application. Swallowing a capsule of licorice root won't help a sore throat. Licorice must coat the throat, which means consuming the powder, sipping the tea, or taking small, frequent doses of an extract.

Dosage is a controversial topic among herbalists. Some herbalists use drop doses. In contrast, practitioners of traditional Chinese medicine usually administer herbs in large doses. Some people react quickly to small doses, and others need larger amounts to effect a change. Finding the dose that works for you may require some experimentation. Consult Chapter Eleven for more information about formulas and dosages.

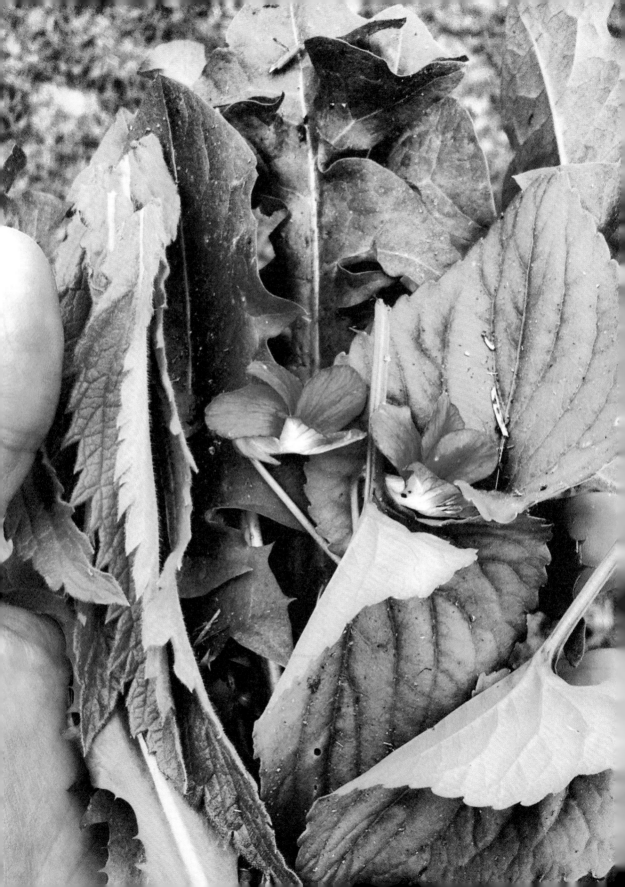

CHAPTER TWO

Herbal Preparations

UNDERSTANDING THE MANY WAYS TO PREPARE AND USE HERBS

Whether you decide to make your own herbal medicines, or to purchase ready-made herbal products, it helps to understand the many ways herbs can be prepared and administered. Each of the following methods are appropriate for certain herbs and situations. Each has its advantages and disadvantages. So, let's start with an overview of the subject.

FRESH HERBS

The most basic way to use herbs is to use the fresh plant material. Herbs can be harvested from the wild or grown in a garden. Some fresh herbs, like garlic, ginger, basil, and other culinary herbs, can even be purchased fresh from the grocery store. Using herbs in this manner is not unlike using fresh fruits and vegetables. We know that the fresher the produce, the more nutritional value it tends to have. The same thing is usually, but not always, true for medicinal plants. The fresher the plant material, the more medicinally potent it tends to be.

There are exceptions to this. Some herbs can be too potent, or even mildly toxic, when fresh, but mellow in action with drying or aging. The laxative herb *Cascara sagrada* is a good example of this. It is violently emetic and cathartic when fresh, meaning the fresh bark will make a person throw up and get severe diarrhea. Cascara must be dried and aged for at least a year to mellow its action. The general rule, however, is that fresh plant material is always better.

The problem is that very few herbs are available fresh all year round. So, to be able to have year-round availability, fresh plant material must be processed in some way to preserve it, either by drying the plant material, or by extracting it in some kind of medium to preserve it.

You can learn more about using fresh herbs in Chapter Three.

Drying is the oldest and easiest method of preparing herbs for storage. It preserves most plant constituents well, so most medicinal qualities of plants are still retained. Dried herbs can be easily stored by placing them in an airtight container and keeping them away from light, heat, and moisture, all of which break down plant material. Most dried herbs will retain their potency for at least 1–2 years, some longer than that.

Generally speaking, flowers, leaves, and other delicate plant parts deteriorate faster after drying than do harder plant parts like barks and roots. Aromatic herbs deteriorate the most, as essential oils evaporate over time and are lost, so it is best to use aromatics within about 1 year. On the other hand, astringent barks and roots may be potent for 10 years or longer.

Dried herbs can be used in a variety of ways. As explained below, they can be used in bulk form or made into capsules or tablets. You can learn more about drying herbs and using them in dried form in the "Harvesting and Drying Herbs" section of Chapter Three.

DRIED HERBS

Bulk dried herbs are easily obtained from a variety of suppliers in packages ranging from a couple of ounces to a pound or more. Depending on the herb, you may be able to get the dried herb in several forms, the most common being powdered, cut and sifted, and whole. The term "cut and sifted" means that the plant material has been cut into small pieces and sifted to keep the pieces at a relatively uniform size.

If you are going to store the herb for a while, we recommend you get cut and sifted or whole herbs rather than powders. The more surface area that is exposed to the air, the faster the plant material tends to degrade. This is especially true for aromatic herbs, as essential oils dissipate more rapidly from powders. If you need to powder the herb later, you can do so with a good grinder.

Dried herbs can be used in numerous ways. Various powdered herbs can be mixed into food and consumed or made into topical preparations like poultices. Herbal powders can also be made into capsules or tablets. Dried herbs can also be used for teas or for making various herbal extracts.

CAPSULES

Capsules have become a very popular way of taking herbs because they are an easy and convenient dosage form. Dried herbal powders are placed in gelatin capsules, so the herbal powders can be swallowed. One of the major advantages of capsules is that they are tasteless. This makes them particularly valuable for nasty-tasting, bitter or acrid, herbs. You are also getting the whole plant material, complete with the plant fibers.

Most gelatin capsules are made from animal by-products, which may be an issue for vegetarians or vegans, but all-plant vegetarian capsules can be purchased, too. If you're willing to put a little effort into it, you can even purchase the capsules and the powders and fill your own capsules.

Capsules do have some drawbacks, however. First, capsules make it harder to regulate dosages, especially with stronger botanicals. When taking an alcohol tincture you can adjust the dose by drops, but it's hard to take ¼ or ½ of a capsule. So, herbs like lobelia, black cohosh, and other strong-acting or mildly toxic botanicals are best taken in a liquid dosage form to allow more precise dosing. Conversely, if you need several teaspoons of an herbal powder (such as psyllium hulls or slippery elm) for an effective dose, that's a lot of capsules to swallow.

The inability to taste and smell the herb also makes regulating dosage more difficult. Your sense of taste and sense of smell are sentinels that are designed to help you regulate what you put into your body. Although refined foods trick these sentinels with flavoring agents, sugar, salt, and processed fats, consumption of all-natural foods is well regulated by your senses. Once you've eaten a certain amount of a natural food like apples or carrots, you suddenly find it's very difficult to eat more. Your body says enough is enough.

The same is true of taking an herbal tea or extract. Even if the taste is unpleasant you'll be able to make yourself take a certain amount, but once you have enough in your system, the body resists and it's tough to make yourself take any more. Thus, taste and smell help you regulate the precise dose your body needs, something you can't do with capsules.

There is one other fairly unknown disadvantage to using capsules (and tablets). Herbs have a primary action that works via the senses to have an immediate effect on the body via the nervous system. For instance, as soon as spicy food or pungent herbs like capsicum are detected by your taste buds, there is an almost immediate warming sensation in the body. There may be a flushing of the face and perspiration forming on your forehead. You may also notice some increased sinus drainage or mucus clearing from the lungs.

These are not reactions based on digesting, absorbing, and utilizing constituents in the plant. They are nervous system reactions that occur because of the input from your senses. If you swallow those same pungent herbs in a capsule, these primary effects will not occur. You will only get the secondary effects that come after the body has absorbed the plant constituents. Secondary effects occur anywhere from 15 minutes to many hours after you take the herb.

Certain benefits of herbs depend almost entirely on primary effects. For example, the taste of bitter stimulates digestive secretions, such as hydrochloric acid in the stomach. Because of this, simple bitters, like gentian, have been used as digestive tonics to improve digestive function when taken in liquid form 15–20 minutes prior to eating. You cannot get the same response by taking gentian in a capsule.

Likewise, in order to induce perspiration, diaphoretics like yarrow work best when taken as hot infusions, or by taking extracts with ample amounts of warm water. Swallowing yarrow in a capsule will not have the same effect.

Primary effects are one of the reasons many herbs seem to work faster when taken in a liquid form. Another reason is that it takes time for the body to break down a capsule, rehydrate the dried powders, and absorb the plant constituents. Liquid herbs are available for immediate absorption.

One way to maintain the primary effects of an herb, while still taking them in capsules, is to break open several capsules of herb powder, then dump the contents into the container with the capsules. Put the lid on the container, and rotate the container slowly in several different directions to coat the capsules with the powder. This way, when you take a capsule, you will taste a little of the herb powder so you can activate the taste receptors on your tongue and gain the benefits of the primary effects, while the majority of the herb is ingested without having to taste it.

TABLETS

Although tablets are more frequently used for nutritional supplements than they are for herbs, some herbs are available in tablet form. It is still the preferred dosage form for many patent Chinese herbal products. To make tablets, herbal powders are mixed with a substance that acts as a binder. They are then rolled or pressed to form the tablets.

In China, they make round herbal tablets by putting herbal powders into a rotating drum. A syrup is then drizzled into the drum, which causes the herbal powders to stick together, forming small round "tablets." These are then sorted by size and dried. In the United States, the powders are generally mixed together and then pressed to form oblong-shaped tablets.

Pressed tablets are often coated with something to help protect them from moisture and preserve them. The coating is often a clear vegetable shellac.

Capsules and tablets have pretty much the same advantages and disadvantages. Again, you can avoid the nasty tastes, but it's harder to regulate dose. Depending on the binders and coatings used, tablets can be harder to digest than capsules. People have been known to pass tablets largely intact. Furthermore, fillers, binding agents, and coatings may not be listed on the label.

LIQUID HERBS (EXTRACTIONS)

As soon as you harvest a plant, some of its components start to break down. Because humans lack the enzyme cellulase necessary to break down the cell wall structure of plants, it could be argued that even if you are munching on a freshly picked plant you're not getting the full medicinal activity. This is why we typically extract herbs into some form of liquid for medicine, traditionally using water to make infusions (teas) and decoctions.

The liquid you use to extract the herb is called the solvent or menstruum. Menstruum is an old alchemical term for a substance that dissolves a solid. The solvents or menstruums we will discuss in this book are water, syrup (water and sugar), alcohol, glycerin, vinegar, and oil. Industrial processes used to make standardized extracts may also make use of chemical solvents like acetone.

Every menstruum has particular constituents it is very effective at extracting and other constituents that it doesn't extract well. Water is a poor solvent of resins, but a great solvent for carbohydrates; alcohol is a great solvent for many medicinal constituents, but is a poor solvent of mucilage; and glycerin by itself (without heat and water) is a poor solvent of most constituents except volatile oils.

What follows is an introduction to preparations made with the solvents we'll discuss in this book. More information about solvents and solubility can be found in Chapter Five, and instructions on how to make these various extractions can be found in Chapter Six.

WATER EXTRACTIONS

Water is the oldest extraction medium for herbs and is still one of the simplest and easiest ways to convert herbs into liquid form. There are two basic water extractions—infusions and decoctions.

Infusions are also known as herbal teas or tisanes (a French term). They are usually made by pouring boiling water over an herb and allowing it to steep for a determined length of time before straining. There are also cold infusions, where you just soak the herb in water, as in making a sun tea. Infusions are generally used on more delicate plant parts like flowers and leaves They are primarily used for aromatic and more pleasant-tasting herbs.

Decoctions are different from infusions, because the herb is simmered in the water. They are made by bringing water to a boil, adding the herbs, then reducing the heat and simmering them for a determined period of time. Decoctions draw out constituents that do not release from the plant material as readily. Decoctions extract more minerals, tannins, and bitter principles than infusions.

Both infusions and decoctions are inexpensive and easy to make. They are also an effective way to take most herbs. They can be stored in the refrigerator for several days and consumed as needed, and because one is sipping and actually tasting the plant, it is easy for the body's senses to help regulate the appropriate dosage.

Teas and decoctions do not work well for nasty-tasting herbs, and some constituents are not water soluble. So, they don't work great in every situation, but they are one of the most basic of all herbal extractions.

SYRUPS

A syrup is a water-based extraction, made in the same way as a decoction, but is done with a mixture of water and a sweetener, typically raw sugar or honey. The ratio is usually 50% sugar or honey and 50% water. Syrups are a good way to cover up the taste of bitter herbs and are usually used as cold and cough remedies. They are nourishing and moistening and are an excellent dosage form for sore throats, coughs, and digestive upset.

Honey has healing properties of its own and adds to the medicinal value of the syrup. However, honey should not be used for children under the age of one.

Syrups are an excellent dosage form for children and the elderly, but their high sugar content is problematic with diabetes or other situations where sugar needs to be avoided. Syrups also have a short shelf life. Refrigerated, they can last for about one month. However, the shelf life of a syrup can be extended by adding alcohol.

ALCOHOL EXTRACTIONS (TINCTURES)

Alcohol is an excellent medium for extracting herbs, and alcohol extracts or tinctures are the most popular dosage form used by professional herbalists. Alcohol is an excellent solvent for most herb constituents and can be used to make tinctures from either fresh or dried plants. Alcohol preparations have the longest shelf life of any herbal extract, so they can be stored for years, in most cases, without losing potency.

Alcohol extracts are great for more potent or potentially toxic botanicals, as dosages can be regulated by the drop. Taking herbs as liquids allows the senses to regulate the dose via the taste. It also rapidly delivers herbal constituents into the bloodstream, making tinctures a fast-acting dosage form. Alcohol tinctures are also a great dosage form for applying herbs topically.

There are a few drawbacks to alcohol extracts. In large doses, alcohol is a toxin to the body. However, the amount of alcohol in a dose of tincture is fairly small. If you assume a dose of 1 milliliter with an average alcohol content of 50%, that's only ½ milliliter of alcohol per dose. In one glass of commercial orange juice there is as much as 1½ milliliters of naturally occurring alcohol. Because we are exposed to small amounts of alcohol in foods, the liver has pathways to detoxify alcohol and turn it into sugar. We also recommend avoiding alcohol preparations with children under two. In acute situations or emergencies, we have used alcohol preparations with young children, but it is best to remove some of the alcohol before administering the herb. You can do this by bringing an ounce of water to a boil. Remove it from the heat and add the alcohol extract. Letting this stand for about 5 minutes allows the heat to evaporate about 15% of the alcohol. It takes almost 4 hours of simmering alcohol in water to remove all of the alcohol. Adding hot water, or simply diluting tinctures in water, makes them more appropriate for use with young children.

For many herbs, tinctures are the preferred preparation. However, some people's religious beliefs prohibit the use of water, and tinctures aren't recommended for children, or for recovering alcoholics or people with liver disorders.

Alcohol doesn't extract all constituents, and some herbs are much better in other menstruums.

GLYCERIN EXTRACTIONS (GLYCERITES)

Glycerin is used less frequently than alcohol as an extraction medium, but it is gaining in popularity. Glycerin is a semiclear, nontoxic, sweet-tasting liquid produced from vegetable or animal fats. Fats are composed of fatty acids and glycerin (also known as glycerol), and our digestive process breaks fats down into these two components. This means glycerin is something our body processes every time we eat fats.

There are both advantages and disadvantages to using glycerin instead of alcohol to make herbal extracts. One advantage is that glycerin is nontoxic and may be used by young children, alcoholics, and other people who can't use alcohol. A disadvantage is that glycerites are generally not as potent as tinctures, so larger doses are required.

Another advantage of glycerin is that it tastes sweet, so it can be used to mask the bitter taste of many herbs. In this sense, a glycerite is similar to a syrup; however, unlike syrups, glycerites do not spike blood sugar levels in most people. Glycerin is not a sugar and is metabolized via different pathways, so it doesn't appear to raise blood sugar levels in healthy people. Some research indicated that diabetics, however, may still need to be cautious when using glycerites.

Alcohol is a better preservative than glycerin and is also less expensive. However, glycerites have a reasonably long shelf life. We have extensive experience in making glycerites and have found that properly made glycerites have a shelf life of at least 3 years. We've even had glycerites that were still effective after 10 years or more.

A disadvantage of glycerin over alcohol is that heat must be used in making glycerites. Without heat, glycerin is a poor solvent. It is also more difficult to make fresh plant glycerites. So, plant compounds damaged by heat or drying will not be effectively extracted using glycerin.

Glycerin has some therapeutic properties of its own. It is antifungal and antimicrobial. It is also soothing and emollient, so glycerites are very good for applications where tissues need to be soothed and moisturized. Glycerin will not extract resins or oils, so use alcohol to extract resinous or oily herbs. It is also difficult, if not impossible, to make a glycerite preparation of most mucilaginous herbs, but these don't extract in alcohol either.

HERBAL VINEGARS OR ACID TINCTURES

Vinegar is not widely used as an extraction medium, but it is useful in some applications. An herbal extract made with vinegar is usually known as an herbal vinegar or acid tincture. This method is most commonly used with culinary herbs for use in cooking or as a salad dressing, although some medicinal plants have also been made into acid tinctures.

Vinegar preparations are generally not as therapeutically strong as alcohol or glycerin preparations, as vinegar is not a great solvent for many herbal constituents. It also has a shorter shelf life, and the flavor of vinegar extracts is very disagreeable to some people. Others love the taste of vinegar and may find this a very appealing extraction medium.

There are two applications where vinegar is very good. The first is in extracting minerals from herbs that contain calcium and other alkaline minerals. The second is for extracting aromatic and pungent herbs, as in making Fire Cider.

OIL EXTRACTIONS

Some herbs may be extracted in some kind of oil or fat, such as olive oil, coconut oil, or lard. Oil extraction is done to create remedies for topical application or to be used as a base for making salves and ointments.

Oil is a very poor solvent for most herbal constituents, which is why some formulas for making ointments and salves begin with a water- or alcohol-based extraction to which oil is later added. There are, however, some plants that extract well in oil, such as St. John's wort flowers and mullein flowers.

Herbal oils are very soothing, softening, and emollient, making them good for minor skin problems such as abrasions, burns, rashes, and dry skin. They should not be used on new cuts or wounds, however, because the oil can trap bacteria in the wound and help the infection to spread.

SPECIALIZED PREPARATIONS

In addition to the basic methods for preparing herbs that we've listed above, there are some additional, more specialized preparations of which you should be aware. Most of these preparations are industrial applications beyond what the average person could make at home. Nevertheless, you should be aware of these preparations and their uses.

LIQUID CAPSULES

An interesting new technology in making herbal products is to put herbal extracts into softgel capsules. This dosage form provides some of the benefits of capsules combined with some of the benefits of liquid extracts. These products can be very effective, but they are more costly than capsules or extracts. At this point, only a few herbs are available in this form, and it is not a dosage form you can make at home.

STANDARDIZED EXTRACTS

Quality herbal products have always been standardized, meaning that the way they were produced was consistent; that is, made according to some standard manufacturing process. Herbal products that were part of the United States Pharmacopoeia in times past were manufactured to USP standards. This designation still appears on some over-the-counter products at the drugstore.

Standardization meant that the material was harvested correctly and verified as being the correct plant part. The raw material also met specific quality control standards. The material was then extracted using the same proportions of herbal material and menstruum each time. The tincturing or processing time was also standardized to a specific period of time.

Today, the term "standardized" usually has a very different meaning. Modern standardization started in 1992 as a result of laws in Germany that required manufacturers to standardize their products to create a guaranteed potency of a particular constituent. This form of standardization grows out of the orthodox scientific view that herbs owe their efficacy to specific chemical compounds, usually referred to as "active constituents."

Many people think that the standardization movement is a step forward for herbal medicine, but the people who tend to be most resistant to it are professional clinical herbalists. These people, who have the most practical experience with herbs, often find that these standardized extracts don't work as well as whole herbs. In fact, standardization flies in the face of traditional herbal wisdom, which says that the whole is greater than the sum of the parts.

Whole plants contain thousands of chemical compounds put together in extremely complex ways. Most herbalists believe that the synergy of these compounds often creates a better effect than any single compound or group of compounds in the plants. In contrast, a standardized extract uses various solvents to isolate or at least concentrate specific compounds considered to be "active," leaving other compounds, which may have synergistic effects, behind.

So, standardized extracts are more like modern pharmaceutical drugs than whole herbal products. This does not mean they are not useful; it just means they should not be viewed as the equivalent of the actual herb. One cannot extrapolate that a single compound or group of compounds found in a plant will have all of the actions of the original herb.

Examples of this type of extract include curcumin, a compound from turmeric, and berberine, an antimicrobial compound found in plants like goldenseal or Oregon grape. These types of extracts have the same relationship to medicinal herbs that vitamin and mineral supplements have to food. They are not equivalent.

Standardized extracts have their place. In fact, some botanicals need to be used in this manner for proper safety and dosage. For example, all the research done on the benefits of ginkgo biloba was done on a standardized extract. The whole leaf was not used in traditional herbal medicine and does not have the benefits of the standardized extract.

Standardization can be used to reduce toxicity in botanicals that may have other compounds that are undesirable. It can also make dosing of strong botanical compounds more precise, such as using the acetogenins from paw paw as an anticancer remedy.

There are a number of problems with these products that the consumer should consider. First, standardization increases the cost of herbal products to the consumer, without necessarily resulting in a more effective product.

Second, there is not always agreement as to which compounds should be standardized, and compounds left behind may also be therapeutically valuable. For example, a curcumin-free extract of turmeric was found to still have anti-inflammatory properties, demonstrating that it isn't just the curcumin in the turmeric that is anti-inflammatory.

Furthermore, modern standards are not created by an objective third party like the United States Pharmacopoeia, nor are they based on clinical experience from practicing herbalists. The standards are created by the pharmaceutical and nutraceutical companies, often reflecting research done on the constituents rather than the whole herbs.

There is also the issue of the chemical solvents that are used to selectively extract and concentrate active constituents at the expense of others. Are traces of these compounds still present in the product?

In summary, standardized extracts create a more specific, more medicine-like action by providing a standardized level of specific plant constituents. Although this may help with dosage regulation and consistency, the product is no longer an herb. Just as an orange and a vitamin C pill are very different, a whole herb is very different from a standardized extract. The synergy of ingredients found in the original plant is lost, which in many cases means the product may not be as effective as the less-expensive whole herb.

ESSENTIAL OILS

An essential oil, also known as a volatile oil, is a concentrated extract of the volatile constituents in herbs. These are the compounds that evaporate from a plant to give it its characteristic aroma. We discuss aromatherapy in more detail in Chapter Ten, but here we will just introduce them.

Like a standardized extract, an essential oil is not the same as the herb from which it comes. It is a concentrated component of the herb, but does not contain all of the other compounds found in the plant. Again, this is important to understand, as many people will attribute therapeutic properties to an essential oil that are found only in the actual herb.

Essential oils are highly concentrated substances, which means they do not have the same degree of safety that a whole plant has. Essential oils can irritate sensitive skin or mucous membranes. Many are toxic and should never be used internally, and even oils that are generally recognized as safe (GRAS) may have toxic properties when ingested in larger quantities (with an essential oil, one drop is a fairly large dose).

Like the taste of a plant, the aroma of essential oils has a very direct and immediate impact on body functions via the nervous system. This means that it is usually not necessary to ingest an essential oil to obtain its benefits. The safest way to use them is to smell them or dilute them and use them topically.

These highly concentrated substances have a fairly long shelf life, tend to be antiseptic and healing, and are useful for emotional healing and mood alteration. Their growing popularity attests to their benefits, and to the marketing of companies selling them. Making essential oils at home requires specialized equipment, with basic setups starting at $500 or more. Many people find that the art of distilling essential oils is a fun and worthwhile investment. Some oils in the marketplace may be extracted or adulterated with chemical solvents, so it is very important to seek out both quality oils and education on how to use them safely.

SELECTING THE BEST DOSAGE FORMS

Table 1 offers some general suggestions for selecting the best dosage forms for the twelve major categories of herbs. Of course each herb is unique, so for more specific information about the best dosage forms for specific single herbs, consult Chapter Thirteen.

Herb	Fresh Plant	Dried Bulk	Capsule/Tablet	Infusion/Decoction	Alcohol Tincture	Glycerite
Aromatic	Excellent	Fair	Fair	Fair	Good	Excellent
Pungent (Spicy)	Excellent	Good	Fair to Good	Fair	Excellent	Good to Excellent
Fragrant Bitter	Good	Good	Poor	Good	Excellent	Poor to Good
Acrid	Poor	Fair	Poor to Fair	Good	Excellent	Good
Simple (Nonalkaloidal) Bitter	Excellent	Good	Poor	Good	Excellent	Poor to Good
Alkaloidal Bitter	Fair to Poor	Good	Fair to Good	Good	Good	Good
Astringent	Excellent	Good	Good	Excellent	Poor to Fair	Excellent
Salty	Excellent	Good	Good	Fair		
Decoction: Excellent	Poor to Fair	Poor to Good				
Sweet (Tonic)	Good	Good	Poor to Good	Good	Excellent	Excellent
Mucilant	Excellent	Excellent	Good	Good	Poor	Poor
Sour	Excellent	Good	Good	Good	Good	Excellent
Oily	Excellent	Excellent	Poor to Fair	Poor	Poor to Fair	Fair

TABLE 1   Best Dosage Forms

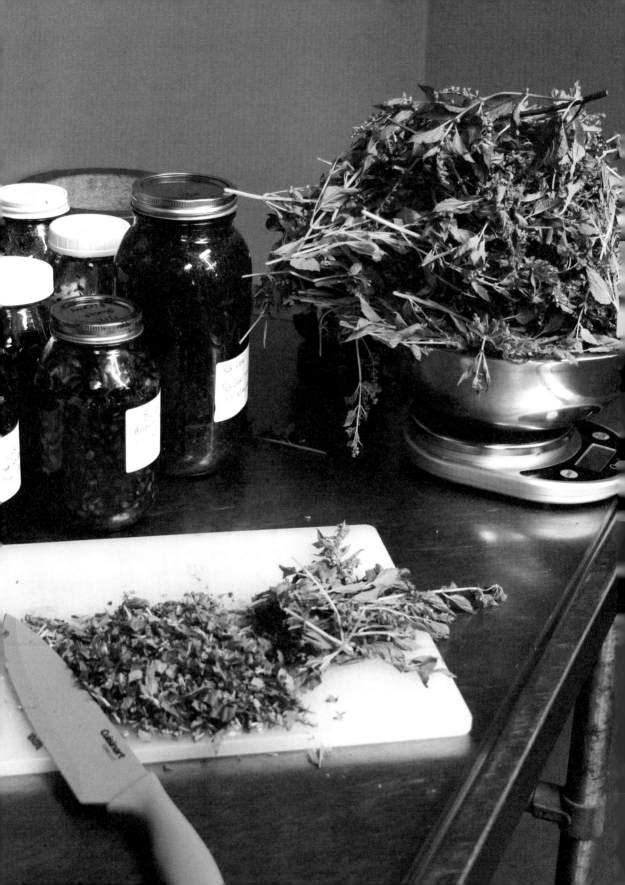

CHAPTER THREE

Using Fresh Plants

HARVESTING, DRYING, AND USING FRESH HERBS

Nature freely provides medicines that can help you solve your health problems and stay healthy. You don't need to go to the wilderness to find these healing plants. Most common lawn and garden weeds have medicinal value. Many medicinal herbs can be found at garden nurseries, and you can plant them in your yard or grow them in pots as houseplants. There are even a few fresh medicinal herbs at your local grocery store.

It isn't necessary to harvest your own herbs in order to make your own herbal medicines, but it is fun and empowering. It deepens your connection with nature so that you start to see it as an ally, filled with living things ready to share their gifts with you.

This book isn't a gardening book or a plant identification guide, but we want to acquaint you with some of the basics you'll need to know to obtain your own medicinal plants. We'll start with growing them yourself, discuss harvesting them from the wild, and finish with talking about some of the ways you can use fresh plants as medicine.

GROWING HERBS

Throughout history, it was common to have a few medicinal herbs in the kitchen garden. Many herbs, especially culinary herbs, are easy to grow. If you have limited space, you can grow your herbs in a planter box or another small container.

You can find basic culinary herb plants at most local nurseries, and some plants that are sold as flowers or vegetables are also medicinal. Start by looking for basil, cilantro, dill, fennel, garlic, oregano, parsley, rosemary, sage, and thyme. Mints, such as spearmint or peppermint, are usually easy to grow and spread like weeds if you don't contain them. You can be exotic and grow orange mint, pineapple mint, chocolate mint, and ginger mint.

Medicinal flowers like yarrow, roses, calendula, or chamomile can easily be planted in a garden. Herbs like borage, bee balm, catnip, and horehound are easy to grow. Searching online for herb plants and seeds will yield even more possibilities. If you have the space, get a good book on growing herbs and plant a medicinal garden for yourself.

WILDCRAFTING HERBS

Ralph Waldo Emerson said that weeds are plants "whose virtues have yet to be discovered." If you have a yard, there are probably many medicinal plants already growing on your property, and if they are not on your property, they are probably growing around the neighborhood.

Before heading out into the wilds to learn to identify medicinal plants, start by becoming acquainted with the medicinal weeds growing in your own backyard. Common medicinal weeds that may grow nearby include burdock, dandelion, red clover, plantain, mullein, and wild lettuce.

Before you start harvesting anything, you need to make sure you have properly identified the plant. It is easy to get some plants confused with other plants, especially in plant families such as the carrot family. Plants should be identified by their Latin names rather than their common names, as the same common name is often given to more than one species of plant.

On rare occasions, people have consumed toxic plants by accident and died from it (although usually you'll just get very sick). If you are not absolutely sure of the plant, don't harvest it. Look for books on local plants at your local bookstore. Most plant identification books do not contain information about how to gather and use the plant, and most herbal guides don't have good information on identification, so you'll want to consult both herb texts and field guides. Have several of each on hand when identifying new plants.

If you want to gather any herbs other than common garden weeds or those you have grown yourself, take a series of herb walks with a skilled herbalist or take a few classes in field botany. Learn to identify the poisonous plants in your area so you do not confuse any other plant with them.

ETHICAL WILDCRAFTING

The overharvesting of certain medicinal plants has resulted in some plants becoming rare or endangered. Check with United Plant Savers (www.united-plantsavers.org) for a list of plants that are at-risk, overharvested, and suffering from habitat loss, and do not harvest those plants.

Even if the plant you want is not endangered or at-risk, it's important to follow some simple guidelines to ensure that these plants will be there for generations to come: Gather medicinal plants only where the plants are abundant. Never take more than 10% of the plants in a given area. Always leave plenty of plants so that nature can replenish the supply.

It helps to know the plant's reproductive habits before you harvest it. A plant that reproduces from underground rhizomes should be thinned, whereas a plant that reproduces from seeds should be gathered sporadically, with flowers left to turn to seed. When possible, gather leaves, seeds, and flowers, which grow back easily, rather than barks and roots, the loss of which may kill the plant. Harvest bark with respect for the needs of the tree, and preferably from recently downed branches or prunings.

When harvesting roots and bulbs, replant the crown portion of the root or rhizomes and fill in holes so you don't leave gaping holes in the earth. When you harvest plants on a hill, leave the plants at the top of the hill untouched to help replenish the downhill slope.

Many indigenous traditions teach that you should ask the plants for permission before gathering them and leave an offering in exchange for the plant. Sit with the plant in a quiet, meditative state for at least 15 minutes before harvesting it. Think about what use you want to make of the plant material, and ask the plant for permission to gather it.

Native people often looked for what appeared to be the "eldest" plant in the area or plant "tribe." They would make an offering of cornmeal or tobacco to this "grandfather" plant, asking permission to harvest some of the tribe.

Even if you choose not to gather plants in these traditional ways, gather the plants in a reverent, thankful manner. Honor the fact that these living plants are giving their lives or part of themselves to help you and others heal.

HARVESTING AND DRYING HERBS

Make sure the plants you gather have not been sprayed with chemicals, and that they are not growing next to busy streets where they are exposed to exhaust fumes. Don't harvest plants from other people's property without their permission. If you are harvesting from government land, make sure you know what the laws and regulations are (it's illegal to harvest plants from national parks in the United States).

Harvest only one species of plant at a time to avoid confusion. Individual plant parts like leaves are easy to get mixed up. Label everything carefully as soon as you get it home.

Know what you will be using the plant for before you gather it. Harvest only the part of the plant that you intend to use medicinally, and gather only as much as you need. Try not to gather from wet ground, where your footprints can damage the soil and make future growth more challenging; wait for a stretch of good weather before collecting in wetland areas. Leave the area in better shape than it was when you found it.

Dry or process herbs into an extract as quickly as possible. If you have to wait, keep the plant material cool until you're ready to dry or process it.

HARVESTING AT THE RIGHT TIME

Like fruits and vegetables, herbs have a season and time of day when they ripen and are at peak strength. Harvest herbs when they are at the peak of maturity and the concentration of active ingredients is highest.

Here are some general guidelines; consult other herbal texts for more specific information. Barks are usually harvested in the spring (and in the morning) because that is when the sap is rising and the bark is most active. This is also the time to harvest young stems, buds, and leaves.

Flowers are usually harvested during the day when the energy of the plant is the most yang, or outward. Flowers are best harvested shortly after they open. (Flowers that open at night should be gathered in the evening when they start to open.) Essential oils rise up the stems and concentrate in flowers in the early morning hours, then dissipate as the day wears on.

As the plant dies back in the fall, the energy and nutrient stores are returned to the root. Roots, therefore, are usually gathered in the fall, and are often more potent when gathered in the evening hours when the plant is pulling its energies downward again.

HARVESTING THE RIGHT PARTS OF AN HERB

Many plants have different uses depending on the plant part. It is important to know which part of the plant you want. Although one part of the plant may be completely safe, other parts may be toxic.

Elder flowers and elder berries are both antiviral. Elder flowers are used to treat topical irritations of the skin, and are used internally as a mild refrigerant to relieve fevers and reduce inflammation. Elder berries are used as a potassium-rich food, and can be added to slippery elm gruel to treat wasting conditions. Elder berries are also used to enhance tonic cardiovascular herbal blends, and have a mild decongestant effect. Elder leaves are astringent and are used primarily as a topical preparation, whereas the bark is bitter, astringent, and mildly toxic, suitable for use only by experienced practitioners.

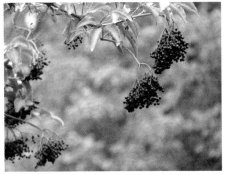

Photo by Nicole Conner

Using the wrong part of a plant can cause toxic reactions, from simple stomach upset to coma and even death. The fruit of the tomato and the tuber of the potato are edible and nutritionally dense, but the leaves and stems of these plants are toxic. The reverse can also hold true: Leafy parts of some plants are edible, whereas the fruit or seeds are toxic.

SPECIFIC HARVESTING DIRECTIONS

Here are some more detailed guidelines for harvesting various plant parts. Again, these are general guidelines. Each herb has its own unique characteristics. As you learn more about each plant, you will also discover the best time to harvest it.

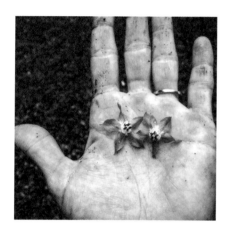

Flowers

Harvesting flowers varies from plant to plant, because different plants flower at different times of the year. Sometimes the part used is the bud; in this case, collect the flowers just before they open. Blossoms should be harvested when they are fully open, just as they reach the peak of their strength, but before they start to turn (wilt, waste, or dry out). Shortly after this, the blossom will begin to wilt at the edges and go limp, and the vibrancy of the color will start to fade.

It is usually best to harvest flowers in mid- to late morning after the dew has dried. Cut or pick them carefully. If the stems are woody, like lavender, it is easiest to use clippers and harvest the stem along with the flowers. If the stem is large or fleshy, remove the flowers from the stems before drying. Keep fresh flowers loose and in open containers so they do not congeal and mold. Remove obvious dirt, soil, and insects, and spread the flowers on a paper-lined tray or newspaper to dry. Flowers should be dried in a well-ventilated area away from sunlight and excessive heat; paper sacks suspended from the ceiling make great drying units. When the flowers are dry (when they crumble when rubbed between your fingers), store them whole in dark, airtight containers.

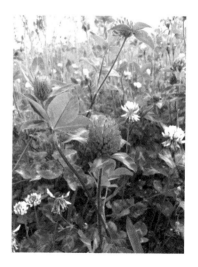

When the plant part used is the flowering herb, leaves and stems are gathered along with the flowers. Tie bunches of stems together with string or twine, and hang them upside down to dry. Dry them away from direct sunlight and excessive heat.

Leaves and Aerial Parts

Leaves are usually best when harvested in the early and mid-summer when their chlorophyll and their aromatic and medicinal constituents are at their peak. Collect leaves in the morning after the dew has evaporated. As the day warms up and photosynthesis gets under way, essential oils are concentrated in the leaves and evaporate in midday heat. Harvest the leaves after some warmth has drawn up the oils but before they have been released in the heat.

Gather leaves when they are tender and showing new growth, either before the flower buds appear or after seeding when new fall growth appears. Treat all leaves gently, taking care not to bruise or crush them. Pick only healthy whole leaves that are not torn, discolored, or insect infested.

According to Nicholas Culpeper's *English Physician and Complete Herbal,* "The leaves of such herbs as run up to seed are not so good when they are in flower as before"(p. 200). Upon flowering, the plant's priorities change and its energy goes into reproduction. At this point the leaves can become bitter and sometimes astringent. Whether you gather the leaves before the plant flowers or after will depend on what components you are looking for.

Pick the succulent leaves of sorrel, bistort, good King Henry, angelica, and all salad herbs when young. Succulent herbs are not typically harvested for drying and should be frozen in cooked food or preserved in oil or vinegar.

Large leaves such as burdock and mullein can be harvested and dried individually; smaller leaves, such as mints, are best left on the stem. Gather the leaves of deciduous herbs just before flowering, and gather evergreen herbs, such as rosemary, throughout the year. If you are using all of the aerial parts, harvest when there are both flowers and seed heads on the plant. Treat all leaves gently, taking care not to bruise or crush them. Pick only healthy whole leaves that are not torn, discolored, or insect infested.

There are several ways to dry leaves. Tie them in small bunches of about 8–12 stems, depending on the size of the stems, and hang them upside down

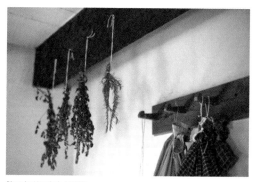

to dry. When the leaves are brittle to the touch, but not so dry that they turn to powder, rub them from the stem onto paper to dry, and discard the stem, if the stem is not required. Leaves can also be spread on screens or placed loosely in small paper bags and hung to dry. Dry leaves away from sunlight. Store in airtight containers when dry.

Seeds

Seeds should be harvested late in fall before the weather turns wet or the snow starts to fall. The plant should be thoroughly dead and dried up when you harvest the seeds. Some seeds, such as poppy and oat, are harvested when they are green due to the concentration of certain medicinal alkaloids. (Note that the use of green poppy seed is illegal.)

The best time of day to harvest the seeds of a plant is midmorning. Pick seeds on a warm, dry day when the seeds are fully ripe but before they have fallen off the plant. The seeds should be tan, brown, or black, not green at all, and they should be hard, with paper-dry pods.

Harvest the entire seed head with about 15–25 centimeters (6–10 inches) of stalk. Hang seed heads upside down over a paper-lined tray or in a paper bag away from direct sunlight. Seeds will usually dry within 2 weeks. Keep all seeds separate and remember to label and date everything.

Roots and Rhizomes

Most roots are gathered in the late fall when the aerial parts of the plant have wilted and before the ground becomes too hard to dig easily. In the fall, the fluids and vitality of the plant drop into the roots or rhizomes. There are exceptions to this rule: Dandelion root, for example, should be gathered in the spring before it becomes too bitter and woody.

Dig up annuals when their growing cycle has been completed at the end of the year. Pick perennial roots in their second or third year of growth or later, when the active components have developed. Because sap rises and falls with the sun, gather roots in the early morning or late afternoon while most of the potency of the plant is in the root.

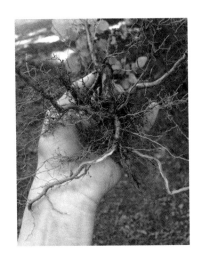

In most cases you should wash the roots thoroughly to remove soil and dirt. Use an old toothbrush to scrub small roots. Most roots, such as horseradish and comfrey, can be scrubbed clean and have their fibrous hairs removed. Others, such as valerian, should not be stripped of their tiny root hairs, as their precious constituents are contained in the epidermal (surface) cells. For these roots, brush the dirt off with a dry toothbrush or wash very gently.

Roots can be difficult or even impossible to cut when dry, so chop large roots into small pieces while still fresh. Spread the pieces of root on a screen or a tray lined with paper, and dry in a warm place away from direct sunlight. Some succulent roots like dandelion and burdock need a bit more heat than normal to kill off small insect eggs; these do best cut into small pieces when fresh, and then dried at 150° in a food dehydrator, or in the oven on the lowest setting with the door propped open. Some roots reabsorb moisture from the air, so discard them if they become soft.

Sap and Resin

The best time to harvest resin from a tree is in autumn when the sap is falling. Sap is usually harvested in the spring when it is rising. In either case, make a deep incision in the bark and wait for the resin or sap to leak out. Sap can be collected by drilling a hole and collecting the sap in a cup or bucket tied to the tree. Sometimes a sizable bucket is needed: a large amount of birch sap, for example, can be collected overnight at certain

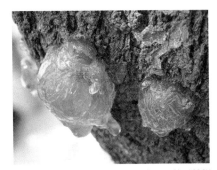

times of year. If you tap (drill) a tree, place a wood cork in the hole after you're done to prevent insects from invading the tree.

You can squeeze sap from latex plants like wild lettuce or desert poppy into a container. Some saps are corrosive (including celandine and fig sap), so wear protective gloves before squeezing. To harvest aloe, slice along the center of the leaf and peel back the edges, then use the blunt edge of a knife to scrape the gel from the leaf.

Fruits

Harvest fruits only when they are completely ripened. This can be anywhere from summer to late fall, depending on the plant. One of the best indicators that a fruit has ripened is how easily it can be harvested from the plant. The fruit should almost fall off as it is touched, and should not have to be pulled with force from the stem that attaches it to the plant.

Harvest berries and other fruits just as they become ripe, before the fruit becomes too soft to dry. Lay them out on covered screens to dry. Turn fleshy fruits frequently to help them dry evenly, and get rid of fruit that show signs of mold. A dehydrator is an excellent way to dry medicinal fruits.

Bark

Both outer and inner bark should be harvested in the late fall, winter, or early spring. This is when they are the most potent, and, depending on where you live, there should be no bug or pest invasion during that time of year. To minimize the damage to the tree, harvest in the autumn when the sap is falling back into the roots. As spring approaches and the fluids rise in the plant, the tree will heal any damage (including the stripped bark). For most plants this is the only time they can heal without environmental complications.

Outer bark is the part of the bark that people cut into when they carve their initials in a tree. The inner bark is the thin layer underneath the hard outer bark that still adheres to the tree. Collect bark from young branches or trunks. Look for recently downed trees before harvesting bark from live ones. When working with live trees, it is best to saw off a branch and then strip it. Bark will peel off easily in wet weather. Be careful to cut carefully so the bark does not tear down the trunk, exposing the tree to insect invasion. If you are harvesting a small amount of bark, take small, lengthwise strips from one of the branches; if you cut around the circumference of the tree you will kill it. Brush off the bark to remove moss or insects, and break or cut the bark into small pieces (1–2 inches square), lay them out on a tray, and let dry.

Sometimes twigs can be used instead of bark. The pruned branches of fruit trees such as peach and apple can be put to good use as herbal medicine.

Bulbs

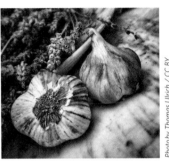

Harvest bulbs after the aerial parts have wilted. Collect garlic bulbs quickly; they tend to sink downward once the leaves have wilted and may be difficult to find. Garlic and onions are examples of medicinal bulbs.

USING FRESH PLANTS

Fresh plants can be used in a number of ways. You can chew the fresh herb and eat it, or add it to soups, stews, or other dishes. You can also extract fresh herbs in water (infusions and decoctions), alcohol, glycerin, or vinegar. Here are some specific preparations that can be made from fresh herbs.

FRESH PLANT POULTICES

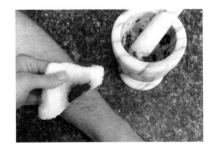

Fresh herbs can be mashed and applied directly to the skin for burns, insect bites, bee stings, cuts, and other minor injuries. You can also chew the plant material a little, crushing it with the teeth and mixing it with saliva, to form a fresh plant poultice. (Spit poultices contain lots of unhealthy bacteria from the mouth and shouldn't be used on broken skin.) Examples of fresh herbs that can be used as poultices include the following:

- Plantain (bee stings, insect bites, snake bites, burns, minor cuts and abrasions; dirty wounds containing sand, dirt, grit, or other impurities)
- Lily of the valley (draws out slivers and pus)
- Yarrow (cuts, bruises, crushed tissues, insect bites)
- Grindelia (bee stings and insect bites, cuts, infected wounds)
- Jewelweed (poison ivy)

INSTANT PASTES AND OINTMENTS

Fresh herbs can be made into pastes and ointments. Make a paste by mixing crushed fresh herbs with a little honey or glycerin. These can be eaten or used as a base for a poultice. You can make an instant ointment by mashing fresh herbs into butter, ghee, or oil.

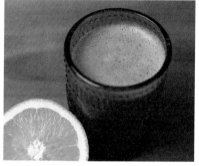

Photo by Natalie Gi / CC BY

GREEN DRINKS

Green drinks are prepared with a blender. Pour fruit juice (pineapple juice is delicious) into a blender, add fresh herbs, and blend the mixture. Strain and drink. Drink green drinks within a couple of minutes to guarantee the full potency of all of the plant's nutrients and constituents. Plants that can be used to make green drinks include dandelion greens, plantain, parsley, wheat grass, and barley grass.

JUICING

Herb juices are commonly made with parsley, garlic, and onions, and fruits such as lemons and limes. Juicing fresh herbs separates the plant fiber from the plant fluids. Herb juices can be made with a food processor or a juicer. The most antiquated method for juicing, still used by the more adventurous among us, is the mortar and pestle. Filter the mashed plant material through a muslin cloth and squeeze through a nylon sieve or jelly bag to obtain the juice.

Juicing requires large quantities of fresh herb: A 10-liter bucket of fresh herb may yield only 100 milliliters of juice.

Dehydrated Herb Juice

After the juice has been expressed from the plant fiber it can be dehydrated. Dehydrating must be done with care and cleanliness to avoid microbial contamination. Dry the juice quickly, but not at such a high temperature that the nutritional factors or therapeutic constituents are degraded. Dry juices in a standard food dehydrator using fruit leather trays. If you do not use heat, you can dry juice on waxed paper or glass as well: Spread a thin layer of juice on the waxed paper or glass container and cover with a muslin cloth to prevent mold and keep flies and pests off. Place in a warm place to dry. Once the juice is thoroughly dried, scrape it off, powder it, and package. If kept in a cool, dark, dry place, this type of preparation will keep for about 3–4 months.

RAW GARLIC

While most herbs work well when dried, there are some herbs that are best used fresh. Garlic is one of them. Garlic bulbs are available at any grocery store, and raw garlic is a good remedy to keep around the house. Garlic is often sold in capsules and extracted in oil, but allicin, an antimicrobial constituent found in raw garlic, degrades rapidly into inactive compounds, so fresh is best.

There are many ways to use fresh garlic. For ear infections and earaches, cut a slice of a garlic clove and place it on the outer ear covering the ear canal. Do not put the garlic into the ear canal. If the raw garlic irritates the skin, coat it with a little olive oil before applying.

For an abscessed tooth, cut a slice of garlic, coat it in olive oil, and place it next to the affected tooth to fight the infection. This will temporarily ease the pain and infection; you still need to see a dentist.

Raw garlic works internally against infections in the intestines and lungs, but it has little effect on systemic infections. To get it down, chop raw garlic into small pieces and take it in a spoonful of honey. There is a formula for Garlic Lemon Aid in Chapter Twelve, as well as a formula for Fire Cider, which includes raw garlic.

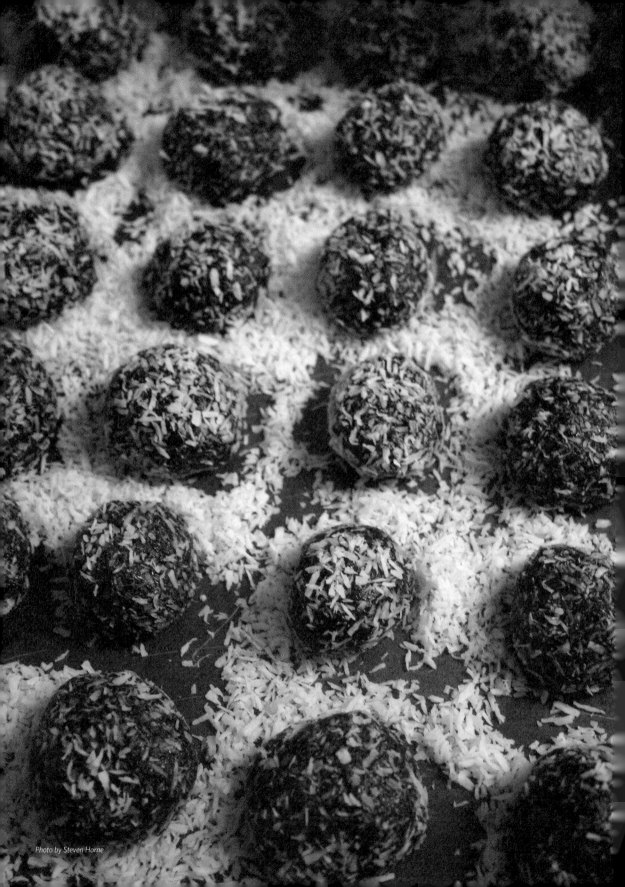

CHAPTER FOUR

Dried Herbs

BULK HERBS, CAPSULES, AND TABLETS

Drying is one of the oldest methods of preparing herbs for storage and use, and is easy to do at home. Most herbs maintain a reasonable potency when dried, whereas some lose potency, and the strength of a few others is enhanced by drying. Dried herbs are often powdered. As they are powdered, plant material is exposed to the air, which causes more constituents to be lost. This means that powdered herbs lose potency faster than herbs that are cut and sifted or whole. Powders may be encapsulated or tableted, and both powders and bulk dried herbs can be used to make extracts and various topical preparations.

PURCHASING DRIED HERBS

When you purchase bulk herbs you depend upon the supplier to ensure that the herb was properly identified and harvested. Be discerning when you choose an herb vendor.

We favor organically grown or wildcrafted herbs. Organically grown herbs are grown without chemical pesticides, herbicides, or fertilizers. Wildcrafted herbs have been gathered from the wild, so unless they are harvested near roadways or farms, they won't have chemical pesticides, herbicides, or fertilizers.

Using cultivated herbs contributes to plant conservation because doing so does not deplete wild stands of plants. On the other hand, plants that grow in their native habitat may be more potent than herbs that are cultivated. Many of the medicinal compounds in plants are produced in response to environmental stress, so a wild-grown plant may have higher concentrations of medicinal compounds than a cultivated plant.

Dried herbs may be whole, sliced, cut and sifted, or powdered. As mentioned above, the more surface area that is exposed to light and air, the quicker plants deteriorate. Keep your herbs whole or cut and sifted until ready for use. A small coffee grinder will reduce most cut and sifted herbs (with the exception of very hard roots and barks) to powder, or you can use a Vitamix, as discussed in Chapter Five.

QUALITY CONTROL ISSUES

When purchasing herbs, here are the quality control issues of which you should be aware. Cheaper brands are not necessarily a good buy. Even today there is adulteration in herbal products. Some products contain the wrong plant species. Others include plant parts that are not considered medicinally valuable. Therefore, purchase from companies that ensure they use the right species and parts of the plant.

Make sure that plants are being harvested at the right time of the year. Potency may also vary with the location where the plant was grown.

It is also important that herbs be harvested sustainably. Avoid companies that are supporting wildcrafters who are endangering species of medicinal plants.

Cleanliness of the plant material is also important. Is the herb free of dirt and insect parts? Is it also free of pesticides and herbicides, heavy metals, and other chemical contaminants? This is especially important for herbs coming from heavily polluted countries like China. Remember that just because an herb is organic doesn't mean that it's free of dirt or insect parts.

These are all reasons why we recommend you stick to purchasing herbal products, including bulk herbs, only from reputable manufacturers. See Appendix Two for a list of suppliers we recommend.

USING DRIED HERBS

Bulk dried herbs can be used in a variety of ways. They can be extracted as discussed in Chapter Five or used in topical applications as described in Chapter Eight. They can also be encapsulated or tableted or made into herbal nut butter balls. The following are some of the dosage forms you can make using bulk dried herbs.

CAPSULES

The herb industry received a huge boon when herbs began to be put into capsules. Encapsulated herbs are easy to consume, and they are one of the most popular ways of taking herbs in the United States today. Encapsulated herbs rarely act as quickly or effectively as traditional teas and tinctures, but for some unpalatable herbs needed in high doses they are very convenient.

Many capsules are made from animal by-products (gelatin) and may not be suitable for people on strict vegetarian diets, but there are an increasing number of products being made with all-vegetable capsules. Most companies that encapsulate herbs add materials like magnesium stearate to lubricate their machinery. For most people the addition of minute amounts of magnesium stearate doesn't cause any problems, but some people with sensitive digestive tracts should avoid it. Several companies, including Pure Encapsulations and Thorne, don't use magnesium stearate.

Home capsule filling machines can be bought for around $30, or you can fill capsules by hand. To do this manually, you need a saucer or flat dish, empty capsules, and the powdered herb you want to encapsulate. Pour the powdered herb into the saucer. Separate the two halves of the capsule case and scoop the powder into both sides of the capsule. Fit the two halves of the capsule together. Store the finished capsules in a cool place in a dark glass jar or container.

Different capsule sizes hold different amounts of herb powder, and machines are more efficient than hand filling. Hand filling a size 00 capsule will result in 200–250 milligrams of powdered herb per capsule. Machine-filled capsules usually hold 45 milligrams of herb powder per a standard size 00 capsule.

TABLETS

Before capsules became popular, many herbs were sold in tablet form. Herbal tablets can still be found in the marketplace. Tablets have the same advantages as capsules, but they can be harder to digest. Some tablets are made with fillers to bind the herbs together, and these ingredients aren't always disclosed on the label.

Tablets contain powdered herbs mixed with filling agents, binding agents, flowing agents, and disintegration agents. Filling agents are designed to make each tablet the exact same size. A binding agent is an ingredient that holds the tablet together. Sticky botanicals such as slippery elm and acacia gum are sometimes used as binding agents. Flowing agents are added to help the herbs go through the numerous manufacturing processes smoothly. Compounds such as magnesium stearate are often used as flowing agents. Most people won't have issues with magnesium stearate, but some people do seem sensitive to it.

Disintegration agents make the tablet dissolve once it is in the digestive system. Corn and potato starch are commonly used as disintegration agents. Cellulose compounds will make the tablet disintegrate after around 15 minutes in a digestive tract. Some mechanisms rely on the pH of the stomach and are therefore dependent on adequate stomach acid for breakdown.

Because of the shape, smell, and taste, tablets are often coated with a thin clear vegetable shellac, a color-coded dye substance, or a sugar coating.

Tablets are made with high-speed machinery. They are not practical to make at home, but you can mix herbal powders together in the same way you would to form a bolus (see Chapter Eight) and form the mixture into small round balls. Lay the balls on a flat surface and allow them to dry for a few days so that they harden slightly. These herbal pills can be swallowed like tablets. If allowed to thoroughly dry, they will store for a few weeks in an airtight container.

HERBAL NUT BUTTER BALLS

Herbal nut butter balls, popularized by herbalist Rosemary Gladstar, are a fun way to prepare tonic and nutritive herbs for consumption. Herb balls allow a higher dosage than what you can get from a few capsules or tablets. It's also a delicious way to prepare herbs for children.

16 ounces (1 pint) almond butter, peanut butter, or other nut butter
1½ cups maple syrup or honey
6–8 ounces powdered herbs
½ cup cocoa powder
Chopped nuts, raisins, or shredded coconut (optional)

Mix the ingredients together and roll them into balls. Roll the balls in coconut or in cocoa powder to coat them so they are less sticky.

Tonic and adaptogenic herbs like maca, astragalus, ashwagandha, ginseng, eleuthero, licorice, ginkgo, hawthorn, reishi, shiitake, and codonopsis all work well in this formula. You can also use herbal spices like cardamom or ginger for flavoring.

For even more ideas, look up "Rosemary Gladstar's Zoom Balls" online, or get her great book *Rosemary Gladstar's Herbal Recipes for Vibrant Health*.

TOPICAL USE OF BULK HERBS

Always apply herbs as close as possible to the problem. If you have a problem with your toe, put comfrey right on the toe. This simple concept forms the basis for treating many problems, and is often more effective than ingesting an herb and expecting it to act systemically. When herbs don't work, it is often as much the fault of improper application as it is poor choice of herbs.

There are a number of ways to apply herbs to the tissues that need them. Poultices, plasters, suppositories, and more are discussed in Chapter Eight.

USING MUCILAGINOUS HERBS

Highly mucilaginous herbs are best used in bulk. They do not work well as any form of extract. The water-soluble fibers they contain are known as mucilage, which does not extract in alcohol, vinegar, or oil. Mucilage is water soluble, but it absorbs the water, turning it into a slippery, slimy, unpalatable mass. So, although small amounts can be made into teas, syrups, and glycerites, the herbs simply work better when taken in bulk form.

Three popular herbs that fall into this category are slippery elm, marshmallow, and psyllium hulls. Slippery elm is on the United Plant Savers at-risk list, and marshmallow is a fully interchangeable and inexpensive alternative. Taking the bulk powder is the best way to obtain the benefits of marshmallow, because an effective dose is about a heaping teaspoon or more, which is difficult to obtain by taking capsules. Fortunately, its bland, slightly sweet taste is not unpleasant.

Marshmallow does not readily mix with water, so it's easiest to mix it with juice in the blender. For example, add a heaping teaspoon of marshmallow to a cup of apple or orange juice and blend them together. You can drink it right away before the mucilage absorbs the water and turns the liquid slimy. However, if you're trying to coat an irritated esophagus, let the mixture turn gelatinous before drinking it.

Marshmallow may also be mixed with applesauce or a hot cereal such as oatmeal.

Another herb that is best used in bulk is psyllium hulls, a bulk laxative. A therapeutic dose can be anywhere from ¼ teaspoon to 2 heaping teaspoons. This makes taking it in capsules impractical. It also is impossible to make an extract of it, again because the mucilage in it is not soluble in alcohol, vinegar, oil, or glycerin. Psyllium rapidly absorbs water, turning into a slimy, gelatinous mass that is not very appealing.

The best way to take psyllium is to mix it into a cup of water or juice (apple is the best). Stir it until it becomes suspended, then drink it before it has a chance to gel. When taking psyllium, start with a small amount (¼–½ teaspoon) and then work up to 1–2 teaspoons daily. Psyllium can also be blended with other herbs. See the Gentle Fiber Blend in Chapter Twelve for directions on making your own.

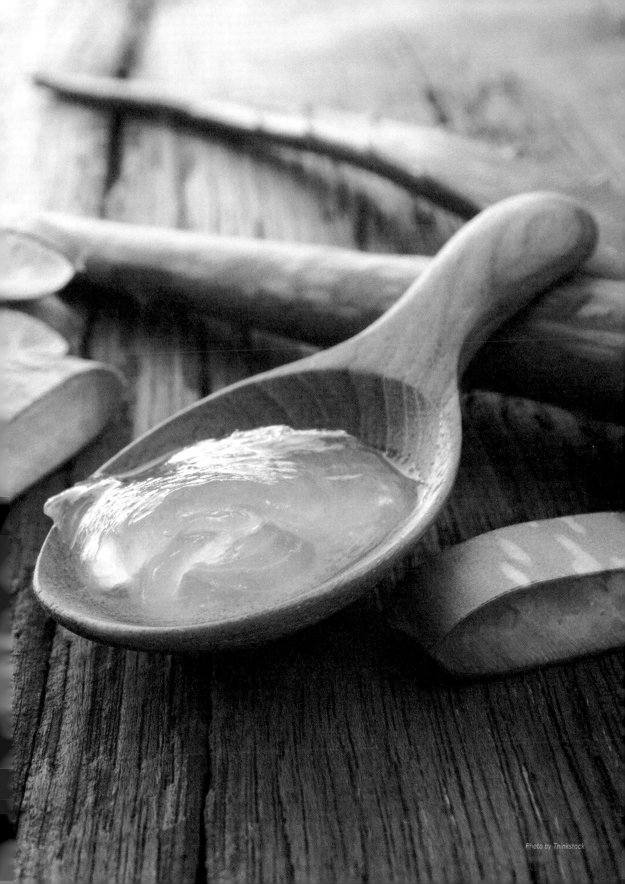

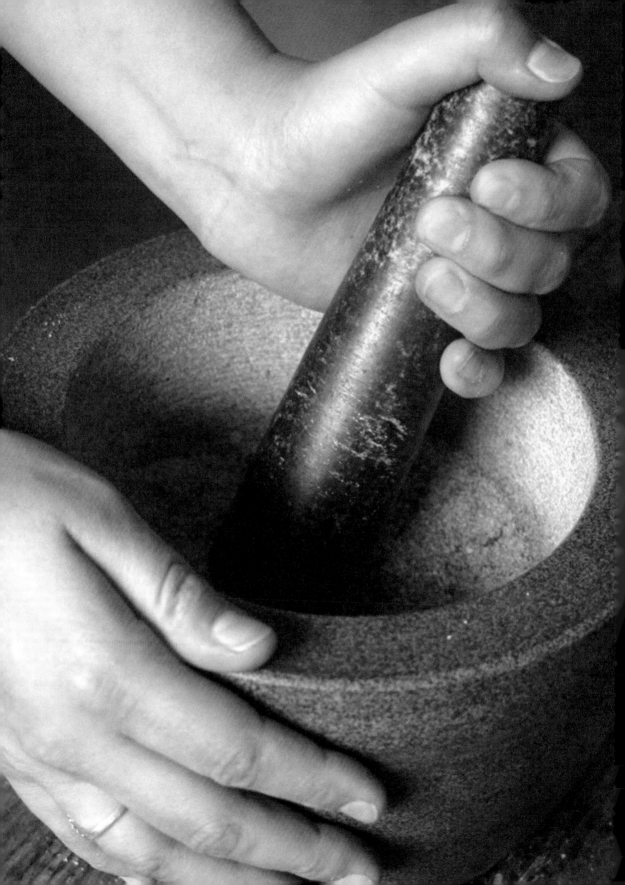

CHAPTER FIVE

Introduction to Extractions

TERMS, EQUIPMENT, SOLVENTS, AND CALCULATIONS

This chapter covers the basic terms associated with extracting herbs, the equipment you'll need, how to determine which solvent you should use, and how to determine potency.

EXTRACTION TERMS

Herbalism has its own unique language. It is the language of our art, and like many professions that use jargon, it invokes a bit of nostalgia and appreciation for the rich history of herbalism. Many of the terms we use in herbal medicine making date back to ancient times and are part of a rich heritage that teaches us how to turn crude plant material into effective herbal medicines. Here are some of the important terms to know.

Garbling is the process of removing stems, diseased plant parts, and critters from freshly harvested plant material. This improves the quality of the medicine being made. Try it by yourself with good music playing in the background and you might find that magical Zen-like state that just seems to make everything better.

Menstruum or solvent: Menstruum is an old alchemical term for a substance that dissolves a solid or holds it in suspension. The modern scientific term is solvent. Although many herbalists confine the term "menstruum" to alcohol extractions, technically anything that you use as a solution to extract the herbs is a menstruum, including water, alcohol, glycerin, vinegar, and simple syrups. Menstruums are measured in fluid volume. The choice to use metric units (liters, milliliters), fluid ounces, or the more standard US measures (cups, pints, quarts) is a personal one. Choose one and stick with it.

Marc is the solid matter (plant material) in your preparation. This marc is mixed with the menstruum for extraction. After the extraction process, the plant material is called the exhausted marc. Marc is measured by weight. Again, you can use metric or US measures; just make sure you use the same standard of measurement for the marc that you're using for the menstruum.

Solubility is the ability of the menstruum to extract various constituents from a plant into a liquid form. Solubility depends on many factors, including the polarity (electrical charge) of the substance, pH, temperature, and the presence of other constituents or compounds in the plant. Solubility is difficult to determine, but herbalists have the cumulative experience of other herbalists as well as some science to determine the best solvents for particular plants. We'll cover this in greater detail later in this chapter.

Maceration is a way to make tinctures. Macerating herbs means you soak the marc in the menstruum for a set period of time that varies from process to process. Maceration allows the menstruum to become saturated with constituents from the marc.

The **maceration container** is a leak-proof container, usually glass but sometimes stainless steel, that is used in the maceration process. Glass canning jars are commonly used by home medicine makers. They come in a wide assortment of sizes (half pints, pints, quarts, and even half gallons) and are relatively inexpensive. When using mason jars place a single layer of parchment paper between the lid and jar to keep your extract from interacting with the metal in the lid. Many solvents can cause metal corrosion, which will adversely affect your extract.

Succussion is an old word for shaking. Maceration extracts are succussed to ensure complete contact between the marc and the menstruum. In dry herb macerations, succussion is an essential part of the process. Agitation moves particles that clump at the bottom of the container back into contact with the menstruum. Succussion isn't normally required for fresh herb macerations; the high-proof alcohol used in fresh plant preparations dehydrates the plant cells, pulling all of the constituents out of the plant and into solution.

Decanting is the process of pouring off the menstruum from one container to another, often through a filtering cloth or paper, without disturbing the sediment at the bottom of the container.

Precipitation occurs when solid particles fall out of solution in a tincture or extract. This most commonly occurs when a tincture hasn't been filtered properly, or when the extract is exposed to light or drastic temperature changes. Precipitation will occur in most tinctures as they age, but if you've made the tincture or extract properly, it should not occur for many years. Mild precipitation can be fixed by decanting the tincture into a clean container. If massive precipitation occurs along with a change in color or taste, it's time to discard the tincture and start again.

MEDICINE-MAKING EQUIPMENT

In order to make herbal medicines, you'll need some equipment. Here are the items we recommend.

Jars. You will need jars—lots of them—if you get into medicine making. An assortment of mason jars is helpful: half pint, pint, and quart jars are all most home medicine makers need. If you're making medicine for an herbal practice, invest in half-gallon mason jars. One-gallon pickle jars work nicely for larger batches of tinctures. Gallon mason jars are no longer manufactured but can be found occasionally on eBay.

Rubber spatulas in an assortment of sizes will help get every last bit of medicine out of your jars.

Mortar and pestle. Although this seems like an antiquated tool, a mortar and pestle still comes in handy in medicine making. Most of the small marble sets are appropriate for displays and powdering small amounts of resins like myrrh. You can use larger sets to powder small batches of tea concentrates. (They are also good for powdering small amounts of whole spices for cooking.) If you have to powder roots and barks by hand, a tall cylindrical mortar and pestle is best.

Every herbalist should powder a pound of burdock root with a mortar and pestle at least once in their life, just for the experience. Okay, maybe not a whole pound, but it's well worth it to learn how to use a mortar and pestle to powder small batches of herbs as part of the experience of making your own medicines.

Coffee grinders are the home herbalist's best friend when it comes to powdering herbs. Buy them new or get them cheaply at thrift stores. They have to be babysat while you use them, and even then they don't last for a long time, but that's better than spending thousands of dollars on a commercial herb grinder.

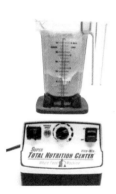

Vitamix. A Vitamix with a dry blade is even better than a coffee grinder. The adjustable-speed Vitamix has been around since about 1995, and although the look changes every few years, the motor stays the same. The dry blade container makes quick work of all but the hardest roots. The old-school Vitamix 3600 with the metal containers can grind hard roots, but can't powder as well as the models that support a dry blade container. The 3600 model is wonderful for making fresh plant extracts. In a pinch you can put your plant material and alcohol into a Vitamix, leave it running for an hour, and produce a passable tincture. (The constant agitation speeds up the maceration process, and the heat from the motor produces a hot ethanol extract.) The new Vitamix models have polycarbonate containers, which tend to get scratched by hard herbs. Keep one container dedicated to herb grinding and another for food.

Both the newer and older models can be found on eBay for $60–$150. At one time, Vitamix 3600 metal containers were produced without the juice spout, but they are impossible to find now. Disassemble and clean the juice spout after each use to prevent cross-contamination of herbs.

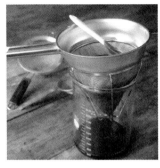 **Strainers and filters** in a variety of sizes are essential to good medicine making. Winco makes a stainless steel 8-inch bouillon strainer that can be found on Amazon for $23. After an initial straining with a fine mesh strainer, pour the tincture through an unbleached paper coffee filter or two. Don't get cone filters with glued bottoms; the glue might be soluble in high-proof alcohol. Place the coffee filters, or lab filter paper if you must, into the cone strainer to filter.

You can also filter with paint strainer bags, available at most hardware stores, or with muslin tea bags. In either case, suspend the bag from the mouth of a jar. The lid band for the canning jar will fit snugly over the bags to hold them in place. Extra-fine gold mesh coffee filters are also nice, and can be reused much longer than cotton bag filters. Extracts made with cut and sifted herbs can be strained using several layers of unbleached, natural cheesecloth or organic cotton or flannel cloth. Don't use stainless or gold mesh filters to strain resinous herbs. It is exceedingly difficult to clean a metal mesh filter that was used to filter boswellia gum.

Mixing bowls. A dedicated set of stainless steel or glass bowls in a variety of sizes is essential. We prefer the stainless steel bowls with a pour spout, but even plastic bowls will work in a pinch.

Herb press. An herb press isn't necessary for the beginning herbalist or home medicine maker, but if you make medicines long enough you'll tire of squeezing herbs by hand, which is time-consuming and inefficient, and leaves a lot of good medicine behind in the marc.

A potato ricer is a nice starting herb press, and is much cheaper than most herb presses. Keep the batch size fairly small to avoid overexertion and cursing. The Norpro 469 Deluxe Cast Aluminum Jumbo Potato Ricer is the one we use. We've only broken one between us, and that took years of use. It is well worth the $30.

If you are pressing batches of herbs larger than a quart, and you can afford it, upgrade to a good hydraulic or screw press. One of the best herb presses is an 1890s Enterprise sausage stuffer, wine press, and cider press. It's more effective than most of the herb presses available on the market, and it looks really cool. The Enterprise name has changed to Chop-Rite and they still make replacement parts for the old models, which can be found on eBay for $150–$300, and you can find them at garage sales and flea markets for a lot less.

If you know how to weld, you can modify a 1-ton hydraulic ball bearing press into an herb press for less than $200. That's a lot cheaper than the thousands-of-dollars hydraulic herb presses that are sold commercially. Large hydraulic presses are not efficient for batches that are smaller than 5 gallons.

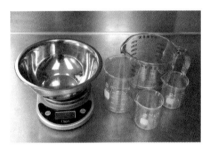

Scale. Buy a scale that measures in grams in addition to ounces and pounds. For the average herbalist a $20 kitchen scale from a big box store is as accurate as you need. To be more precise, buy a triple beam scale with a big basket, or buy a 100-gram tester weight to make sure your scale is balanced.

A **digital thermometer** helps manage temperatures for oil extracts or when cooking off alcohol from glycerin extracts. If you have the budget, get an infrared thermometer; if not, a digital candy thermometer works well.

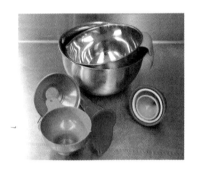

Measuring cups are helpful when making weight-to-volume extracts. Graduated cylinders are great when you need precise measurements. Glass graduated cylinders look good on shelves, but the first time you break a $40 Pyrex cylinder you'll invest in a few cheap polypropylene ones (the solvent only comes into contact with the plastic momentarily) You can get a seven-piece polypropylene set with cylinders ranging from 10 to 1,000 milliliters for less than $35 from Amazon or a lab supply store.

Funnels in a variety of sizes are helpful in pouring liquid extracts and powders from container to container. Canning funnels are great, and you can check out your local automotive or kitchen supply store for a bigger variety of sizes.

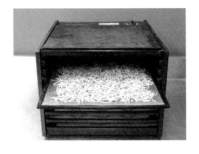

Dehydrator. Although not essential, a dehydrator is a useful tool for an herbalist. Dehydrators dry small batches of herbs quickly, and can be used to dehydrate herbal extracts to make tea concentrates and fluid extracts. It's also a wonderful investment if you want to dehydrate food like flaxseed crackers, fruit leathers, kale chips, or jerky.

A horizontal dehydrator, like the one pictured here, is a good addition to your apothecary, but even a cheap vertical dehydrator is better than no dehydrator. (A space heater and a fan are not quite as efficient.)

PICKING A SOLVENT AND EXTRACTION METHOD

Throughout history, and especially since the 1600s, herbalists, alchemists, and physicians have been experimenting with various methods of extracting herbs. One of the great pioneers of this science was John Uri Lloyd (1849–1936), who was widely regarded as the best pharmacist of his time and the maker of the highest-quality herbal extracts in history. Lloyd approached every plant differently, using up to eight solvents on one plant to extract what he considered the essence of the plant.

Every menstruum has particular constituents that it extracts effectively and other constituents that it doesn't extract well. Water is a poor solvent of resins, but a great solvent for carbohydrates; alcohol is a great solvent for many medicinal constituents, but is a poor solvent of mucilage; and glycerin by itself (without heat and water) is a poor solvent of most constituents except volatile oils. Oil and fat can be used as menstruums to make extracts, but these are normally only used externally. Steam and carbon dioxide are used to extract essential oils.

Commercial manufacturing and home extractions often use mixtures of menstruums (water, alcohol, glycerin, or vinegar). Standardized extracts may involve the use of chemical solvents to concentrate specific constituents, but that is not necessary for herbal products made at home.

Some molecules, like water, are polar. That means that, just as a magnet has a north pole and a south pole, the molecule has a positively charged region and a negatively charged region. This means that polar molecules can attach to both positively charged elements and negatively charged elements. Water is highly polar, which is why it is a nearly universal solvent. On the other hand, a non-polar molecule will be more electrically neutral and therefore a less-effective solvent.

Water and glycerin are polar molecules; water is the most polar of the two. Alcohol is also polar and can be used to extract polar constituents when the percentage of alcohol in water is low. A higher alcohol content is better for extracting nonpolar constituents. Fats and oils are nonpolar solvents.

Constituents that are best extracted using water, glycerin, or lower per-centages of alcohol include carbohydrates (sugars and starches), mucilage and gums, most glycosides, and water-soluble vitamins. Some alkaloids can be extracted with polar substances. Oil and higher percentages of alcohol are bet-ter at extracting essential oils, terpenoids, carotenoids, fat-soluble vitamins, lipids, resins, and most alkaloids.

Chapter Thirteen lists numerous single herbs and suggests a number of ways to prepare them. Table 2 provides a basic guide to the best extraction medium for the major categories of herbs. The primary constituents of each category of herb are listed in parentheses.

POTENCIES

A critical consideration when extracting any herb is how much liquid to use in proportion to herbs. This ratio depends on how potent you want your prepa-ration. The commonly accepted way to standardize the potency of a formula is to calculate the ratio of the amount of herb to the amount of solvent. This is written with the amount of herb first and the amount of liquid second (1:5).

	Solvent				
Herbs	*Water*	*Alcohol*	*Glycerin*	*Vinegar*	*Oil*
Aromatic Herbs (essential oils)	Fair	Good	Excellent	Good	Excellent
Pungent Herbs (alkamindes)	Fair	Excellent	Excellent	Good	Excellent
Pungent or Resinous Herbs (resins)	Poor	Excellent	Fair to Good	Poor	Excellent
Aromatic Bitters (sesquiterpene lactones and triterpenes)	Good	Excellent	Poor to Fair	Poor	Poor
Simple (nonalkaloidal) Bitters (diterpenes, glycosides)	Good	Excellent	Fair to Good	Poor	Poor
Alkaloidal Bitters (alkaloids)	Good	Good	Fair to Good	Good	Poor
Acrid Herbs (resins, alkaloids)	Good	Excellent	Good	Fair	Poor
Astringent Herbs (tannins)	Good	Fair	Excellent	Fair	Fair
Salty Herbs (minerals)	Excellent	Poor	Fair	Poor to Fair	Poor
Sweet or Tonic Herbs (polysaccharides, saponins, glycosides)	Excellent	Good	Good	Poor	Poor
Demulcent Herbs (mucilage and gums)	Good	Poor	Fair	Poor	Fair
Sour Herbs (organic acids)	Good	Good	Excellent	Fair	Poor
Oily Herbs (oils)	Poor	Fair	Fair	Poor	Excellent

TABLE 2   **Basic Categories of Herbs and the Best Solvents**

Amounts are always measured by weight, not by volume, as the weight of various solvents is different. When measuring water, weight and volume are closely related. One fluid ounce of water weighs about 1 ounce. Sixteen fluid ounces of water (which is 1 pint or 2 cups by volume) weighs about 1 pound (16 ounces by weight). The same applies in metrics. One liter of water weighs 1 kilogram, and 100 milliliters of water weighs about 100 grams. The exact weight of the water depends on its temperature and other factors, but for home preparations these differences are not critical.

As shown in Table 3, alcohol has the same weight-to-volume relationship as water, but other extraction mediums, such as vinegar, glycerin, and oil, do not. Once again, these differences are not so critical that you can't measure the liquids by volume.

Substance	Weight per Gallon	Weight per Quart	Weight per Pint
Water	8 lb (128 fl oz or 16 cups)	2 lb (32 fl oz or 4 cups)	1 lb (16 fl oz or 2 cups)
Alcohol	8 lb (128 fl oz)	2 lb (32 fl oz)	1 lb (16 fl oz)
Vinegar	8.4 lb	2.1 lb	1.05 lb
Glycerin	10.5 lb	2.51 lb	1.25 lb
Olive Oil	7.6 lb	1.9 lb	0.95 lb

TABLE 3   Weights of Various Solvents

Amount of Herb	Amount of Menstruum
1 ounce	8 ounces (1 cup)
1 pound	8 pounds (1 gallon)
100 kilograms	800 liters
1 kilogram	8 liters

TABLE 4   1:8 Weight-to-Volume Extraction Ratio

Most home preparations are between 1:2 and 1:10 in potency. Table 4 shows the amount of menstruum needed to make a 1:8 potency with various amounts of herb.

The strength of the extract depends partially on the density of the herb you are extracting. It is usually easy to make a 1:4 or 1:5 extract of heavy pieces of bark or roots at home. When making a Simpler's maceration with lighter fresh plant materials like dill weed or chamomile flowers, you're more likely to end up with a 1:8 or even 1:10 extract, unless you really pack the plant material into your jar.

Table 5 shows some standard potencies.

Ratios are important in determining dosage. A 1:2 extract will be four times stronger than a 1:8 extract, which means you'll need to take four times more of the 1:8 extract to get the same results as you would taking a 1:2 extract. You can read more about dosages in Chapter Eleven.

These guidelines are based on the assumption that you are extracting all of the available constituents from the plant material, but plants vary greatly in their chemical composition. Plants that are wild and plants that are harvested when they are under environmental stress tend to be more chemically active than cultivated plants. Some plant constituents in the same plant can vary by up to 10,000% within a 2-week period. While we advocate using

Potency	Ounces of Herb to Add per Quart of Menstruum	Strength
1:2	16	very strong
1:4	8	strong
1:5	6.4	standard
1:6	5.2	weak
1:10	1.6	very weak, often used for toxic botanicals

TABLE 5   Standard Weight-to-Volume Ratios

weight-to-volume ratios to help determine potency, we also suggest tasting tinctures and extracts and comparing them to previous batches. You might also compare them to commercial extracts or to the extracts of other herbalists. Assess the taste, smell, texture, and visual appearance of each preparation to determine its potency.

WORKING WITH ALCOHOL

Different herbs extract better in different percentages of alcohol. Proof is a measurement of the percentage of alcohol in an alcoholic solution and is double the percentage of alcohol: 80 proof is 40% alcohol, and 160 proof is 80% alcohol.

Most home tinctures are made with a weak solution of 40% alcohol like brandy. Some herbs need to be extracted with a higher alcohol content. A moderate-strength solution can be made with 60% alcohol, and a strong solution with 80% alcohol.

The strongest alcohol solution commonly available is grain alcohol (the brand Everclear is the most widely available), which is usually 190 proof or 95% alcohol. You can purchase large quantities (55 gallons) of organic cane or grape alcohol for about the same price as Everclear. Consider going in with other herbalists and splitting an order. Organic cane or grape alcohol has a smoother taste and a more pleasant action than grain alcohol.

Unless you are making a fresh plant extract, 95% alcohol needs to be diluted to reach the desired concentration. If you have 95% alcohol and need 40% alcohol, put 40 parts of alcohol in a container and add enough water to make 95 parts. (A part is any volume of liquid measurement that you choose, such as 1 fluid ounce.) To dilute 95% alcohol to 60%, put 60 parts of alcohol in a container and add enough water to make 95 parts. Tables 6, 7, and 8 will help you with these conversions.

Now that we've gotten all the technical stuff out of the way, we can get to the fun part: Making your own herbal extracts.

Alcohol Proof	95% (190 Proof)	90% (180 Proof)	80% (160 Proof)
Amount of Alcohol	40 ml or fl oz	40 ml or fl oz	40 ml or fl oz
Amount of Water to Add	55 ml or fl oz	50 ml or fl oz	40 ml or fl oz
Total Amount of Solution	95 ml or fl oz	90 ml or fl oz	80 ml or fl oz

TABLE 6 Weak Solution (40% Alcohol)

Alcohol Proof	95% (190 Proof)	90% (180 Proof)	80% (160 Proof)
Amount of Alcohol	60 ml or fl oz	60 ml or fl oz	60 ml or fl oz
Amount of Water to Add	35 ml or fl oz	30 ml or fl oz	20 ml or fl oz
Total Amount of Solution	95 ml or fl oz	90 ml or fl oz	80 ml or fl oz

TABLE 7 Medium Solution (60% Alcohol)

Alcohol Proof	95% (190 Proof)	90% (180 Proof)	80% (160 Proof)
Amount of Alcohol	80 ml or fl oz	80 ml or fl oz	80 ml or fl oz
Amount of Water to Add	15 ml or fl oz	10 ml or fl oz	none
Total Amount of Solution	95 ml or fl oz	90 ml or fl oz	80 ml or fl oz

TABLE 8 Strong Solution (80% Alcohol)

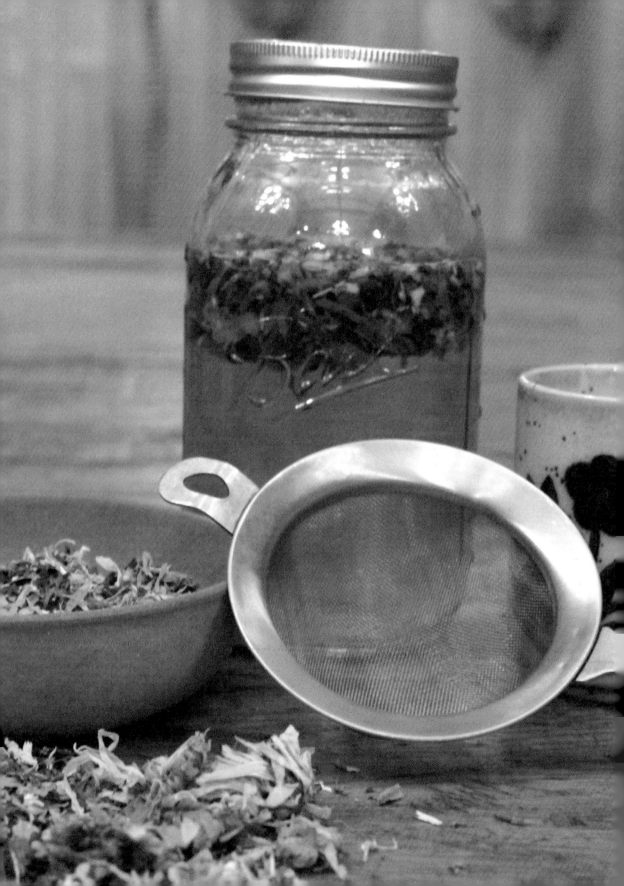

CHAPTER SIX

Making Basic Extracts

EXTRACTING HERBS IN WATER,
ALCOHOL, GLYCERIN, AND VINEGAR

M aking your own herbal extracts is enjoyable and educational. The process of extracting herbs will teach you a lot about different kinds of herbs and help you understand how to use them better. You'll learn how to use your own senses to understand the effects herbs have on the body, especially if you taste what you make during the process (like a good chef does with her food).

The key to making good extracts is to start with high-quality plant material. You don't have to start with fresh plants to make high-quality extracts, but you can't make good extracts out of a bag of 5-year-old, dried-out, cheap, imported herbs either. Use only reputable suppliers, or look for independent herbalists who sell or barter cultivated or wildcrafted plants from their region. Check out Appendix Two for companies that sell high-quality herbs and for groups that facilitate the swapping or selling of herbs from independent bioregional herbalists.

Once you have the plant material you need, you can turn it into liquid extracts using a variety of solvents and extraction methods.

WATER-BASED EXTRACTIONS

Water extraction is the oldest and most basic method for making herbal medicine.

INFUSIONS

Herbal teas are easy to make and are a good start to learning to use herbal remedies. A hot or cold infusion can be made from fresh, dried, or powdered herbs. An infusion is sometimes called a tisane, which is a French word for tea. Teas are cheap, simple, and effective, and require only a short time to prepare.

Infusions are a pleasant way to take some herbs, but are less palatable when the herb has a disagreeable flavor. Many constituents, especially the more bitter and astringent principles, are not released into the water in a simple tea but need to be extracted by more potent infusions or decoctions. Aromatic principles are lost if the container is left uncovered while the herbs are steeping.

Infusions are used for topical applications as rinses, compresses, and foot soaks. An infusion may have a single ingredient or many. It may be taken hot or cold, inhaled as a vapor, used to perfume a pillow, or enjoyed in a bath.

Hot Infusion

Hot infusions are best for leaves and flowers whose medicinal properties, including vitamins and volatile oils, are easily released into water. To make a hot infusion, pour boiled water (boil water, take off the heat, and wait 30 seconds) over the herb. Cover the container. Use a canning jar, a covered pan, or a china, glass, or enamel teapot, and the purest water you can get. Let the infusion steep for at least 15 minutes, depending on the desired strength (see below), then strain the infusion into a cup. Drink it lukewarm or cool, but take it hot to break up a cold or cough. Teas can be sweetened with honey or raw sugar, or flavored with herbs such as lemon verbena or spearmint. Make infusions fresh each day, or refrigerate unused tea for up to three days.

Water with a high lime content (very hard water) can impede the extraction of active constituents. Adding a little vinegar or lemon juice will help with the extraction of alkaloidal bitters, such as plants with berberine, or minerals like calcium.

Some herbs take up more space than others and have to be packed down into the steeping container. The more surface area that is exposed, the more potent the tea, so don't be afraid to chop the herb finely or even powder it before making tea.

Most people steep tea a few minutes. This isn't enough time when using plants for medicines. Here are the different steeping times depending on what strength you need.

Weak Infusion Use 15 grams of herb per liter of water, or ½ ounce per quart. The steeping time varies depending on what part of the plant is used. Steep leaves for 1 hour, flowers for 30 minutes, crushed seeds for 15 minutes, and bark and roots for 4 hours.

Standard Infusion Steep 30 grams of herb in 1 liter of hot water, or 1 ounce per quart, for 30–60 minutes. Strain well, pressing as much water out of the herb as possible, and drink the tea. Use within a day. Cut the formula down if you are drinking less than a liter of tea daily; use 15 grams of herb to 500 milliliters of water (½ ounce per pint).

This medicinal infusion represents about 1 gram of herb for every ounce of tea and is much stronger than normal tea. In most cases, the required dose is significantly less than a whole cup, which is wonderful for those not-so-pleasant-tasting teas.

Strong Infusion Make as a standard infusion and steep for 8 hours.

Cold Infusion

A cold infusion is best for herbs with highly volatile constituents, or constituents that are damaged by heat. Soak 15 grams of herb in 1 liter of cold water (½ ounce per quart) for 8–12 hours. Strain and drink. Make a fresh infusion daily.

DECOCTIONS

When your medicinal plant is tough, as in the bark, roots, rhizomes, seeds, nuts, or woody stems, you need to use the decoction method to extract the plant constituents. Decoct green plant parts if you are trying to extract mineral salts. A decoction is like a tea, except that the herb is simmered in water until some of the liquid has evaporated. Simmering evaporates volatile principles, so the decoction method is not a good technique for aromatic herbs.

Like infusions, decoctions may contain one ingredient or many. They may be ingested hot or cold or applied externally. Make decoctions fresh daily and refrigerate unused tea. A decoction should keep for up to 3 days in the refrigerator.

Standard Decoction

Put 30 grams of herb and 1 liter of water (1 ounce per quart) in a pot, cover, and bring to a low simmer for 10–20 minutes. Turn off the heat and steep for an additional hour.

Strong Decoction

Place 30 grams of herb and 1 liter of water (1 ounce per quart) in a pot, cover, and bring to a low simmer until the water is reduced by half.

Southern Decoction

Place 30 grams of herb and 2 liters of water (1 ounce per 2 quarts) in a pot. Bring to a low simmer for 4 or more hours, until there is about 500 milliliters (about 1 pint) of fluid remaining.

This process allows most volatile oils to escape while extracting more mineral salts, creating a tea with a different medicinal action than standard teas.

SYRUPS (ELECTUARIES)

A syrup is a water extract that is preserved with a sweetener, typically honey or raw sugar. Most syrups are made by simmering the herbs in a mixture of 50% water and 50% sweetener and straining the syrup for use.

Syrups keep longer than water extracts, because the sugar preserves the extraction. The sweet taste covers the nasty flavor of many herbs, such as dandelion, white pine bark, poplar bark, or raw garlic. Try medicinal syrups for anyone who cannot or will not tolerate bitter or strong flavors.

Sweeteners

Honey is a natural sweetener with proven antibiotic and antiseptic properties. Honey is a combination of sugars produced from nectar by the enzyme invertase, which is found in the bodies of bees. Honey contains about 40% fructose, 31% glucose, 18% water, 9% other sugars, and 2% sucrose. The flavor varies depending on the flower source. Honey contains all the vitamins and enzymes necessary for the proper metabolism and digestion of glucose and other sugar molecules. Honey is about 50% sweeter than table sugar, which means that ¾ cup honey adds the same sweetness to a formula as 1 cup sugar. Do not give syrups made with honey to children under the age of one.

Maple syrup is a natural sweetener made by boiling the sap of maple trees. It contains primarily sucrose, the same type of sugar as raw sugar. Maple syrup contains significant amounts of manganese and moderate but notable amounts of zinc. Pure maple syrup is expensive, but makes an excellent medicinal syrup base.

Raw sugar. Syrups can be made using natural sugars like raw sugar, yellow D sugar, or freeze-dried sugarcane juice (Sucanat). These sugars are not as sweet as honey and do not have the same medicinal benefits, but they add their own flavor to the syrup, which may improve the taste of some preparations. Refined sugar is the ultimate naked carbohydrate, stripped of all nutritional benefits, and should be avoided when making syrups if raw sugar, honey, or maple syrup is available.

Making a Syrup

Standard Method Mix sweetener and water in equal parts by heating the mixture slightly. Add the plant material at a ratio of 1:5, or 20% of the volume of liquid by weight. To make 1 pint syrup (16 fluid ounces), mix 1 cup water (8 fluid

FRESH BERRY SYRUP

Heat fresh berries (such as elder berries, bilberries, hawthorn berries, or rose hips) in just enough water to soften the berries, then press the berries and water through a jelly bag to express the juice, as you would do for making jelly. Measure the amount of berry juice and add an equal amount of honey or raw sugar. This syrup can be bottled or canned like jelly.

ounces) and 1 cup raw sugar or honey (8 fluid ounces). Add about 3.2 ounces (20% of 16 ounces) of herbs. Bring the mixture to a boil, then turn the heat down low and simmer, covered, for 20–30 minutes. Strain the herbs and bottle the syrup.

Simple Method Make a strong infusion or decoction of the herbs. Measure the volume of the decoction or infusion and add an equal amount of honey or raw sugar.

Using Syrups

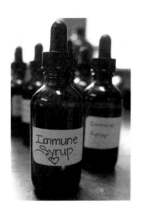

Syrups are great for soothing sore throats, coughs, and most digestive upsets. The high sugar content makes them unsuitable for treating chronic fatigue, nutritive imbalances, or deep-seated chronic disorders like diabetes. Avoid syrups with people who have severe intestinal dysbiosis (an imbalance of gut bacteria that causes gas, bloating, and digestive upset), and use cautiously with hypoglycemia.

Doses for syrups are relatively large (from 1 teaspoon to 2 tablespoons). Syrup stores in the refrigerator for up to a month.

If the syrup develops an off taste, or if mold appears on the top of the syrup, discard it. To preserve the syrup for a longer period, add 20% of an 80-proof alcohol like brandy or rum. Syrups with alcohol added will last for a year or more when refrigerated or canned.

There are several formulas for syrups in Chapter Twelve.

ALCOHOL EXTRACTIONS (TINCTURES)

Water preparations have limited shelf life. To make liquid preparations with a longer shelf life, you need to use a menstruum that has preservative actions. Alcohol has been used to make herbal extracts for thousands of years. The chemical analysis of residue found in clay pots in China confirms that a fermented drink made of honey, hawthorn berry, and grape was being produced between 7000 and 5600 BCE. At around the same time, barley beer and grape wine were being made in the Middle East. There is evidence of alcoholic beverages being consumed as far back as 3000 BCE in Egypt and 2000 BCE in the Americas. Research dating back to ancient Mesopotamia suggests that beer preceded bread as a caloric staple and as a way to preserve grains throughout the winter. There is even literature from the Babylonians and Egyptians warning about the ill effects of the overconsumption of alcohol. Ayurvedic texts from India describe the medicinal effects of alcohol and warn of alcohol-induced disease and intoxication.

The medicinal effects of alcohol are cataloged in many of the oldest written works. The Bible talked about the medicinal use of wine. The Catholic Church and early Protestant leaders taught that alcohol was a gift from God to be used in moderation for enjoyment and health.

In medieval Europe small beer was made and consumed by most households. Water and barley, boiled and then fermented, made a much safer drink than plain water. There are reports of people drinking more than a gallon of small beer daily, which clocks in at around 1% alcohol by volume.

The use of wine as medicine was mentioned in Sima Qian's biography of Bian Que, a Chinese doctor in the fifth century BCE. It is not known if Bian Que used herbs in the making of wine, or if he assigned energetics to different varieties of wine in a manner similar to that of traditional Chinese food theory. According to the Yellow Emperor's Classic, written between 475 and 221 BCE, medicinal wines were made by fermenting herbs along with the fruit. It wasn't until the Qing dynasty in the 1600s that tincturing and infusing wines with medicinal herbs became commonplace.

HERBAL BEERS AND WINES

Historically, bittering agents and flavorings (gruit) used in beers varied throughout the world. Households and geographic areas had favorite combinations of herbs that provided taste and helped with the preservation of the drink. Gruit typically consisted of a number of medicinal herbs, including sweet gale, yarrow, mugwort, ground ivy, and spruce tips.

Herb-infused wines have been used in the Western world at least since Hippocrates. They played a big role in materia medicas prior to the seventeenth century, when distillation became more common. In our opinion, medicinal wines should play a bigger role in modern herbalism than they currently do. There is a wine formula under wild cherry in Chapter Thirteen.

DISTILLATION

Distillation vessels have been found dating back to the first century CE, but most experts think that they were used in the distillation experiments of alchemy rather than to distill alcohol or volatile oils. The discovery of alcohol distillation is a topic of contention. There is some evidence that the Chinese invented it, and other evidence that it was the Italians or Greeks. Most experts believe that the Arabians invented alcohol distillation. The Persian alchemist Jābir ibn Hayyān is credited with inventing the alembic, the precursor to the pot still; and the great physician Ibn Sīnā (Avicenna) refined distillation by adding the cooling coil. It was the German Albertus Magnus (1193–1280) who first clearly described the process for manufacturing distilled spirits.

Distillation and the concentrated alcohol it produced spread slowly in medicine. Herbalists administered herbs as decoctions and wine infusions until the thirteenth century, when Spanish alchemists Arnold of Villanova and

Raymond Lully introduced aqua vitae (water of life, otherwise known as brandy) as a solvent in European medicine. In the sixteenth century, Paracelsus popularized the use of distilled alcohol as a solvent to prepare tinctures. At this point brandy contained at most 70% alcohol. In the early nineteenth century, Aeneas Coffey invented the continuous column still, which led to the production of 94–96% ethanol.

DRIED HERB TINCTURES (MACERATIONS)

The most common way of making a tincture is by soaking an herb in a solution of alcohol and water for 14 days or more. This process is called maceration. Most maceration extracts are done as a cold process, meaning they do not require heat.

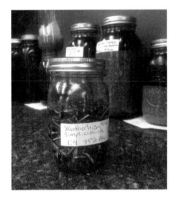

Standard tinctures are made using a weight-to-volume ratio of 1:5 with dried herbs. A quart jar will hold about 150 grams of plant material with 750 milliliters of menstruum. The percentage of alcohol used depends on the plant and the constituents you are trying to extract. For most dry plants an alcohol content of 40–60% is best. The two most common choices for home medicine making are 40% alcohol vodka and brandy and 50% alcohol vodka. Note that the proof is double the percentage of alcohol, so 40% alcohol is 80 proof. In many cases it is more cost effective to buy 190-proof alcohol (95% EtOH) such as Everclear and dilute it with water to the appropriate percentage, as described in Chapter Five.

Some herbs require a higher alcohol percentage than others. Resins and gums should be macerated in 90% alcohol to extract constituents, whereas glycoside-containing herbs like soapwort, mullein, or licorice, or a tannin-containing herb such as witch hazel, might require only 25% alcohol.

Keep the maceration in a dark place. Shake the jar daily for 2 weeks or more. Pour the liquid out through a muslin cloth and squeeze the marc (herbs) until you have removed as much of the extract as possible. Put the finished tincture in an amber bottle or other dark container to protect it from degradation by light.

FRESH PLANT TINCTURES (MACERATIONS)

Fresh plants usually contain significant water content, so most fresh plant tinctures are made with 95% alcohol. High-proof alcohol ruptures the cell walls of plants, bringing the constituents into solution with the alcohol. It is easiest to make a fresh plant tincture by blending the plant material with alcohol in a blender, or you can chop the herb by hand and mix it with alcohol in a jar. Allow the maceration to sit for at least 14 days, then strain and bottle. We have found jars of fresh plant macerations, forgotten in the back of a cabinet for more than 5 years, to be effective medicine. So while 14 days is the minimum time necessary to let a fresh plant maceration sit, the maximum time is whenever you remember to strain the tincture.

If you want to make a fresh plant tincture using a lower percentage of alcohol, you will need to figure out the moisture content of the fresh plant material. This is not necessary for home herbalists unless they are making products for commercial sale.

To determine the percentage of water in a plant, dry 100 grams of the fresh plant in a dehydrator or oven. Weigh the dried plant material. The difference between the fresh weight and dried weight is the percentage of water content: If the herb weighs 70 grams after drying, the plant material was 30% water.

USING ALCOHOL WITH OTHER SOLVENTS

To get a better extract, you can blend alcohol with other solvents. Adding 10% glycerin to an alcohol tincture helps extract volatile oils and stabilizes tannins. It gives the tincture a more pleasant taste, especially when using high-proof alcohol. In plants where the dominant constituents are alkaloids or minerals, add 5% vinegar to extract the constituents more effectively. Add 10% raw sugar or honey to a finished alcohol extract to create an elixir.

GLYCERIN EXTRACTS (GLYCERITES)

Glycerin is an underused menstruum in the herbal world. The sweet taste of glycerin helps to mask bitterness and other disagreeable flavors. Glycerin is a tri-atomic alcohol, not a sugar. This means glycerin does not affect blood sugar levels in healthy people, nor does it cause problems with yeast.

Glycerin is a natural component of triglycerides. Fats and oils are composed of three (tri-) fatty acids attached to a molecule of glycerin (-glyceride). The body breaks down fats and oils to fatty acids and glycerin. It reassembles them to make the body's own fats, or it can metabolize the glycerin and fatty acids for fuel. The conversion of glycerin to glucose produces only carbon dioxide and water.

Glycerin is moisturizing, and it is frequently used in soaps, lotions, and creams. It is also a preservative, inhibiting the growth of bacteria and fungi. Because it is sweet, nourishing, and nontoxic, glycerin is the best menstruum to use in herbal extracts for children or adults who cannot use alcohol.

Glycerin is a polar solvent, but not as polar as water. It does not extract constituents very well unless heat is used during the extraction process, so it is not a good menstruum to use for heat-sensitive herbs.

Glycerin is sticky, so it's not as easy to work with as alcohol. When using it as a menstruum, purchase pure vegetable glycerin that is intended for food use. Glycerin is available from a number of companies that sell bulk herbs and can easily be found on the internet.

HOW GLYCERITES ARE MADE

There are a number of ways to make an herbal glycerite. Here are four methods:

Traditional Method

Edward Shook, author of *Advanced Treatise in Herbology*, was a big advocate of glycerites. He made a strong decoction or infusion and added an equal amount of glycerin as a preservative. The resulting mixture is 50% water and 50% glycerin. In our experience, 10% of extracts made this way develop mold on the top. Increasing the glycerin content to 60% prevents mold growth. You can also add 20% of an 80-proof alcohol to a finished glycerite to improve shelf life of a 50% water/50% glycerin preparation.

Standard Method

Another method for making glycerites is to use the standard method for making syrups, as described earlier in this chapter. Some of the water will simmer off in this process, so start with 55% glycerin and 45% water. Add the herbs to the glycerin–water mixture at a 1:5 ratio. Simmer the herbs for 20–30 minutes, then strain and bottle.

Sealed Simmer Glycerites

Simmering herbs in a pot, even with the lid on, allows many of the volatile oils in the herbs to escape. To make a sealed simmer glycerite, start with a mixture of 60% glycerin and 40% water. Put the herbs and menstruum into canning jars at the standard 1:5 ratio. For pint jars add 3.33 ounces of herbs, and for quart jars add 6.66 ounces of herbs. If the plant material is dense, round these figures up to 4 ounces of herb for a pint jar and 8 ounces for a quart jar. If the plant material is extremely light and you can't get the full amount of herb into the jar, pack it no more than three-quarters full.

Cover the plant material with the glycerin–water mixture, leaving at least ¼ inch of headspace in the jar. Put the canning lid on the jar and put it into a boiling water bath or steam canner. When the water starts to boil (or the steam starts to stream out of the steam canner), start timing the extract. Extract the herbs for a minimum of 15 minutes for leaves and flowers and 30 minutes for denser plant materials like barks and roots. Let the jars cool until they can be safely handled, then strain the contents and bottle them. To use a pressure canner to make glycerites, process the jars at 5 pounds of pressure for 10 minutes for leaves and flowers, and for 15 minutes for barks and roots.

Fresh Plant Glycerites

Glycerin will extract essential oils in fresh aromatic herbs such as peppermint and lemon balm. Stuff a canning jar completely full of the fresh plant material, leaving about 1 inch of headspace. Fill the jar with a mixture of 70% glycerin and 30% water. Put the canning lid on the jar and seal tightly to prevent the essential oils from escaping. Put the jar in the canner or a boiling-water bath and process in boiling water for about 15 minutes. Allow the jar to become cool to the touch before opening and straining out the herbs. The fragrance and aroma of such extracts are absolutely incredible.

NOTES ABOUT COMMERCIAL GLYCERITES

Alcohol can be used as an intermediate if the active constituents are not water soluble. Some glycerites are made commercially by making standard alcohol tinctures, then drawing off the alcohol using a vacuum and gentle heat. Glycerin is added to make a very strong glycerite preparation. Most of the aromatic qualities of the extract are lost during this process.

USES AND APPLICATIONS OF GLYCERITES

Glycerites are great for children, alcoholics, people whose religious beliefs prohibit the use of alcohol, and people who dislike the taste of alcohol tinctures.

We have never seen a glycerite go bad as long as the glycerin content was well above 50% and the product was stored in a cool, dark place. Done properly, glycerites have a shelf life of at least 3 years. Some people refrigerate glycerites just to be safe.

Glycerin isn't as strong of a solvent as alcohol. Whereas the dose of tinctures is usually measured in drops, glycerites are taken in teaspoons. Glycerin is more expensive than alcohol, and the large dose makes glycerites more expensive per dose than alcohol tinctures.

HERBAL VINEGARS

Vinegars have been used for five thousand years as flavor enhancers and food preservers. Vinegars help digest heavy foods and high-protein meals and can be used in condiments, relishes, or dressings. The most nutritious vinegars still contain the mother (a mixture of beneficial bacteria and enzymes) in the bottle; they look slightly cloudy.

HOW VINEGARS ARE MADE

Herbal vinegars are made with apple cider or wine vinegar as a base. To make culinary vinegars, bruise freshly picked herbs and pack loosely in a jar. Cover with vinegar and cap with an acid-proof lid, or place parchment paper between the mouth of the jar and the metal lid. Set the vinegar in a sunny window and shake daily for 2 weeks. Test for flavor. If it is not strong enough, strain the vinegar and repeat the process with fresh herbs. Store as is or strain through cheesecloth and rebottle. (Add a fresh sprig of the herb to the bottle for identification and visual appeal.) Use culinary vinegars in salad dressings, marinades, gravies, and sauces.

You can also make vinegars with fresh berries or flowers. To make a raspberry vinegar, steep 500 grams of raspberries in 1 liter of wine vinegar for 2 weeks, then strain. Berry vinegar can be added to cough remedies or used in gargles for sore throats, and the delightful flavor masks the taste of bitter herbal expectorants. To make floral vinegars, remove the stems and any green or white heels from the petals before steeping. Carnations, clover, elder flowers, lavender, and sweet violets make good vinegars.

Medicinal vinegars are made with high-mineral herbs like horsetail, oat straw, alfalfa, nettles, and even eggshells. Vinegar leaches the minerals out of herbs and eggshells, and can be a great addition to a program for bone building.

Fire Cider, a traditional remedy for cold and flu, is made using vinegar. See Chapter Twelve for a formula.

USES AND APPLICATIONS OF VINEGARS

Herbal vinegars are good for bone building and for use in salads and cooking applications. They help to regulate gut flora and improve function in the digestive tract. Vinegar extracts are generally not as strong as alcohol or glycerin preparations, so they require larger doses. However, they are inexpensive to make and are a great way to incorporate herbs into the diet.

Vinegar is used as an addition to some tinctures to acidify the solution, and is particularly useful if you use hard water or if you are trying to extract alkaloids from the herb.

Because herbal oils are nearly always intended for topical use, we explain how to extract herbs in fat and oil in Chapter Eight, "Topical Preparations."

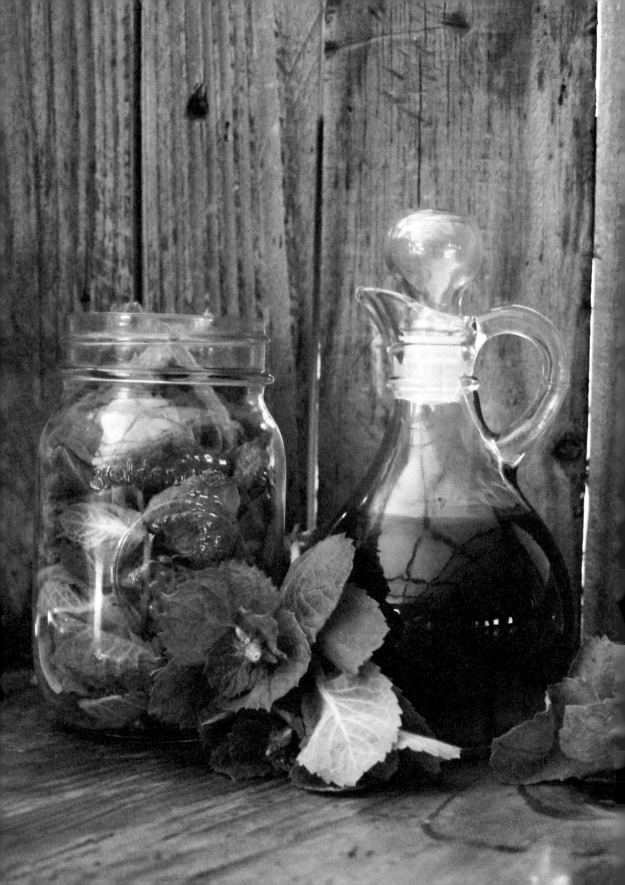

CHAPTER SEVEN

Advanced Extraction Techniques

PERCOLATION EXTRACTS, FLUID EXTRACTS, AND SOXHLET EXTRACTS

The techniques described in Chapter Six produce reasonably good herbal extracts. In this chapter we'll cover making more potent extracts, including percolation extracts, fluid extracts, and Soxhlet extracts. All of these techniques require more equipment and setup than macerations and teas, but they are not so technical that you can't do them at home.

PERCOLATION EXTRACTS

Percolation is the process of passing a solvent (such as alcohol) through plant material. As the solvent drips through coarsely powdered plant material, active constituents of the herb are extracted while inert components of the plant are left behind. Drip coffeemakers are a great example of a percolation extraction. The coffeemaker slowly drips hot water (the solvent) through coffee grounds to produce coffee. Making herbal percolation extracts is a very similar process, usually using a combination of water and alcohol as a solvent.

Percolation extracts became popular in the mid-nineteenth century, and directions for making them can be found in older pharmaceutical texts. Herbalists favor percolation extracts over regular tinctures for a number of reasons:

- Experience suggests that for many herbs percolation results in a more complete and potent extract.
- Percolation extracts are usually ready in 2 days. Macerations take a minimum of 2 weeks.
- Percolations don't require pressing or straining to extract the liquid.
- Percolations allow greater flexibility in deciding the strength of the extract. If you make a 1:3 percolation and decide that you want more tincture, you can pour fresh menstruum through the herb and turn it into a 1:4 or 1:5 extract.

There are some drawbacks to making percolation extracts. You can't use this technique to extract gums, resins, or herbs that contain a lot of mucilage; nor can you percolate fresh plant material. Making a percolation extract requires more hands-on time than a regular maceration or tincture.

It is difficult to describe the process of percolation in words. In addition to the instructions below, you can watch a video demonstration at our website, modernherbalmedicine.com.

EQUIPMENT NEEDED

To make a percolation extract you will need the following equipment:

Percolation cone. Search for "percolation cone" online to find retailers who sell them, or you can make your own. To make a percolation cone, use a glass cutter to cut off the bottom of a thick glass water bottle such as Perrier or San Pelligrino. Keep the screw-top lid so you can control the drip rate of the percolation. You can also use a wine bottle with a silicon stopper and a brass needle valve to control drip rate (instead of the bottle cap).

Wide-mouth, half-gallon mason jar. This jar is used to hold the percolation cone and to collect the finished extract.

Packing rod. You will need a long instrument with a broad end to tamp down the powdered herbs inside the percolation cone. Wooden dowels (muddlers) and large granite pestles work well.

Filter. Use an unbleached coffee filter or cotton balls. These are used on the bottom of the percolation cone to hold the powder inside the cone, and coffee filters are also placed on top of the powdered herbs. Don't use funnel-style coffee filters, which are glued together at the bottom. If you do, the alcohol will dissolve some of the glue and you'll wind up with glue in your extract. Cotton balls can be inserted into the neck of the bottle and are the easiest filters to use.

Weight. A small weight is needed to hold down the top filter. Marbles work very well for this purpose. Early texts called for washed sand, but we don't recommend that. Whatever you use for a weight needs to be clean and nonporous.

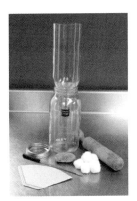

Lid. You will need a lid to cover the top of the percolation cone to prevent evaporation and contamination. A wide-mouth mason jar lid will fit most glass bottles, or you can use a plastic bag secured with rubber bands.

Once you have all of these items, assemble the percolation cone as shown. Now it's time to percolate.

PREPARING THE PLANT MATERIAL

You will need coarsely ground (powdered) dried herb for your percolation. A uniform powder allows the solvent to flow through evenly. If you grind the plant material yourself, pass it through a sieve with at least 30 holes per inch (#30 sieve) to get an even powder.

In any tincture or extract using dried herbs, some of the solvent will remain in the plant material when you are finished. If you put 1,000 milliliters of solvent into a percolation cone without premoistening, less than 900 milliliters will come out. This throws the weight-to-volume ratio off considerably. Before starting the percolation, you need to moisten the powdered herb with a small amount of menstruum.

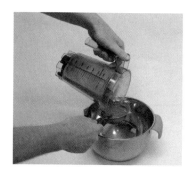

There are two ways to calculate the amount of solvent needed to moisten the plant material. The first method is to weigh the plant material and add 75% of that weight in solvent. For example, 100 grams of plant material requires 75 milliliters of solvent to moisten it, and 100 ounces of plant material requires 75 fluid ounces of solvent.

The second calculation method is more accurate. Pack the powdered plant material into a liquid measuring container to determine its volume, adding a little bit of the herb at a time and tamping it down to ensure it is evenly packed. For instance, 100 grams (or ounces) by weight of plant material might take up 120 milliliters (or fluid ounces) of volume. Add the amount of solvent the herb displaces by volume: In this example, add 120 milliliters or 120 fluid ounces of solvent.

Mix all of the menstruum at once. This includes the desired final volume of the tincture plus the amount you calculated to moisten the herb. If you are preparing a 1:5 percolation with 100 ounces of herb, and the herb takes up 120 ounces by volume, you need 500 ounces plus 120 ounces of total menstruum.

Slowly add menstruum to the plant material to moisten it. When the powder is properly moistened, it should be damp enough that it sticks together

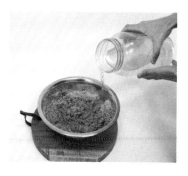

when you pinch it between your fingers, like wet sand. You can always add more liquid, but if you add too much you'll have to add more powdered herbs, which will really throw off your calculations. You may end up with menstruum left over from the amount that you calculated; add this to the rest of the menstruum. If you calculated 120 ounces to moisten the herb and only used 100 ounces, add the remaining 20 ounces to the 500 ounces of menstruum that you are using for the percolation. Once the powdered herb is properly moistened, set it aside in an airtight container for 1–12 hours.

PACKING THE PERCOLATION CONE

Once the powdered herb has had time to properly absorb the menstruum, it's time to prepare the percolation cone.

Learning to pack a percolation cone requires practice. Use the cheapest herbs you can find for your first few tries. Licorice root is a good herb to practice with; not only is it inexpensive, but it packs well, and it's always nice to have on hand.

Step one: Put a filter at the bottom of the percolation cone. Many people use a coffee filter cut to size. Putting two organic cotton balls in the neck of the bottle works just as well and it's a lot easier. After you put the cotton balls in, put your cap on loosely or put your stopper in, leaving your valve open.

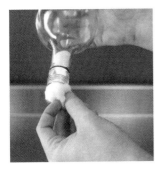 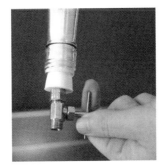 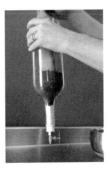

Step two: Fill the cone with the moistened herb powder. Divide the premoistened plant material into three equal parts. Put the first third of the powder in the cone and tamp it down evenly with the packing rod. Add the second third of the plant material and pack it down, and then add the remaining powder and tamp it down too. This is another skill that you will get better at with practice and experience. Don't pack the plant material too tight or too loose: too tight and the menstruum won't be able to get through; too loose and the menstruum won't flow evenly through the powder.

Step three: Cut a coffee filter so that it is slightly larger than the opening to the percolation cone. Set the coffee filter on top of the herb powder to prevent the packed plant material from being disturbed as you pour your menstruum on it. Put the washed weight on top of the filter to hold it in place.

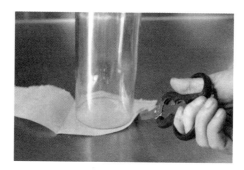

Step four: Set the percolation cone in the mason jar or in the stand, and add the menstruum to the cone. Cover the top of the percolation cone with a lid. Allow the menstruum to seep through the plant material and cotton balls so that it drips a few times. Then tighten your cap or close your valve. Letting the menstruum flow all the way through forces out air, and prevents an air bubble from burping up through your packed herb powders. Let this sit (macerate/digest) for 24 hours.

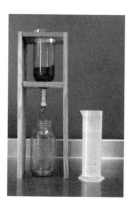
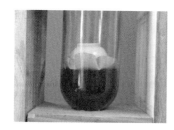
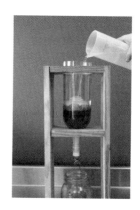

Step five: After 24 hours, slightly loosen the cap of the percolation cone to allow a slow, steady drip of menstruum. About 1 drip every 3–5 seconds is ideal. Let the menstruum percolate through the marc until the menstruum stops flowing out of the percolation cone.

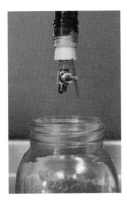 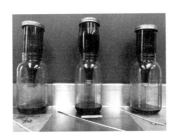 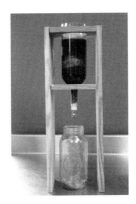

Step six: Let the extracted liquid sit for 24 hours to allow precipitates to settle to the bottom. Decant the liquid, leaving the precipitates behind, and bottle the finished tincture.

RE-PERCOLATION AND DUAL PERCOLATIONS

Some of the old pharmacy texts recommend running the finished tincture back through the plant material a second time. This dual extract throws the weight-to-volume ratio off slightly and there isn't a good formula to account for the difference. Dual extraction seems to increase the potency of the extract for many herbs, but doesn't make a difference with others. Experiment and decide for yourself if these extra steps are worth it.

Step seven: Once all of the menstruum has run through the percolation cone, set the extracted liquid aside in a covered container and put the percolation cone into a fresh mason jar. Remove the cap at the bottom of the cone and slowly pour boiled water through the cone. When the liquid dripping out of the cone is clear and tasteless, remove the cone and set it aside.

Step eight: Put the water extract that percolated through the cone into a stainless steel or enamel pot. Simmer over low heat until the liquid is reduced by 90% of its original volume (1,000 milliliters of water extract would be reduced to 100 milliliters, or 100 fluid ounces to 10 fluid ounces).

Step nine: Add the concentrated water extract back to the original percolation extract and mix them together. Let the mixture sit for 24 hours, then decant the liquid, leaving the precipitates behind. Bottle the finished tincture.

FLUID EXTRACTS

Fluid extracts are tinctures that are concentrated to a ratio of 1:1. They are made by percolation, with some added steps.

To make a fluid extract, use the standard 1:5 weight-to-volume ratio but increase the volume of alcohol by 20%. If the herb is normally extracted using 50% alcohol, this means increasing the percentage of alcohol to 70%. The added alcohol makes up for the water that will be added later during the process.

Set up the percolation and allow the equivalent of 75% of the weight of the herb to percolate through. If you used 100 grams of herb, you would allow 75 milliliters to percolate through; if you used 10 ounces of herb, that would be 7.5 fluid ounces. Set this liquid aside.

Continue percolating the remaining menstruum, then loosen the cap on the percolation cone and flush the marc with boiling hot water. Transfer the remaining percolated menstruum and the water to a shallow pan and evaporate in a food dehydrator or in an oven on low heat until the liquid is reduced to 25% of the volume of herb. Using the above examples, that's 25 milliliters or 2.5 fluid ounces. Combine this 25% reduction with the 75% percolated menstruum that you set aside earlier. You now have a 1:1 fluid extract.

FLUID EXTRACTS STEP-BY-STEP

Here's a step-by-step guide to making a 1:1 fluid extract of calendula.

Step one: Calendula is normally tinctured using 70% alcohol. Add 20 to 70% to get 90%. Prepare a menstruum that is 90% alcohol and 10% water.

Step two: Calculate the amount of menstruum based on a 1:5 ratio. For example, 5 ounces of calendula would need 25 fluid ounces of menstruum. (The final product will yield 5 fluid ounces of a 1:1 fluid extract of calendula.)

Step three: Calculate 75% (by volume) of the weight of the herb. For instance, 75% of 5 fluid ounces is 3.75 ounces. Measure out 3.75 ounces of water and pour it into the jar you will be using to catch the percolated menstruum. Use a permanent marker to mark the water level on the outside of the jar, then empty the water from the jar. (We'll call the marked jar Container A.)

Step four: Set up the percolation cone and start the percolation process, using Container A to catch the percolated liquid. When the liquid in Container A reaches the line that you marked in step three, tighten the cap on the percolation cone to stop the flow. Transfer the 3.75 ounces of liquid into another container (Container B) and set aside.

Step five: Return Container A to its place under the percolation cone and continue the percolation. When the menstruum has finished dripping through, loosen the cap on the cone. Flush water-soluble constituents out of the marc by pouring boiling hot water through the percolation cone until the water runs clear.

Step six: Calculate 25% of the desired final volume of the fluid extract. In our example, 25% of 5 ounces is 1.25 ounces. Follow the instructions in step three to mark this volume on a shallow container (Container C).

Step seven: Transfer the liquid from Container A to Container C. Put Container C in a food dehydrator or an oven set on the lowest temperature. Check the liquid frequently until it has evaporated to the mark you made, leaving you with 1.25 fluid ounces of extract.

Step eight: Combine the liquids from Container B (3.75 fluid ounces) and Container C (1.25 fluid ounces). You now have 5 fluid ounces of an extract made from 5 ounces of calendula, which means you have a 1:1 extract. Congratulations! You have made a fluid extract.

Only a few herbs respond well to concentration without changing the relative ratio of constituents, and most herbs are not given in such a big dose that concentration is necessary. Some herbs that do work well as fluid extracts include Corydalis yanhusuo, calendula, turmeric, Echinacea angustifolia root, eleuthero, licorice, black walnut, passionflower, Jamaican dogwood, willow bark, prickly ash, kava kava, dandelion, and barberry.

SOXHLET EXTRACTION

The Soxhlet extractor is a piece of lab equipment that was developed in 1879 to facilitate the continual extraction of plant material and create very concentrated extracts. In a Soxhlet extractor, the menstruum is boiled, evaporated, and allowed to condense. As it condenses, it drips through the plant material to extract constituents. This extract returns to the heated container, where it is boiled, evaporated, and condensed again to drip through the plant material and extract more constituents.

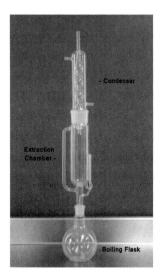

A Soxhlet extractor with a 500 milliliter boiling flask will hold about 100 grams of plant material. One run through the extractor will produce a standard 1:5 tincture. If you replace the exhausted marc with 100 grams of fresh plant material and extract that using the original menstruum, you get a 1:2.5 extract. Repeat the process a third time to get a 1:1.25 extract.

It takes a day or two for a Soxhlet extractor to make such a concentrated extract, but once you've set it up it requires only occasional monitoring.

MATERIALS FOR MAKING SOXHLET EXTRACTS

A high-quality, American-made Soxhlet extractor can set you back $500. You can sometimes find cheaper, Chinese-made Soxhlet extractors on eBay for less than $100. Cheaper glassware means thinner glass, which means you'll have to be more careful when handling it. With the less-expensive glassware, you can set up a complete Soxhlet extractor for around $200. You should be able to find all of the components on the internet. Here's what you'll need.

- A **lab stand** to hold the Soxhlet extractor, with a heavy base for stability. Look for a cast iron support ring stand.
- **Lab clamps** to secure the Soxhlet extractor to the lab stand. Get the kind with three prongs.
- A **submersible recirculating pump** is used to pump ice water into the condenser at the top of the Soxhlet extractor. A submersible pump like a fish tank pump that can pump 3.8 liters is sufficient.
- A **DC power supply** to run the pump (unless you get a 110-volt pump).
- **Plastic tubing** to connect the pump to the condenser on the Soxhlet extractor. You can get tubing from any hardware store. Make sure to get **hose clamps** as well.

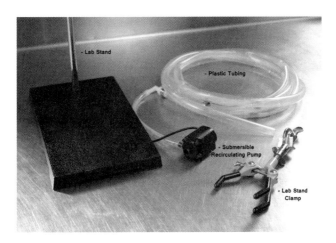

- An **insulated container** to fill with ice water and connect to the tubing.

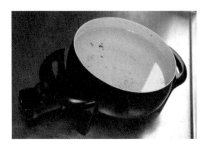

- A **heat source** to put under the Soxhlet extractor to boil the menstruum. The safest (and most expensive) option is a heating mantle with a magnetic stirrer. Prices start at $200. A $20 fondue cooker filled with vegetable oil will hold the temperature within a few degrees of where you want it.

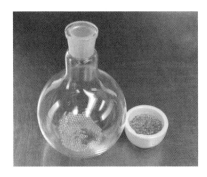

- **Boiling stones** ensure an even boil of the menstruum. They go in the boiling flask that holds the menstruum. Look for stones that are 4–6 millimeters in diameter.

- A digital or laser **thermometer** to monitor the temperature of the oil bath in the fondue cooker.

SOXHLET EXTRACTION STEP-BY-STEP

Step one: Prepare the heat source. If you are using a fondue cooker, fill it with vegetable oil. (Oil doesn't evaporate, so it requires less watching than a water bath.) The oil can be reused to make multiple batches of extracts. It will start to smell rancid after a few uses, but you can add 1 drop rosemary essential oil to mask the smell.

Step two: Moisten the plant material using the same method described for percolations earlier in this chapter. Allow the moistened powder to sit for at least 4 hours before beginning the extraction.

Step three: The plant material goes in the middle section of the Soxhlet extractor. Put a filter at the bottom of this middle piece. Try different types of filters: Some options include lab filter paper, organic unbleached cotton balls, and organic unbleached facial cleansing pads.

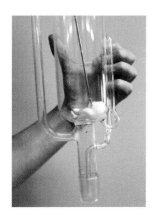

Step four: Spoon the moistened plant material on top of the filter in the middle piece of the Soxhlet extractor. Clamp the middle piece of the Soxhlet extractor to the lab stand.

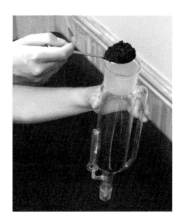

Step five: Fill the flat-bottomed boiling flask 80% full with the menstruum. This can be straight alcohol or a mixture of alcohol and water. Add a teaspoon of boiling stones to the flask.

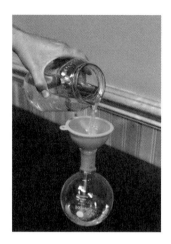

Step six: Grease all of the joints on the Soxhlet extractor with a thin layer of shea butter, cocoa butter, or a natural oil. Lubricate both of the pieces that are joined together to prevent the pieces of glass from getting irreversibly stuck together.

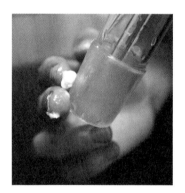

Step seven: Slide the boiling flask into place below the Soxhlet extractor, and fit the joints together. Lower the Soxhlet extractor into the oil bath or heating mantle. Attach the condenser to the top of the extraction chamber. (Make sure the joints are greased!)

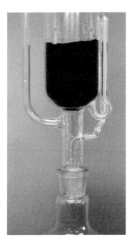

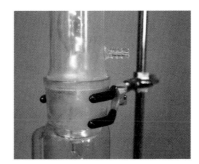

Step eight: Connect the plastic tubing to the condenser. The input line attaches at the bottom of the condenser, and the output line attaches at the top. Use hose clamps to secure the tubing connections.

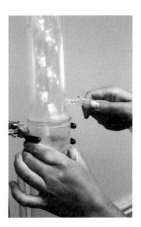

Step nine: Put the loose end of the output line from the condenser in an insulated container filled with ice water. Run a line from the insulated container to the input line of the water pump. Connect the input line from the condenser to the output line of the pump. Turn the pump on to start circulating ice water through the condenser.

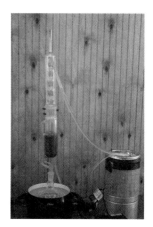

Step ten: Turn the heat source on. If you are extracting alcohol-soluble constituents, set the temperature at 195°. To extract both alcohol- and water-soluble constituents, set the temperature at 220°. Check the temperature occasionally while the Soxhlet extractor is running, adjusting as needed to keep it within 5° on either side of the optimal temperature.

Step eleven: Check the ice water bath every few hours, adding ice packs as needed to keep the temperature below 45°.

Step twelve: Once the menstruum runs clear through the reflux tube, turn the heat source off and let everything cool down. Disassemble the Soxhlet extractor and replace the exhausted plant material with fresh material. Set the exhausted marc aside in a separate container and keep it covered in the refrigerator until the extraction is complete.

Step thirteen: Put the Soxhlet back together and start the oil bath again. Repeat the process. You can do this as many times as you need to until you reach the desired concentration.

Step fourteen: To extract water-soluble constituents, put all of the exhausted marc into a pot and decoct it. Strain the decoction and then simmer it to concentrate it down to about 2 ounces. Add this back to the alcohol extract to produce the finished Soxhlet extract.

Soxhlet extraction in some cases doesn't produce better tinctures than percolation or maceration. It seems to work best when a plant has difficult-to-extract alcohol-soluble compounds and lipids. Calamus, angelica, lemon balm, spearmint, and blue vervain all make exceptional Soxhlet extracts.

Making percolation extracts, fluid extracts, and Soxhlet extracts is more complicated than making a standard alcohol tincture, but these techniques produce more potent extracts, so you get more value from the same amount of plant material and you can use smaller doses. Don't be afraid to experiment.

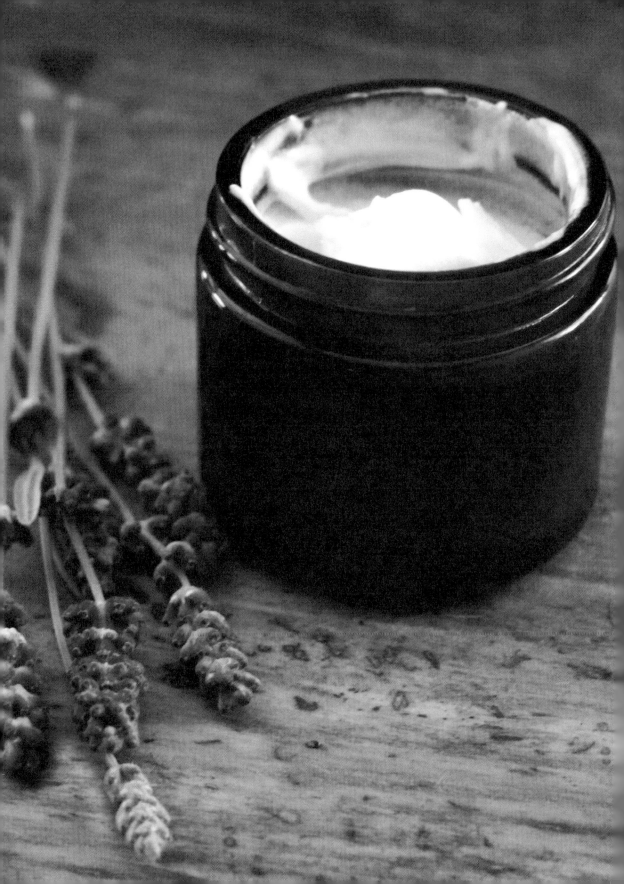

CHAPTER EIGHT

Topical Preparations

OIL-BASED EXTRACTIONS, TOPICAL APPLICATIONS, AND LOCAL APPLICATIONS

There are many topical (local) applications of herbs. In this chapter we discuss how to make oil- or fat-based extractions and turn them into salves, ointments, lotions, and other topical preparations. In the second half of the chapter, we discuss techniques for applying bulk herbs and various extracts topically.

OIL-BASED HERBAL PREPARATIONS

Oil-based preparations of herbs are suited for minor skin problems like abrasions, burns, rashes, and dry skin. Be careful with new cuts or wounds, especially if the wound is deep; oil can trap bacteria and help them spread. For active infections, direct application of herbs in a poultice or indirect applications like compresses and soaks work best.

Compresses are made by soaking a cloth in an herbal tea or decoction and applying the cloth to the affected area; soaks are done by submersing an area in an herbal tea or decoction (compresses are covered later in this chapter, and soaks are discussed in Appendix One). After a couple of days of healing, if the wound shows no sign of infection, salves are more convenient than poultices and compresses. Salves work really well for the proliferative and remodeling phases of tissue healing.

EXTRACTING HERBS IN OIL OR FAT

In an oil extract (*olea medicata* in Latin), herbs are macerated in a fixed oil to extract constituents that are soluble in fats. Olive oil, grape seed oil, almond oil, peanut oil, and apricot oil are commonly used to make herbal oils. In the past, herbs were frequently extracted in saturated fats such as lard or butter. Oil isn't a great solvent on its own. Using gentle heat or an intermediate solvent like alcohol produces a better oil. Making an herbal oil is the first step to making an oil-based salve, as described later in this chapter.

Herbal Oils (Oil Extractions)

There are three primary methods for creating an herbal oil. The first is similar to making a tincture, the second is like making a low-temperature decoction, and the final method uses intermediate solvents to produce the oil.

Cold Extraction Pack herbs loosely in a glass jar. Add enough oil to barely cover the plant material. Put the jar in a warm, dark area for 14 days, shaking or stirring daily, then strain and bottle the oil.

Most oils made with fresh plants will grow mold due to the water content of the plants. Two herbs that can be used fresh to make herbal oils are mullein flowers and St. John's wort flowers. Gather the flowers and place them loosely into a jar. Cover them with oil and macerate for 14 days as described above.

Some herbs commonly infused in oil after drying include garlic, lobelia seeds, and poke root. Other plant materials should be dried for about 48 hours and extracted using the hot extraction method.

Hot Extraction The 1898 King's American Dispensatory recommends maintaining heat between 122° and 140° to produce medicinal oils. You can use the lowest setting on a slow cooker or oven, which will hold the temperature at about 150°. Extracting at 150° rather than between 122° and 140° won't damage the plant compounds, but oils that are heated above 150° tend to go rancid faster than otherwise. To keep the temperature within the range given by King's American Dispensatory, prop a wooden spoon against the door of the oven to keep it slightly ajar. If you are using a slow cooker, you can have an electrician wire a light dimmer into the power cord to control the temperature more precisely. Use a thermometer to monitor the temperature.

To extract herbs in a slow cooker, put them in the crock and add enough oil to barely cover the herbs (approximately 1 gallon of oil to 1 pound of herbs). Turn the slow cooker on low and let the herbs steep overnight, or for 8–12 hours. Let the oil cool, then strain and bottle it.

If you are using an oven, use a large enamel pan to hold the herbs. Cover them in oil. Set the oven to the lowest temperature and prop the oven door open with a wooden spoon for ventilation. Keep the herbs in the oven for 8–12 hours, allow the oil to cool, then strain and bottle.

To make a hot extract using fresh plants, keep the plant material in the oven or crock until all the liquid is cooked out of the fresh plant material and the herbs are crispy.

Using Intermediate Solvents To make a more potent oil, you can use high-proof alcohol as an intermediate solvent. Measure the amount of plant material by weight and add 75% of that weight in 95% alcohol to the plant material. For 200 grams of plant material, use 150 milliliters of 95% alcohol, and for 16 ounces of herb add 12 fluid ounces of 95% alcohol. Let this sit for 24 hours, then add the oil at a 1:5 ratio and apply gentle heat for 8–12 hours as described above. All of the alcohol will evaporate. For a 1:5 oil extraction of 200 grams of plant material, you need 1,000 grams by weight of oil, or 5 pounds of oil to 1 pound of herbs. This kind of precise measurement is not necessary for making herbal products for use by family and friends.

SALVES, OINTMENTS, AND BALMS

Salves are semi-solid medicinal preparations made of an herbal oil base that is solidified with beeswax or candelilla wax (a vegan alternative). Salves can also be called ointments. Herbal salves are used for scrapes, burns, skin irritations,

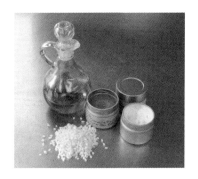 and other skin conditions. They are used to carry herbs directly to the tissues that need them, or to deliver compounds like volatile oils to a referred site (like massaging a salve into the upper back and chest to affect the lungs). Some salves act as drawing agents to pull splinters and glass out of skin.

To make a salve, make an herbal oil as described above. Use a 6:1–8:1 ratio of oil to beeswax, depending on how hard you want your salve. For softer salves use less wax, and for harder salves use more. That's around 30 grams (1 ounce) of wax by weight for every 170–220 milliliters (6–8 ounces) by volume of oil.

Wax pellets and grated wax are easier to melt than chunks of wax. (Use hot water to melt the wax off the grater.) Melt the beeswax in a jar or can that is dedicated to melting wax so you don't have to deal with getting wax off the sides of a pot. Fill a large pot halfway with water and set a few canning jar rings on the bottom of the pot. Set the container full of beeswax on the canning rings so that it does not touch the bottom of the pot. Simmer the water over medium-high heat to melt the wax. While the beeswax is melting, warm up the oil in a nonreactive stainless steel or enamel pot. When the wax is completely melted, pour the hot wax into the warm oil.

Another way to make salves is to pour beeswax pellets or grated beeswax directly into the hot oil. Stir regularly for about 20 minutes until the wax is completely melted. Keep an eye on the wax to keep it from bursting into flames.

Once the oil and wax are blended together, remove them from the heat. Stir the liquid salve as it cools to make sure that the wax and oil do not separate. As the mixture cools, it will begin to turn translucent, at which point it is ready to put into jars. Add heat-sensitive ingredients like essential oils, vitamin E, and lanolin at this point, if desired.

Cleaning up equipment that was used to make salve is tedious. Wipe down the equipment with paper towels while the salve is still liquid, and be prepared to wash everything in very hot soapy water a few times to get the equipment completely clean.

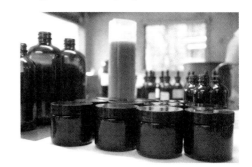

There is a basic salve formula in Chapter Twelve to get you started.

Balms are made with more beeswax than salves are: 30 grams (1 ounce) by weight to 80–110 milliliters (3–4 ounces) by volume of oil. The beeswax creates a protective barrier on the skin.

LOTIONS

Lotions are mixtures of oil and water that are used to moisturize dry skin. Water and oil do not naturally mix and must be emulsified. Emulsifiers are also known as surface active agents or surfactants, which will cause oil and water to stay mixed. For example, when blended with oil, the lecithin in egg yolk creates the stabilized emulsion known as mayonnaise.

Commercial lotions usually contain highly processed chemical emulsifiers. Emulsifying wax is a reasonably safe chemical emulsifier, or you can make an emulsifier.

Lotions need to include a preservative to prevent mold and bacteria growth. Rosemary essential oil and vitamin E oil are both antibacterial, and can be added to extend the shelf life of your lotions to well beyond 6 months.

To make a lotion, melt the following ingredients together in a pan:

2 parts of a liquid fixed oil (grape seed oil, olive oil, or almond oil)
1 part of a solid fixed oil (cocoa butter, coconut oil, mango butter, or shea butter)
1 part emulsifier

Stir in 4–6 parts of one of the following: an herbal infusion, aloe vera juice, or a hydrosol like rose water. Add 1 drop rosemary essential oil for every 110 milliliters (4 ounces) of liquid, and add 1 milliliter of vitamin E oil per 240 milliliters (8 ounces) of liquid. You can blend the mixture by hand with a whisk if

HOMEMADE EMULSIFIER

80% beeswax
10% borax
10% liquid lecithin

This emulsifier will not keep for long and needs to be made fresh with each batch of lotion.

you happen to be an Olympic level athlete. For us mere mortals, a stick blender or a strong countertop blender works a lot better.

BUTTERS

Body butters are a whipped blend of saturated oils (solid at room temperature) and monounsaturated or polyunsaturated oils (liquid at room temperature). Body butters aren't usually made with water (although they can be), so they last longer than lotions and have a creamy-smooth feel without the hassle of adding an emulsifier. (If you use a hydrosol or aloe vera gel to make body butter, you will need to add an emulsifier.)

To make a butter, use:

7 parts by weight of a solid fixed oil
3 parts by weight of a liquid fixed oil

Slowly melt the oils together in a double boiler. Remove the oil from the heat, add essential oils, and let the oil cool to room temperature. Whip the mixture into a buttery consistency with a hand or stand mixer. Refrigerate for 30 minutes and whip again. See Chapter Twelve for a sample formula.

MASSAGE OILS

Massage oils are made with carrier oils with essential oils added for fragrance and therapeutic action. Depending on the person and the oils used, massage oil can have a relaxing or stimulating effect on the mind and spirit. Massage oils help to relieve stress and tension by their effect on nerve endings, the mind, and muscles. Oils and massage can improve skin cell growth and accelerate the elimination of wastes through the body's lymphatic system. See Chapter Ten for more information on using essential oils.

OTHER TOPICAL APPLICATIONS

Alcohol tinctures, glycerites, teas, and decoctions can be used topically.

LINIMENTS

Liniments are made in the same way as macerated tinctures, but with rubbing alcohol instead of drinkable ethanol. This cuts down on cost. It also makes the liniment toxic for internal use; many use regular alcohol tinctures topically as liniments to avoid the risk of poisoning. Label liniments that are made with rubbing alcohol to prevent accidental ingestion. Menthol crystals or wintergreen add a nice smell, increase the anti-inflammatory properties of the liniment, and help prevent accidental ingestion. The Antispasmodic Tincture in Chapter Twelve makes a good liniment.

COMPRESSES AND FOMENTATIONS

A compress is a cloth pad soaked in an herbal extract and applied to the skin. Most compresses are applied warm, but cold compresses have their applications. Compresses are used to ease pain or accelerate the healing of wounds or muscle injuries. Cold compresses are used for headaches, burns, bites, and stings. Infusions, decoctions, and tinctures or glycerites diluted with water may be used for a compress. The pad may be soft cotton or linen, a cotton ball, or woven gauze.

To prepare a compress:

- Submerge a clean piece of soft cloth in a warm infusion or other herbal extract.
- Squeeze out the excess liquid.

- Place the pad against the affected area.
- When the pad cools or dries, repeat the process.

Fomentations are compresses that cover a larger area of the body. Soak a cloth in hot tea and apply it to the affected area. Herbs that make good compresses and fomentations include chamomile, elder flowers and leaves, yarrow, and calendula.

POULTICES AND PLASTERS

A plaster or poultice (also known as a cataplasm) is a mixture of dried or fresh herbs moistened with water or oil and applied externally. It is similar to a compress, but plant parts are used rather than a liquid extraction. Generally a poultice implies a hot treatment, whereas a plaster is applied at room temperature. Smash or chop fresh herbs and apply them directly to the affected area. If you're using dried herbs, boil them for up to 5 minutes or mix them with a small amount of boiling water. Apply the poultice or plaster in between layers of gauze to prevent messes.

Poultices should be applied as hot as can be tolerated. Use a gauze bandage covered with a warm cloth over the poultice.

Good herbs for making plasters and poultices include slippery elm, comfrey leaf and root, marshmallow, flaxseed, white oak bark, psyllium seeds, plantain, lily of the valley, pine gum, lobelia, calendula, yarrow, goldenseal, and aloe vera. In addition to herbs, you can use fine clay and activated charcoal in plasters and poultices. There is a basic poultice formula in Chapter Twelve.

Prickly pear cactus (nopal, *Opuntia ficus-indica*) is a great herb to use as a poultice. Its actions are similar to those of aloe vera gel. Most ethnic grocery stores sell nopal pads with the spines removed; if you harvest a fresh prickly pear pad, you will have to remove the spines yourself. Prickly pear cacti have two types of spines: large fixed spines and small, hair-like glochids that can work their way into the skin, causing general irritation and misery. Remove the glochids from the pads by scraping them off with a knife; if you roast the pads over an open flame first, it becomes much easier. Cut the pads in half vertically to expose the gooey inside, warm the pads, and apply them directly over wounds and burns. The goo can be scraped out, dehydrated on a fruit leather tray, then powdered and reconstituted as needed.

LOCAL APPLICATIONS

These are applications made to specific parts of the body, such as the rectum, vagina, mouth, nose, eyes, and ears.

SUPPOSITORY, PESSARY, OR BOLUS

A suppository is used to insert herbs rectally or vaginally. A pessary is another word for a vaginal suppository. A bolus is administered orally.

To prepare a suppository or pessary, melt cocoa butter on low heat, preferably in a double boiler, and stir in finely powdered herbs. The last thing you want to do is insert rough, scratchy plant material in a sensitive area, so make sure the herbs are very finely powdered.

Add essential oils, if desired, and pour the herb-infused cocoa butter into a suppository mold and let it cool. Wrap each suppository individually with waxed paper and store it in the refrigerator. Insert rectally or vaginally depending on need. Use suppositories within 7–10 days, or keep in the freezer for up to 6 months.

To make a bolus, mix a binding herb like marshmallow or comfrey root with other herbs to form a stiff paste. Shape the paste into pieces the size of large pills and wrap with waxed paper. Boluses must be used immediately.

Herbs for suppositories and boluses include comfrey root, marshmallow, Oregon grape, and cranesbill (geranium).

Making a Suppository Mold

To make a suppository mold, wrap a pencil, a slim marker, or the handle of a wooden spoon in several layers of aluminum foil. Slide the foil off and seal one end of the foil mold. Make several of these and stand them together in a can or jar. When the suppository mixture is ready, fill each tube and freeze for 3 minutes. Remove the foil and slice the suppositories into pieces 2 centimeters (¾ inch) long.

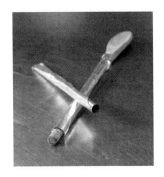

GARGLES AND MOUTHWASHES

Herbal gargles and mouthwashes are used for sore throats, laryngitis, tonsillitis, irritated throats, dry coughs, and bad breath. Make a decoction or mix tinctures or glycerites with water.

Suggested Ingredients for Herbal Mouthwashes and Gargles

Antiseptics and disinfectants: Myrrh, barberry, thyme, clove
Astringents: Bayberry, white oak bark, sage, calendula
Demulcents (for dry, irritated throats): Licorice, slippery elm, marshmallow
Flavoring agents: Spearmint, peppermint, anise, fennel, licorice, clove, cinnamon
Stimulants: Capsicum (used in very small amounts), ginger, thyme

HERBAL SNUFF

A snuff is used to dry up excess mucus in the sinuses or to shrink nasal polyps. Take a pinch of powdered herb in the palm of your hand. Use your other hand to hold one nostril closed while you inhale the powder through the other nostril. Repeat with the other side. Be prepared for a few sneezes and copious drainage.

Herbs that are used for sinus snuffs include bayberry bark, goldenseal, and yarrow.

TOOTH POWDER

Tooth powders can tone bleeding gums and strengthen tooth enamel. Use tooth powders with a toothbrush or with short sticks made from rosemary stems.

Herbs for Tooth Powder

Horsetail (strengthens tooth enamel)
White oak bark (tones bleeding gums)
Black walnut (tones bleeding gums)
Calendula (tones bleeding gums)
Myrrh gum (antiseptic)
Elecampane (antiseptic)

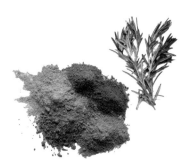

EYEWASH

Herbal infusions can be applied as drops, as eyewashes, in eyecups, or in a compress for sore, red, tired eyes or for eye infections. Use only freshly made teas to avoid the risk of infection. Herbs for eyewashes include agrimony, chamomile, eyebright, and red raspberry.

EAR DROPS

Earaches and ear infections can be very painful. Herbal ear drops reduce inflammation, fight infection, and reduce pain in the ear. Make sure the eardrum is intact before putting anything into the ear.

Warm a bottle of oil or tincture in a pan of hot water until the oil or tincture feels warm, but not hot, on the inside of your wrist. Drop 5–10 drops in the ear and use a cotton ball to prevent the oil or tincture from leaking out. Herbs that are used for ear drops include garlic, mullein, and St. John's wort. Tea tree, lavender, or lemon essential oils can be diluted 1:20 in olive oil and applied as above.

CHAPTER NINE

Other Preparations

CONCENTRATES, LOZENGES, AND TRADITIONAL CHINESE METHODS

This chapter covers some interesting techniques for preparing herbal medicines. These include powdered concentrates, lozenges, and hot alcohol extraction. We also discuss some of the Asian techniques used to prepare herbs. As you become more skilled at making your own herbal medicines, these are some techniques you can use to expand your skills.

POWDERED CONCENTRATES

These are techniques for taking herbs that have been extracted using water or alcohol and turning them back into powders. These powders are very potent and require much lower doses than bulk herb powders or regular capsules.

TEA CONCENTRATES

Tea powder concentrates are a great way to concentrate the water-soluble constituents from a plant extract. The idea, in a nutshell, is to make a strong decoction, reduce the decoction (concentrating it), then dry the decoction into a powder that can be easily administered in a beverage, as a capsule, or as a powder.

Concentrated powders are great for children or adults who are unlikely to drink a cup of bad-tasting tea, and for those who can't take tinctures. Any herb that can be decocted works well as a tea concentrate.

Here's the step-by-step way to make a tea powder concentrate.

Step one: Slightly moisten ground herb powder (if dry) or freshly minced herb (if fresh) with 95% alcohol. If alkaloids are the primary constituent you are trying to extract, use a mixture of equal parts alcohol and apple cider vinegar to moisten the plant material. Let the marc soak for 1 hour.

Step two: Add 1 part herb to 32 parts water. So, 1 ounce of herb would be added to 32 ounces (1 quart) of water. Simmer the herbs and water for 2–4 hours on very low heat.

Step three: Strain the decoction to remove the marc (plant material). Then return the liquid to the pot.

Step four: Simmer the remaining liquid down to about 20% of its original volume. So, 20 ounces would be reduced to 4 ounces.

Step five: Remove the liquid from the heat and measure the amount of concentrated liquid. You are going to add a powder to this mixture before drying. Two possibilities are arrowroot starch or some of the herb powder. For example, if you just made a decoction of licorice root, you'd use some fresh licorice root powder.

If you are using arrowroot starch, add 5 grams (⅙ ounce) for every 30 milliliters (1 ounce) of liquid. If using herb powders, add 10 grams (⅓ ounce) of powdered herb for every 30 milliliters (1 ounce) of liquid. Blend the powder and liquid well.

Step six: Thinly spread the mixture of the decoction and powder onto a fruit leather tray and place in a dehydrator. Set the temperature to 120°. Allow the mixture to dry until it is dry and brittle.

Step seven: Remove the dried concentrate from the tray. Grind it into a powder using a coffee grinder or a mortar and pestle. Store the powder in an airtight container away from heat and light.

You now have a concentrated herbal extract in powdered form. You can encapsulate the powder or mix it into water, juice, or honey to consume.

TINCTURE POWDER CONCENTRATES

Tincture powder concentrates are similar to tea concentrates, but are appropriate for herbs with alcohol-soluble constituents. They don't work well for plants whose primary constituents are aromatic oils. Here are the steps for producing tincture powder concentrates.

Step one: Add 5 grams (⅙ ounce) of arrowroot starch or 10 grams (⅓ ounce) of dried powdered herb for every 30 milliliters (1 ounce) of tincture and blend well.

Step two: Spread the mixture thinly on a fruit leather tray. Place in a dehydrator set at 140°. Allow it to dry until it becomes dry and brittle.

Step three: Remove the dried concentrate from the tray and grind using a coffee grinder or mortar and pestle. Store in an airtight container away from heat and light.

Due to the alcohol content, dehydrate tincture powder concentrates in a well-ventilated area away from any sources of flame or spark.

LOZENGES OR COUGH DROPS

You can make lozenges or cough drops out of herbal extracts to ease sore throats and respiratory problems. This is actually a form of candy making and follows the same procedures for making hard candy. Although not completely necessary, candy molds are helpful for making uniform lozenges. It's also helpful to have a good thermometer for checking the temperature. Here are the procedures to follow.

Step one: Make a decoction of the herb or herbs you want to use in your cough drops. Good choices include horehound, wild cherry, white pine, coltsfoot, elder berry, or cinnamon.

Step two: Measure 1 cup of the decoction and add either 2 cups organic raw sugar or freeze-dried sugarcane juice or 1½ cups honey and ⅛ teaspoon cream of tartar. The cream of tartar helps offset the excess moisture in the honey so the candy will harden.

Step three: Heat the mixture in a saucepan on low heat until the syrup reaches the hard-crack stage (about 290°–300°). You can check this by dropping a small amount of the syrup into ice water. If it hardens properly, it is ready.

Step four (optional): Just as the mixture reaches the proper temperature, you can add some essential oils to make the drops more potent. Good oils to consider are eucalyptus, thyme, rosemary, and peppermint. Add about 10–20 drops of essential oils.

Step five: Being very careful not to get any of the syrup onto your skin (it will burn you very badly), pour the hot mixture into your greased candy molds. If you do not have candy molds, you can pour it onto a greased dish. If using the dish method, wait until the candy is halfway hardened, then score the mixture with a knife to create drop-sized pieces. You'll be able to break the candy along the scores after it has hardened completely.

Another option if you don't have candy molds is to fill a pan with powdered sugar. (If you don't want to use refined sugar, powder freeze-dried sugarcane juice in the blender.) Drop little bits of the candy mixture into the powdered sugar. They will form small drops. You can roll the drops in the sugar when they cool to coat them with sugar.

Step six: When the lozenges have cooled, store them in a sealed container. You now have your own homemade lozenges.

HOT ALCOHOL EXTRACT

Certain herbs, such as usnea, can be extracted using alcohol and heat. This is a potentially dangerous method of extraction, because alcohol has a lower boiling point (173°) than water (212°). Alcohol is also very flammable, so keep the extract away from any open flame and keep the temperature well below the boiling point of alcohol (173°) during the extraction process.

The safest way to do this is using a mason jar and a crock pot. Put the herbs along with the appropriate mixture of water and alcohol into the mason jar(s). Put lids on them, but do not tighten them completely. Allow a little space for ventilation so that pressure does not build up inside the jar and cause it to break or explode.

Fill the crock pot with water and place the jar(s) into the water. Turn the crock pot on low for 8 hours. Wait until the jar has cooled before opening the jar and straining the extract.

TRADITIONAL CHINESE METHODS

Both Ayurvedic and traditional Chinese medicine developed methods for processing herbs that reduce toxicity, increase their effectiveness, alter their properties, or remove offensive odors. Western herbalism is not as sophisticated in its processing methods. Here are some of the methods used in traditional Chinese medicine.

Steaming and drying: A glutinous and demulcent root such as *Rehmannia glutinosa* (which has a cooling energy) is repeatedly steamed with wine and sun-dried by the Chinese. Korean red ginseng is made by steaming the ginseng roots and then drying them. These processes make the herbs have a more warming energy. Western herbs such as marshmallow and comfrey may be prepared in this manner.

Dry-roasting and stir-frying: Dry-roasting certain herbs will enhance their fire or yang characteristics. Herbs like bupleurum are prepared in this way. Western herbs that are dry-roasted for added flavor include dandelion, chicory, and comfrey roots. In the raw state these herbs have a cooling energy, but when roasted they develop a slightly warmer energy. When a little honey is added to the herb as it is stirred and dry-roasted in a wok, it adds a tonic effect through its sweetness. In traditional Chinese medicine, licorice and astragalus are often dry-roasted with honey.

Soaking in spirits or wine: Herbs that are soaked in grain spirits or wine enter the blood with optimum efficiency and have an escalating energy. The alcohol acts as an usher as well as an energizer to blood circulation. Such preparations are used in traditional Chinese medicine as tonics to treat circulatory disorders such as arthritic and rheumatic complaints.

Processing with salt: In traditional Chinese medicine, a pinch of salt is added to herbs intended to tonify the urinary tract. Salt acts as a carrier for the other herbs in the formula, bringing their action to the kidneys. It also adds a moisture-retaining effect. Salt enhances the descending energy of a formula.

Processing with vinegar: The sour taste generally, and vinegar in particular, has a descending and astringent energy and targets the liver.

Leaching with water: This is done mainly to remove tannic acid and certain toxic substances. Acorns were prepared in this manner by Native Americans.

Sand heating: Certain herbs are roasted by mixing them in sand and heating them in a wok while stirring frequently. This allows a much higher temperature than stir-frying without sand, and the roots will heat more evenly.

Baking: Herbs can be baked with honey, ginger, or other carriers to enhance certain effects. Honey makes herbs more tonic and moistening. Ginger makes them more warming and dispersing, promoting circulation and digestion.

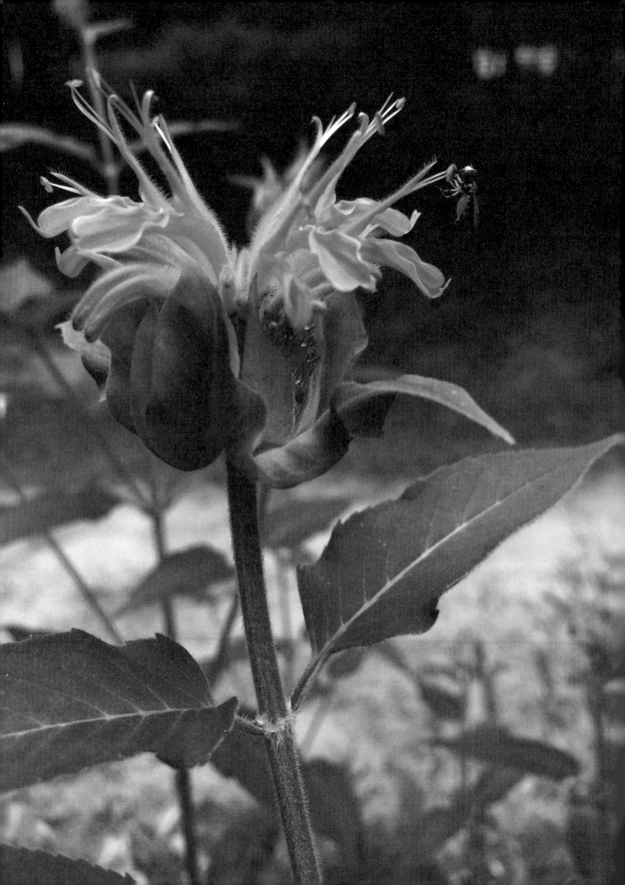

CHAPTER TEN

Aromatherapy and Flower Essences

TWO UNIQUE WAYS TO EXTRACT AND USE HERBS

This chapter covers the use of specialized preparations made from plants—essential oils, homeopathic remedies, and flower essences. These preparations require additional study in order to be able to use them effectively, but we will introduce them here.

AROMATHERAPY

Aromatherapy is a specialized application of plant medicine that uses the volatile compounds from plants known as essential oils. Essential oils are what give flowers and herbs their distinctive fragrances. They are liquids that readily evaporate at room temperature. When we smell something, these volatile compounds are triggering the olfactory receptors in our nose.

Essential oils are derived from the flowers, leaves, stems, seeds, or bark of different plants. Although they are called oils, essential oils are not made of the fatty acids found in fats and vegetable oils. They are complex mixtures of alcohols, terpenes, terpenoids, phenols, ketones, and oxides and are soluble in fats, oils, glycerin, and high-proof alcohol, but not in water.

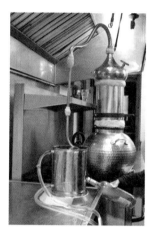 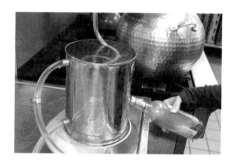

The French chemist who coined the term "aromatherapy," Professor René-Maurice Gattefossé, conducted experiments with essential oils on wounded soldiers during World War I. At that time, the most commonly used antiseptic was phenol, which was good for cleaning hospital floors but not very effective for healing wounds. The soldiers Gattefossé treated had badly infected wounds that often resulted in serious poisoning as the body reabsorbed harmful substances produced by decaying tissue. His work proved that essential oils, particularly lavender, are superior to chemical antiseptics in their ability to detoxify and speed up the elimination of these substances.

Aromatherapy is widely accepted in Europe by the medical profession. In England, for instance, the relaxing aroma of lavender is wafted through the wards to help raise patient morale, which helps patients to heal faster. Before bed, these same patients are given a choice of a tranquilizer drug or an aromatherapy oil massage. The use of essential oils is also gaining popularity in the United States, as more and more companies are selling the oils and promoting their use.

HEALING PROPERTIES OF ESSENTIAL OILS

There are many benefits of essential oils, one of them being that they do not appear to lose their effect with repeated applications. Generally speaking, most essential oils have effects on the nervous and glandular systems and help to destroy harmful microbes. Their effects on the nervous and glandular systems make them mood altering, and this effect takes place primarily through the sense of smell.

The sense of smell is unique because it is wired directly into the brain. Nerve pathways connect the sinus cavity with the olfactory bulb, which is part of the limbic system of our brain. This is a survival mechanism, as smells can alert us to danger or suggest that something may be good to eat.

ESSENTIAL OILS AND MOOD

Odors directly affect the amygdala and the hippocampus, as well as the hypothalamus, the part of the brain that regulates the pituitary gland. This means that smells can directly alter hormone production and affect the autonomic nervous system, which regulates digestion, heart rate, blood pressure, and breathing. This is what gives them their mood-altering effects.

Marketers were the first to capitalize on the ability of fragrances to alter mood. For instance, the Smell and Taste Treatment and Research Foundation tested the effects of various scents on shoppers in stores selling Nike® shoes. The results were surprising: 84% of customers preferred shoes in the scented showroom and were even willing to pay more for them! Soon thereafter, Japanese companies began applying this type of research by using lemon and other citrus scents in their office buildings to stimulate alertness and concentration, thereby reducing errors and boosting productivity.

Because of their effect on mood, essential oils can even help set the mood for intimacy or aid meditation and spiritual awareness. They can also be used in emotional healing work and to aid in the treatment of mood disorders, such as anxiety, sadness, and depression. They can also improve mental alertness, concentration, memory, and cognition.

PHYSICAL HEALING PROPERTIES

Besides having a direct impact on our mind and mood, essential oils have beneficial physical healing properties. As already mentioned, essential oils tend to be infection fighters, possessing various degrees of antibacterial, antiviral, antifungal, and, in some cases, antiparasitic actions. They can stimulate various metabolic processes, which may result in the faster healing of wounds, increased white blood cell counts, improved digestion, enhanced energy production, and increased circulation.

It is not necessary to ingest essential oils to obtain these benefits. Research has shown that essential oils are absorbed through the sinuses and skin and carried through the circulatory system to all the organs. They are then removed from the body via various eliminative organs such as the lungs or the urinary system.

The process takes anywhere from minutes to several hours. You can experience this if you rub the sole of your foot with a slice of raw garlic. It will show up on your breath several hours later. The volatile compounds in garlic are absorbed through the skin, travel through the bloodstream, and are eliminated from the body via the lungs. The organs the body uses to eliminate an oil are going to receive the antimicrobial and stimulating actions of that herb. Because garlic is eliminated via the lungs, but not the kidneys, it helps respiratory infections but not urinary tract infections.

UTILITARIAN USES

Essential oils have utilitarian uses, too. They are often added to products for skin and hair care, such as lotions and shampoos, both for their therapeutic benefits and their emotional appeal. Their disinfectant properties make them useful in mouthwashes, natural deodorants, and disinfectant cleaners for the home. Essential oils can also be used as perfumes and natural air fresheners. Many will also help to repel insects and rodents.

Aromatherapy involves using essential oils in many different ways. For example, they can be added to a fixed oil or massage lotion to be applied to the skin. They can be added to bath water or used in soaks, compresses, fomentations, gargles, and mouthwashes, or diffused into the air for inhalation via a vaporizer or diffuser. For health problems, they are usually inhaled and applied topically, although some may be used internally by professionals if they are highly diluted.

The chaos of modern life and the continual rise of medical costs have inspired many individuals to rediscover aromatherapy as a natural self-help technique.

ESSENTIAL OIL SAFETY

Because the oils used in aromatherapy are available over the counter, some people assume that they are completely safe. They are safe when used properly, but can cause problems ranging from irritation of the skin and mucous membranes to more severe reactions such as liver damage, uterine hemorrhage, and abortion. Consult with a qualified aromatherapist before using undiluted oils, and talk to a health care professional before using aromatherapy if you are pregnant, have high or low blood pressure, or have allergies. The National Association for Holistic Aromatherapy is a good place for finding information on practitioners and education in aromatherapy.

Reports abound about people having serious reactions from using essential oils without proper respect. Thomas has seen several cases of elevated liver enzymes, and one case of colitis, from the internal use of essential oils by untrained individuals. Eventually, if these adverse reactions continue, the FDA is likely to step in and enact strict regulations on the sales of essential oils. To continue to have these marvelous remedies available long term, we must become more conservative in their use, and stop the trend of using them undiluted and internally for problems easily treated by more gentle remedies. Carefully follow the guidelines provided below for safely diluting and using essential oils.

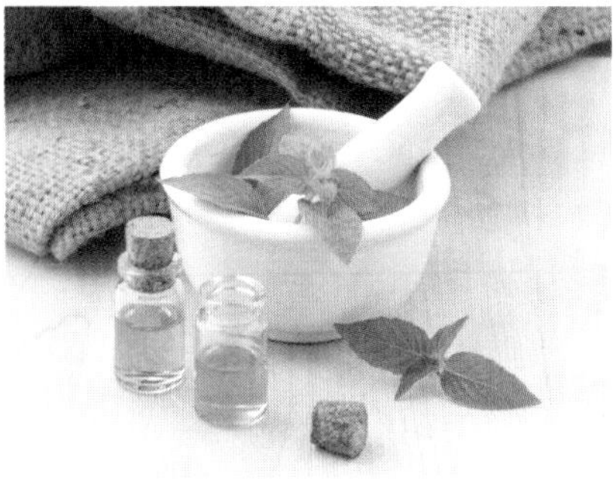

Photo by kerdkanno / CC BY

USING ESSENTIAL OILS

To get started, we want to acquaint you with some basic terms and techniques for using essential oils (EOs). Although they are natural substances, EOs are highly concentrated, which increases their potential for misuse. So, be sure you understand the following terms and basic guidelines for using these powerful natural substances.

Diluting Oils

EOs can be diluted with a fixed vegetable oil (like almond or olive oil) or a natural soap or lotion. EOs can also be added to unscented liquid soap products. Generally, the finished product should be about 2%–3% EOs. For easy reference, use Table 9 to calculate how much oil to add to a liquid for a 2½% and 5% dilution.

Amount of Carrier Oil or Other Liquid	Fluid Ounces	Amount of Essential Oils for 2½% Dilution	Amount of Essential Oils for 5% Dilution
1 teaspoon (⅓ tablespoon)	⅙ fl oz	2-3 drops	4-6 drops
1 tablespoon (3 teaspoons)	½ fl oz	7-8 drops	14-16 drops
2 tablespoons (6 teaspoons)	1 fl oz	15 drops	30 drops
1 cup (16 tablespoons)	8 fl oz	⅕ fl oz (about 1.25 tsp.)	⅖ fl oz (about 2.5 tsp.)
1 pint (2 cups)	16 fl oz	⅖ fl oz (about 2.5 tsp.)	⅘ fl oz (about 5 tsp.)
1 quart (4 cups or 2 pints)	32 fl oz	⅘ fl oz (about 5 tsp.)	1⅗ fl oz (about 10 tsp.)

TABLE 9 Essential Oil Dilutions

Topical Use

The term "neat" is used for oils that can be applied topically in an undiluted form. Oils that are too irritating to be used neat should be diluted as described in the next paragraph. Certain essential oils, such as tea tree or lavender, may be applied neat to wounds to fight infection and stimulate tissue healing and repair.

Other essential oils can be diluted (as per Table 9) into a fixed oil or lotion and applied topically for the treatment of skin conditions. People with sensitive skin may want to dilute even neat oils at least 1:1 (equal parts).

One can also blend oils in this manner for local use; for example, massaging essential oils diluted in a carrier oil onto the neck for a sore throat, the chest for coughs and congestion, the abdomen for gas, bloating, and infection, and so forth. Essential oils make good additions to many of the topical preparations mentioned in Chapter Eight, including salves, balms, lotions, butters, liniments, and other preparations.

Diffusion

Diffusing oils can help to freshen the air, enhance mood, and/or kill airborne microbes to promote healing and prevent the spread of infection. It is a very safe and effective way to use EOs. There are many types of diffusers you can purchase on the market that can be used to disperse essential oils into the air. You can also diffuse oils by bringing a pot of water to a boil on the stove, turning the heat down to a simmer, and adding 5–15 drops of one or more essential oils. Let the water simmer uncovered on the stove for 20–30 minutes to diffuse the oil(s).

Steam inhalation is an excellent method of application for treating problems of the respiratory system, such as colds, coughs, and sinus conditions, and relieving tension and headaches. The aroma goes straight to the brain while the oils pass from the lungs into the bloodstream.

To diffuse oils in this manner, put 5–10 drops of oil in a bowl containing 2 cups boiling hot water. Inhale the steam for 5–10 minutes, keeping your nose about 8 inches above the water. Keep your eyes closed. You can drape a towel over your head to concentrate the steam. Repeat up to 3 times daily.

You can make a portable inhaler by putting a few drops of EO on a handkerchief or tissue and taking deep breaths through the cloth.

You can also make an EO spray to use as an air freshener. To make your own air purifier, fill a spray bottle halfway with distilled water. Blend 30 drops of vegetable glycerin and about 20 drops of EO(s) for every 30 milliliters (1 fluid ounce) of water and then add this mixture to the spray bottle. Shake well and spray as you would any air freshener.

Perfumes

One can also get the benefit of EOs by using them as perfumes. Add 10–15 drops of an EO to ¼ ounce of a massage oil and place in a bottle with a roll-on applicator to apply topically.

Baths and Soaks

To disperse EOs into a bath, first add 8–15 drops of the oils to 1 tablespoon of unscented natural liquid soap like Dr. Bronner's Supermild Baby Soap or Nature's Sunshine's Sunshine Concentrate. Hold this mixture under the faucet while drawing the bath. This will disperse the EOs into the bath water. For a foot or hand soak, use about 4 drops in a teaspoon of liquid soap and add it to a container of water. Aromatic baths soothe muscular aches and pains, skin disorders, circulation problems, tension, fatigue, and insomnia.

Internal Use

There is a big movement, popularized by essential oil companies, to use EOs internally. Although some EOs can be used internally, that is best left to well-trained aromatherapists. In fact, the use of oils internally comes from the French school, where it's primarily medical doctors, trained in aromatherapy, who are using them internally. There are not many instances that the internal use of EOs offers better results than a cup of herb tea, so we don't advise it. If you do decide to use them internally, please only use EOs that are GRAS (generally recognized as safe), and know that even then they should be well diluted to avoid mucosal irritation. EOs that are not GRAS should never be used internally, as they can have harmful effects when ingested. When using EOs internally, you must always dilute them. Because they do not dissolve readily in water, taking them with water is not a good idea, as the oils will float to the top of the water.

You can also add EOs to herbal extracts to increase their potency, mask disagreeable flavors, or improve the taste. Generally speaking, add no more than 1–2 drops per 2 ounces of extract.

FLOWER ESSENCES

Flower essences are homeopathic-like remedies made from the flowers of plants. They help a person find healing on an emotional, rather than a physical or mental, level. Like homeopathy, flower essences are a form of energy medicine, but are not made to the exacting standards of homeopathics. Also, they are designed to affect a person's emotional state rather than their physical symptoms.

Dr. Edward Bach, an English medical doctor and homeopath, discovered how to use flowers for emotional healing and created the first thirty-eight flower essence remedies. Dr. Bach was frustrated by the symptomatic approach of modern medicine. He felt that medical doctors focused too much on the pathology (the disease symptoms) and not enough on the patient.

Bach was a pioneer in understanding gut microflora. He developed homeopathic "vaccines" called Bach nosodes to adjust the friendly flora of the gut to improve health. He also was an advocate of healthy diet and detoxification of the gastrointestinal tract as a route to good health.

As he observed patients, however, he began to notice that certain infections and illnesses tended to go with certain personality traits. He also noticed that a patient's emotional state had a lot to do with their ability to heal. Bach felt that unresolved emotional conflicts within the person created disharmony between the soul and the mind, which eventually led to physical illness. In Bach's mind, health was created by restoring internal harmony, with health being "the true realization of what we are; we are perfect; we are children of God."

Bach wanted to create a system of healing that wouldn't destroy living things and that would be gentle and effective in nature. In his search he found that homeopathic preparations of flowers could guide a person to greater emotional balance. He called these preparations flower essences, and more than eighty years later millions of people have benefited from Bach's remedies. Also, since the time of Dr. Bach, many more flower essences have been discovered, so that today, there are hundreds of flower essences from dozens of suppliers that can help a person with just about any emotional issue one might face in life.

HOW FLOWER ESSENCES WORK

To understand how flower essences work, we need to understand that plants have to overcome challenges, just like we do. They may encounter extremes of temperature or moisture, harsh weather conditions (such as wind or rocky soil), and attacks by insects and animals. Plants, like people, have a "personality," characteristics that help them rise above these challenges. The plant personality is found in its energy pattern, which can become apparent when we study how the plant grows and the form it takes in meeting its life challenges.

Just as associating with a person with positive personality traits can help you learn how to meet life's challenges in a constructive way, so can associating with the right plant energies. As Matthew Wood says in his book *Seven Herbs: Plants as Teachers,* every healing plant is the embodiment of a conflict in the environment that the plant has successfully overcome. By capturing the "vibration" of the plant's personality through the flower, you can take that vibration into your own being and "learn" how to experience that same emotional energy. The plant "teaches" us on a vibrational level how to cope with life in a happy, peaceful, and loving manner.

Flower essences are made by soaking flowers in pure spring water, usually in the sunlight, and then preserving the strained water with brandy. The resulting mother tincture is then diluted in a homeopathic-like manner to imprint the plant's vibration into the flower essence remedy.

When we take the flower essence, it floods our body with a positive vibration that can break through emotional blocks and help us to become more aware. This increased awareness helps us make constructive changes in our lives, which, in turn, helps us find our way back to a balanced emotional state of inner peace and happiness.

MAKING FLOWER ESSENCES

You can make your own flower essences using the following process.

Step one: Obtain flowers from the plant at the peak of blooming. Place them in a glass bowl filled with clean spring water. Allow them to soak in the sunlight for 3–5 hours. If the plant blooms at night, gather the flowers at the height of their blooming and soak them (preferably under a full moon) for the same 3–5 hours.

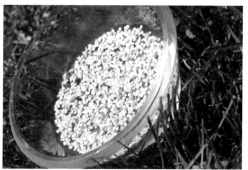

Photo by kerdkanno / CC BY

Step two: Pour off the water into a storage container, straining out the flowers. Preserve the flower water with an equal amount of brandy. This produces the flower essence mother tincture.

Step three: Prepare a second bottle filled with a mixture of water and brandy. This bottle needs to be only about 20–25% brandy. To this bottle, add 5–6 drops of the mother tincture for each ounce of water in the new bottle. Put the lid on this bottle and shake it vigorously up and down against the palm of your hand about 10 times. This creates the stock bottle, the preparation the practitioner keeps on the shelf.

Step four: Dilute the stock tincture in the identical manner as described in step three to create a dosage bottle. The dosage bottle is what the practitioner gives to the client. You can add about 1–5 different flower essences to the dosage bottle.

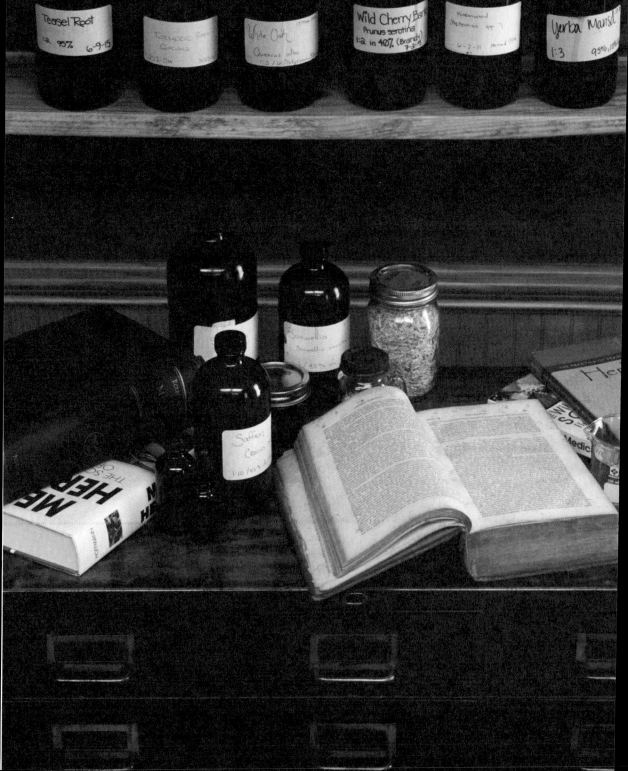

CHAPTER ELEVEN

Formulas and Dosages

DESIGNING HERBAL FORMULAS AND USING HERBS EFFECTIVELY

This chapter covers two very critical considerations in herbalism—how to combine herbs together effectively and how to determine the effective dose. These topics are important because they help a person get the results they want from herbal remedies. We'll cover the principles of herbal formulation first and how to determine dosages second.

PRINCIPLES OF HERB FORMULATION

It is frustrating for an experienced herbalist to see books that describe the actions of herbal combinations by listing all the properties of the individual single herbs they contain. Such information gives the illusion that by taking this particular formula one can derive all of the benefits of each herb in the product as if each herb were being taken separately. This is simply not the case.

Just as the action of a single herb is different from the individual actions of its constituents or so-called active ingredients, the total action of a formula is different from the action of its individual herbs. It is no different from the effect of cooking with foods; a complete dish is different from its individual ingredients. The ingredients blend to form a new creation.

Even if you're not going to design herbal formulas, you may take more than one herb at the same time. When you do this, you are creating a formula, because the herbs interact with each other. Basically, some herbs will enhance or increase the activity of each other, whereas other herbs will counteract or diminish each other's effects.

This is largely based on simple common sense. For instance, if one mixes an herb that stimulates the peristalsis of the colon with an herb that restrains the peristalsis of the colon, one cannot claim that the mixture will cure both diarrhea and constipation. Quite the contrary: the contradictory actions may result in the formula being good for neither.

FORMULAS VERSUS SINGLES

Herbs can be used as single remedies in much the same way that homeopathic remedies are. Each herb has a unique combination of actions and properties, and when a person's overall symptom picture very closely matches that of a single herb, very powerful effects can be created using single remedies.

Using herbs in this manner requires a great deal of knowledge and skill, however. Most herbalists give their clients more than one remedy, which means they are creating a custom formula for the client. So herbs are more often used in combinations than they are as singles.

Most herb books focus primarily on single herbs, but ironically, it's harder for a beginner to see results with single herbs than it is with well-crafted herbal formulas. It can be likened to the difference between using a rifle and a shotgun to hit a target. Using single herbs is like using a rifle. It has a lot of power, but you have to know how to aim it properly to hit the target.

A formula, on the other hand, is like a shotgun. You may not hit the target with as much concentrated force, but your aim doesn't have to be as good.

This is because an herbal formula combines many herbs that work on multiple causes of a problem. Using St. John's wort, an herb that is often used for depression, as an example, we would find that St. John's wort would help a person's depression only if it is the kind of depression that St. John's wort works best on (depression related to anxiety and intestinal problems).

However, if we mix several herbs together that work on several different underlying causes of depression, a person is more likely to get at least some benefit. This is partially because the formula is composed of herbs that address multiple potential root causes of a problem. It is also partly because the synergy of the ingredients often enhances the basic action, and because the multiple ingredients tend to counteract some of the other effects of the single herbs, which also lessens the chance of the remedy throwing the body out of balance in other ways.

To paraphrase Michael Moore, a famous southwestern herbalist, single herbs have subtle and deep actions. Combinations tone down those subtleties to a gray background noise and leave the predominant effects of the herb intact. The literature of the Eclectics, a group of medical doctors who used herbs in the nineteenth century, emphasized utilizing the subtle effects of the herbs and matching all of a person's problems to one herb. However, in actual practice, they frequently resorted to tried and true formulas.

Traditional Chinese medicine (TCM) also relies heavily on formulas. Basic formulas are used for certain situations, with the ingredients being modified to fit individual needs.

CREATING HERBAL FORMULAS

People unskilled in herbalism often create "kitchen sink" formulas, where they simply blend together everything that has been historically used for a particular health problem, thinking that this will be highly effective. This does not take into account the idea of herbal energetics, however. The principle of energetics tells us that some herbs will enhance each other's effects, whereas some herbs will counter each other's effects. So, randomly mixing herbs together does not always yield more effective results.

Herbal Formulas and Energetics

Herbal energetics refers to the ability of herbs to move the body's energies in specific directions. We use a model of energetics based on six tissue states and six basic directions of action. Without going into great detail, here are the basics.

First, herbs can affect metabolism in two general directions. Cooling herbs reduce irritation and excess heat (inflammation and fever). Warming herbs relieve depression and cold (underactivity of organs and tissues). Warming herbs and cooling herbs have opposite actions, which means they tend to restrain each other's effects. We use the term "neutral" to describe herbs that are neither warming nor cooling.

Second, herbs affect the balance of minerals and fluids in the body. Drying herbs treat stagnation and water retention, drying up excess fluids, reducing swelling, shrinking swollen lymph nodes, and otherwise tightening tissues by removing excess moisture. Moistening herbs restore flexibility and tissue function in atrophy, which means they are used when tissues are dry, hard, brittle, or inflexible. Again, these two actions move the tissues of the body in opposite directions, so they tend to counteract and restrain each other. We use the term "balancing" to describe herbs that help to bring tissues back to normal from either stagnation or atrophy.

Third, herbs can affect muscle tone, relaxing the body to promote flow and secretion, or tightening tissues to reduce flow and secretion. Relaxing herbs ease muscle spasms and improve the flow of energy and fluids by easing constriction. Constricting herbs stop leakage by toning up tissue relaxation.

Finally, we use the term "nourishing" to describe herbs that work primarily by providing nutrients that help the body heal itself and restore normal function. These herbs tend to not move the body's energies strongly in any direction, although they might be slightly warming or cooling, or slightly moistening or drying.

So, the first step in creating an herbal formula is to decide the primary energetic you want the formula to have: warming or drying, cooling or moistening, relaxing or nourishing, and so forth. To get this effect, combine herbs into a formula with a similar energetic.

Body Systems and Properties

In addition to considering energetics, you can also design formulas to target specific organs and body systems. Because herbs have affinity for organs and tissues, you can blend herbs to support the structure and function of specific body systems. For example, you can create digestive formulas, respiratory formulas, nervous system formulas, or a formula targeted specifically to the liver, heart, or brain.

Herbs also have certain properties, meaning they affect the structure and function of the body in specific ways. By blending herbs with similar properties, you can create a synergistic effect, making the formula have very specific healing actions. For instance, you could create nervine formulas, diuretic formulas, alterative or blood purifying formulas, or hepatoprotective formulas.

In contrast, herbal formulas will be less therapeutic and more nourishing in their effects when herbs are combined in ways that cancel out their energetic effects and properties. This prevents the formula from having a specific action or moving the body's energies strongly in any direction.

A Plan for Designing Formulas

We use a system for creating herbal formulas based on four major components. It is not necessary to use all four components in any formula, but we usually create formulas using at least 2–3 of them. These components are key herbs, supporting herbs, balancing or harmonizing herbs, and catalysts.

Key Herbs A key herb is one that has the primary action you want the formula to have. So, if you want the formula to have primarily an energetic action, you choose a single herb that has a very strong energetic. For example, if you want a warming formula, you might choose an herb like capsicum or ginger.

You can also choose a key herb based on organ affinity. So, if you want your formula to be focused on the heart, you might choose hawthorn as a key herb. If you want your formula to be a liver formula, you might choose milk thistle.

You can also choose a key herb that has a specific property you want. For example, if you want to create a stimulating diuretic formula, you might choose juniper berries as a key herb. If you want the formula to help a person go to sleep, you might choose hops or scullcap as a key herb.

Your key herb can have a combination of any or all of the above. For example, hawthorn is well known as a heart herb and has cooling and toning effects on the heart. So, you could use it as a key herb for a formula designed to reduce cardiac inflammation and to tone or strengthen the heart.

Think of the key herb as the king or emperor of the formula; it directs the action of the other ingredients. Generally speaking, a formula will have only one or possibly two key herbs.

Supporting Herbs Supporting herbs are like the advisers to the king or emperor. They may have a similar action to the key herb(s) or may somehow enhance the action(s) of the key herb. A supporting herb may also be used to "fill in" effects wanted in the formula that are not supplied by the key herb(s). So, in the previously mentioned idea of using hawthorn in a heart formula, you might add motherwort to calm the heart rate.

Balancing or Harmonizing Herbs These are optional ingredients in any formula. They help to harmonize the action of the whole formula. Balancing or harmonizing herbs may reduce an undesirable side effect of the key herb. For example, cascara sagrada tends to cause intestinal cramping. To counteract this, you might add an antispasmodic like lobelia to the formula.

You might also add a balancing herb to help counteract a disagreeable flavor in the key and/or supporting herbs. For instance, licorice root is often added as a balancing herb in bitter formulas, as it adds a sweet flavor that reduces the bitter taste.

Traditional Chinese herbalists nearly always use balancing herbs in their formulas. They add just a small amount of herbs that have exactly the opposite effect as the key herb(s) in order to make the formula more balanced. In other words, if they are creating a warming formula, they add a small amount of cooling herbs to balance out the warming nature of their key and supporting herbs.

Catalysts These are herbs that help activate the formula or make it work more quickly. In Western herbal formulas, these are usually small amounts of an aromatic or pungent herb like capsicum or ginger. John Christopher used lobelia and capsicum in small amounts as catalysts in nearly all of his formulas. Traditional Chinese herbalists often use licorice root or ginger as catalysts. We often use aromatic herbs as catalysts in our formulas.

Determining Parts Once you have selected all the herbs for the formula, use them in parts as follows:

1–2 key herbs (8–16 parts per herb)
2–4 supporting herbs (4–8 parts per herb)
0–3 balancing herbs (2–4 parts per herb)
0–2 catalysts (1–2 parts per herb)

Parts are measured in weight, so a part could be a milligram or an ounce in making a small batch, or a kilogram or a pound in making a large batch. So, for example, we might make a formula with proportions as follows.

8 ounces key herb
4 ounces supporting herb 1
4 ounces supporting herb 2
2 ounces supporting herb 3
2 ounces balancing herb 1
1 ounce balancing herb 2
1 ounce catalyst

If you examine many of the formulas we have included as examples in Chapter Twelve, you will gain greater insight into how to use this system to create effective formulas. We recommend that you learn to adjust formula ingredients by tasting the formula, just as a good chef always tastes the food he is preparing. You can adjust proportions to get just the effects you want, as well as to improve the overall flavor and appeal.

DETERMINING DOSAGES

Part of learning to use herbs correctly is learning how to dose them properly. Herbalists use a broad range of dosages, from single-drop doses of tinctures to bulk doses of herbs in near food quantities.

Because of this, dosage, especially of tinctures, sometimes becomes a point of contention in Western herbal medicine. Some professional herbalists favor large doses (5 milliliters), whereas others use drop doses (1–5 drops), of most common tinctures. We believe that both drop doses and substantial doses have their place in herbal medicine, and we've listed both types of doses with specific herbs in Chapter Thirteen.

The theory is that small doses of tinctured plants contain the essence, or energetic signature, of the plant. When matched to a person correctly, they act in a subtle yet powerful way through an unknown mechanism of action. On the other hand, substantial doses of herbs act through their chemical constituents to influence physiology and pathology.

THE DROP

Although the dosages for many tinctures are given in drops, the drop was never a good way to measure fluid volume. The size of a drop varies depending on the size of the dropper, the technique used to produce the drop, and the density and surface tension of the liquid. In pure water there are about 20 drops per milliliter, in pure alcohol there are about 60 drops per milliliter, and in pure vegetable glycerin there are about 12 drops per milliliter. Most tinctures are a mixture of alcohol and water (a hydroalcoholic extract). For a standard low-proof tincture (25%–40% EtOH) you can assume around 22–28 drops in 1 milliliter. For a high-proof tincture (80%–90% EtOH) there are around 35 drops per milliliter. These differences in drop size led English pharmacists in 1809 to adopt the minim as an alternative to the drop. The minim is measured in a graduated pipette called a minimometer. A minim is described as exactly 61.611519921875 microliters.

Knowing the exact number of drops in a milliliter or even a minim is not really necessary in modern herbalism. The only time dosing by the drop is important is if you are taking a low-dose (toxic) botanical. Low-dose botanicals should be made according to an official dispensatory and dosed as that dispensatory advises. We prefer either The Dispensatory of the United States of America by Remington, Wood, and colleagues (1918) or King's American Dispensatory (1898). Drop doses of low-dose botanicals are most often added to a large volume of water and given in teaspoonful doses, making them safer than if they were given in direct drop doses.

DOSING STRATEGIES FOR ADULTS

We have included the standard adult dosages for all of the formulas and single herbs in this book. When purchasing commercial herbal formulas or single herbs, assume that the recommended dose on the bottle is for an average weight person of around 150 pounds.

Lower-range dosages are used for people who are smaller than average or who react with sensitivity to herbs and supplements. Use higher-range doses for larger people or people who are less sensitive to herbs and supplements. You can also adjust the dose upward if the results you're getting aren't strong enough or the condition is more severe.

Develop your intuition when dosing herbs by paying attention to your own body, especially when using liquids. Generally speaking, a formula will be tolerable (or even taste good) only as long as you need it. As soon as you have taken enough, the taste changes and you will not want any more. (An exception to this is digestive tonics: although you might not like the bitter taste to begin with, most of the time you begin to tolerate or even enjoy it within a few days.)

DOSING STRATEGIES FOR CHILDREN

Many herbalists calculate children's dosages by age, but calculating by weight is just as easy and probably a bit more accurate.

Clark's Rule (for children ages two to seventeen)

Divide the child's weight in pounds by 150 (which is the weight that is assumed for adults when calculating adult doses) and multiply the result by the adult dose to find the equivalent child's dosage.

$$(\text{Weight in pounds} \div 150) \times \text{adult dose} = \text{child's dose}$$

If the adult dose of a tincture is 5 milliliters and the child weighs 30 pounds, divide the weight (30) by 150: 30/150 = ⅕. Multiply ⅕ times the adult dose (5 milliliters) to get 1 milliliter.

Fried's Rule (for children under two years old)

Divide the age of the child (in months) by 150. Multiply the result by the adult dose.

$$(\text{Age of child in months} \div 150) \times \text{average adult dose} = \text{child's dose}$$

If the adult dose of tincture is 2 milliliters and the child is one year (12 months) old, divide the age of the child (12 months) by 150 to get 0.08. Multiply this by the adult dose (2 milliliters) to get 0.16 milliliters for the child's dose.

In a normal hydroalcoholic (water plus alcohol) extract there are around 25 drops per milliliter. Multiply 0.16 times 25 to get 4 drops per dose.

EXPECTED RESULTS

It doesn't take forever to see results. The following are general guidelines for when you should begin to see improvement if you are on the right track.

With acute illnesses, small, frequent doses work best. Dose every 15 minutes up to every 2 hours. You should see improvement within 1–3 hours.

Subacute illness happens when you don't treat an acute illness and it lingers. Dose every 2–4 hours or 4–8 times daily. You should see improvement within 24–48 hours.

Chronic illness is illness that has been around for more than a week or two. When dealing with chronic conditions, dosing is usually 2–4 times daily. Some improvement should occur within 7–10 days.

Degenerative illness occurs when the body is extremely run-down. Dosing strategies are similar to those for chronic illness, but it takes as long as 1–3 weeks to see any significant improvement.

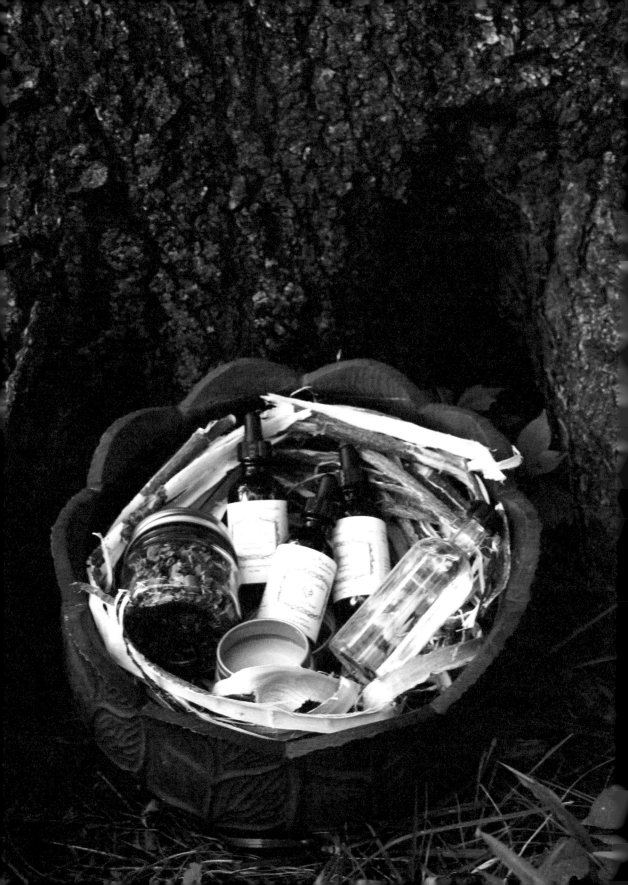

CHAPTER TWELVE

Sample Formulas

SOME OF OUR FAVORITE FORMULAS

The following are some sample formulas designed using the principles outlined in Chapter Eleven. When reading a formula, keep in mind that a part can be anything from a liquid ounce to a pound depending on how big a batch you want to make. In most formulas, start by making a small batch using 1 ounce to equal 1 part.

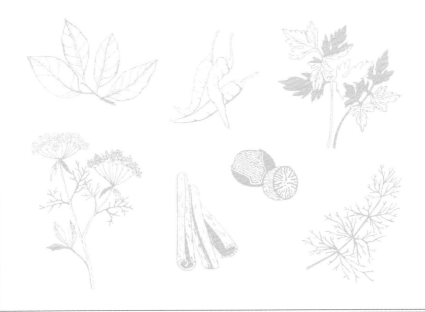

LIQUID FORMULAS

These are formulas designed to be made as infusions (teas), decoctions, tinctures, glycerites, or other liquid preparations.

ANTIALLERGY FORMULA

This formula reduces allergic reactions in cases of hay fever, red and itchy eyes, watery sinus drainage, and frequent earaches. Mix together:

4 parts eyebright (key herb)
4 parts nettle leaf (key herb)
2 parts goldenrod (supporting herb)
2 parts burdock root (supporting herb)
1 part blessed thistle (supporting herb)
1 part bitter orange peel (catalyst)

Prepare from individual tinctures, or macerate at 1:5 in 50% alcohol or as a 1:6 glycerite.

ANTIFUNGAL FORMULA

This is an antifungal formula for oral thrush and gastric or vaginal yeast infections.

4 parts pau d'arco (key herb)
2 parts oregano (supporting herb)
1 part usnea (supporting herb)
1 part reishi mushroom (balancing herb)
1 part black walnut (balancing herb)
½ part thyme (catalyst)

Prepare from individual tinctures or make as a 1:6 glycerite.

ANTISEPTIC GARGLE

This is a basic formula for an antiseptic gargle. Mix together:

1 part myrrh gum (key herb)
1 part bayberry root bark (supporting herb)
¼ part clove buds (catalyst)

Prepare as a 1:6 glycerite. Mix the finished glycerite with an equal amount (by volume) of *Echinacea angustifolia* root tincture.

ANTISEPTIC MOUTHWASH

This is a formula for making your own antiseptic mouthwash.

2 parts peppermint (balancing herb)
1 part myrrh (key herb)
1 part *Echinacea angustifolia* root (supporting herb)
½ part thyme (optional supporting herb)

Prepare from individual tinctures, or macerate at 1:5 in 50% alcohol. Add an equal volume of glycerin to the combination of tinctures along with 1 drop peppermint essential oil for every 4 ounces mouthwash.

ANTISPASMODIC TINCTURE

This tincture can be applied topically to relax muscle spasms and ease pain. It can also be used internally at the first sign of a cold or the flu.

1 part lobelia (key herb)
1 part capsicum (supporting herb)
½ part black cohosh (supporting herb)
½ part blue cohosh (supporting herb)
½ part prickly ash (supporting herb)
½ part clove (catalyst)

Tincture the herbs in 100-proof alcohol at a 1:5 ratio and macerate for 14 days. This formula can also be made using the sealed simmer glycerite process.

ANTIVIRAL FORMULA

Antiviral herbs typically target one family of viruses. This formula is specific to the influenza virus.

4 parts Chinese scullcap (key herb)
3 parts boneset (supporting herb)
2 parts licorice (balancing herb)
2 parts red root (supporting herb)

1 part lomatium (supporting herb)

1 part isatis (supporting herb)

Prepare from individual tinctures, or macerate at 1:5 in 50% alcohol. Take 60 drops (2 milliliters) every hour with fresh ginger juice tea.

BALANCED BITTERS

This is a formula for stimulating digestive secretions in cases of poor appetite or poor digestion. Mix together the following:

2 parts dandelion root (key herb)

2 parts orange peel (key herb)

1 part angelica (supporting herb)

½ part cardamom (balancing herb)

½ part anise (balancing herb and catalyst)

You can optionally add ½ part gentian as a supporting herb to this formula (which will increase its bitterness, but improve its effectiveness). You can also add 1 part peppermint as a supporting and balancing herb to improve the flavor.

Prepare from individual tinctures or macerate at 1:5 in 50% alcohol.

BASIC BLOOD PURIFIER (ALTERATIVE)

This is a basic blood purifying or alterative formula. It is used for eruptive skin disorders, liver problems, and general detoxification. Mix together the following:

4 parts burdock root (key herb)

4 parts red clover (key herb)

2 parts dandelion root (supporting herb)

2 parts yellow dock (supporting herb)

1 part mullein (supporting herb)

1 part parsley (supporting herb)

½ part lobelia (catalyst)

½ part ginger (catalyst)

Prepare from individual tinctures, or macerate at 1:5 in 50% alcohol, or as a 1:6 glycerite.

BRONCHIAL INFLAMMATION AND CONSTRICTION FORMULA

2 parts licorice (key herb)
2 parts wild cherry (key herb)
1 part khella (supporting herb)
1 part lobelia (supporting herb)

This is a useful formula for asthma or relaxing the bronchials in spastic coughing. Prepare as a 1:5 tincture in 50% alcohol.

CHILDREN'S COMPOSITION

This is a formula that has the same effect on children as Herbal Composition and Herbal Crisis do on adults. It is used for colds, flu, fevers, sore throats, upset stomachs, and other acute illnesses. It is antiviral, reduces fever, and stimulates digestion and circulation. It is not as strong a decongestant as Herbal Composition or Herbal Crisis. For serious congestion, also take the Herbal Cough Syrup (Drying) formula listed below.

1 part yarrow (key herb)
1 part elder flower (key herb)
1 part peppermint (balancing herb and catalyst)

This formula works best when prepared as a sealed simmer glycerite. It can also be made into a syrup or tincture or prepared as an infusion. The formula can be modified by adding any of the following ingredients.

½ part chamomile (supporting herb for digestion, nerves, and reducing inflammation)
½ part lemon balm (supporting herb for antiviral effect and balancing herb for flavor)
½ part elder berries (supporting herb for antiviral effect and balancing herb for flavor)
½ part catnip (supporting herb for digestion and fever reduction)

The formula can be used internally at the first sign of cold or flu. Allow children to take as much as they would like in small doses every 15–20 minutes with plenty of water.

COMPOUND WINE OF SOLOMON'S SEAL

This is a tonic formula, beneficial for digestion and structural inflammation.

2 parts Solomon's seal root (key herb)
2 parts plantain leaf (supporting herb)
1 part wild cherry bark (supporting herb)
1 part chamomile flowers (supporting herb)
½ part gentian root (supporting herb)
½ part ginger root (catalyst)

To this, add sherry wine (20% fortified wine) 1:8, bring to a boil, remove from heat, and let steep while covered until cool. Once cool, transfer to a jar and macerate for 3 weeks. Strain and drink 1–2 ounces before meals, 3 times daily. Best kept refrigerated.

DAVID WINSTON'S ANXIETY FORMULA

This formula by David Winston works very well for generalized anxiety disorder. It can be modified for other nervous disorders, as explained below.

2 parts bacopa (key herb)
2 parts motherwort (key herb)
2 parts fresh milky oat seed (balancing herb)
1 part blue vervain (supporting herb)
1 part Chinese polygala (supporting herb)

If the person's mind is racing and they cannot shut their head off at night, add 2 parts Passionflower. If they have muscle tension or spasms or fly off the handle with anger, add 1 part scullcap.

DAVID WINSTON'S DOPAA BITTERS

This formula by David Winston is a pleasant and broad-acting digestive bitters. It enhances digestion, absorption, and elimination and is appropriate for all functional digestive disorders.

2 parts dandelion root (key herb)
1 part orange peel (supporting herb)

1 part angelica root (catalyst)

1 part artichoke leaf (supporting herb)

Prepare from individual tinctures or macerate at 1:5 in 50% alcohol.

DAVID WINSTON'S SAD FORMULA

This simple formula by David Winston is great for seasonal affective disorder, and demonstrates herbal synergy.

1 part lemon balm (key herb)

1 part St. John's wort (key herb)

Prepare from individual tinctures or macerate at 1:5 in 50% alcohol.

ELDER BERRY SYRUP

Pick fresh elder berries and remove as much of the stem as possible. Put berries into a pan, adding just enough water to cover the bottom of the pan. Heat berries on a medium-low burner. As the berries start to steam, mash the berries to release the juice. To increase the amount of juice extracted, puree with an immersion blender. Strain the juice through cheesecloth or a jelly bag. Measure the juice and add an equal amount of honey. Process in pint jars by placing in a boiling water bath for 15–20 minutes (adjusting for altitude). Remove from heat, place new, sterilized canning lids on jars, and let them cool, sealing the jars. They will keep for a year on the shelf, or longer in the refrigerator. Use as pancake syrup or as a tonic for colds, coughs, and viral infections.

FIRE CIDER

This is a great cold and flu remedy made as an herbal vinegar. The formula originated with Rosemary Gladstar. Prepare the following ingredients:

½ cup fresh horseradish root, grated (key herb)

1 medium onion, chopped (supporting herb)

½ cup fresh ginger root, grated (key herb)

¼ cup garlic, mashed (key herb)

2 jalapeño peppers, chopped (catalyst)

1 lemon (zest and juice) (balancing herb)

2 tablespoons dried rosemary leaves (optional balancing herb)

Place all ingredients in a jar and cover with raw apple cider vinegar. Protect the metal lid with waxed paper or parchment paper before putting the lid on the jar. Keep the jar in a dark place and shake daily for 4 weeks. Strain, add honey to taste, and rebottle. As a cold and flu remedy, take 2 tablespoons up to 8 times daily as needed.

GARLIC LEMON AID

This is a simple, but great formula for fighting colds and respiratory infections. It tastes better than it sounds. Peel 1 lemon to remove the yellow part, leaving the white part of the peel intact. Cut the peeled lemon into quarters and place in a blender. Add 1–2 cloves garlic, ⅛–¼ cup honey or real maple syrup, and 1 quart water. Blend until smooth, strain, and drink ½–1 cup at a time throughout the day.

GENTLE FIBER BLEND

This formula is made from bulk herbs. It's a gentle bulk laxative that tones and improves the function of the colon.

   1 part psyllium husk (key herb)
   1 part freshly ground flaxseed (key herb)
   1 part triphala powder (balancing herb)

Take 1–3 teaspoons as needed for fiber. Freeze or refrigerate after making to prevent the oils in the flaxseed from going rancid.

GI INFECTION AND PARASITE FORMULA

This formula addresses severe dysbiosis and amoebic infections.

   4 parts barberry (key herb)
   2 parts black walnut (key herb)
   1 part neem (supporting herb)
   1 part chaparral (supporting herb and catalyst)
   1 part papaya seeds (supporting herb)
   1 part fennel (balancing herb)

Prepare from individual tinctures, or macerate at 1:5 in 50% alcohol, 10% glycerin, and 40% water. Take 5–10 milliliters 3 times daily.

GINGER MAGIC

Juice fresh ginger using a vegetable juicer. Measure the amount of ginger juice and add an equal amount of glycerin (or honey). Then add ¼ of that amount of brandy or spiced rum. So, if you added 1 cup glycerin, you'd add ¼ cup brandy. This is great for settling an upset stomach or for fighting colds and flu. Note: The resins will settle to the bottom of the jar. This formula is helpful because fresh ginger has anti-inflammatory properties that dry ginger does not.

HAPPY FORMULA

This formula works well for stress and stress-induced depression.

    4 parts mimosa bark (key herb)
    2 parts scullcap (fresh tincture) (key herb)
    1 part holy basil (supporting herb)
    1 part hawthorn leaves and flowers (balancing herb)
    1 part rose petals (balancing herb)

    Prepare from tinctures and take 1–4 milliliters 3 times daily.

HERBAL COMPOSITION

Herbal Composition is one of Samuel Thomson's formulas. It is designed to "scour the bowels and remove the canker [mucus]." It is a decongestant, expectorant, and circulatory stimulant and can be used for most acute illnesses. To make it, mix the following herbal powders together:

    4 parts bayberry root bark powder (key herb)
    2 parts white pine bark powder (supporting herb)
    1 part ginger root powder (supporting herb)
    ½ part clove powder (catalyst)
    ½ part capsicum powder (catalyst)

    Prepare as an infusion using 1–2 grams (¼–½ teaspoon) per cup of water. Drink for colds, flu, sweat baths, congestion, etc.

HERBAL COUGH SYRUP (DRYING)

This formula is an expectorant and decongestant formula for damp coughs where there is a lot of mucus production and sinus drainage. It works well in combination with the Children's Composition formula. Mix the following herbs together:

2 parts wild cherry bark (key herb)
2 parts white pine bark (key herb)
1 part spikenard (supporting herb)
1 part elecampane (supporting herb)
1 part yerba santa (supporting herb)
1 part licorice root (balancing herb)
½ part thyme (catalyst)
½ part cinnamon (catalyst)

This blend can also be made as a 1:6 glycerite or syrup, or a 1:5 tincture in 40% alcohol.

HERBAL COUGH SYRUP (MOISTENING)

When the cough is dry and unproductive, the following formula can moisten the lungs and help expel trapped mucus.

2 parts mullein (key herb)
2 parts marshmallow (key herb)
2 parts plantain (key herb)
1 part licorice (supporting herb)
½ part pleurisy root (optional supporting herb)
½ part lobelia (balancing herb and catalyst)

This formula works best when made into a decoction. It can also be made into a 1:6 syrup or glycerite.

HERBAL CRISIS (MODIFIED COMPOSITION)

Herbal Crisis is a modified composition formula designed by Edward Milo Millet. It cuts mucus, stimulates circulation, acts as a decongestant, and fights infection.

Mix the following together:

4 parts bayberry root bark (key herb)
2 parts white pine bark (supporting herb)
1 part goldenseal or myrrh gum (balancing herb)
1 part lobelia or blue vervain or boneset (balancing herb)
1 part ginger (supporting herb)
½ part clove (catalyst)
½ part capsicum (catalyst)

This formula works best when made as a sealed simmer glycerite, although it can also be used as a tea, like Herbal Composition. Use internally for colds, flu, sore throats, respiratory congestion, early stages of infection, or other acute illnesses. The formula can also be used as a compress for insect bites, bee stings, and minor injuries. Use 2 grams (½ teaspoon) per quart of water as an enema solution.

HERBAL MINERAL TONIC

This is a formula of mineral-rich herbs for building the tissues of the body. Mix together the following herbs:

8 parts nettle leaf (key herb)
4 parts alfalfa (supporting herb)
2 parts red raspberry (supporting herb)
2 parts oat straw (supporting herb)
1 part marshmallow (optional supporting herb)
1 part horsetail (supporting herb)
1 part oak bark (supporting herb)

Moisten the herbs in apple cider vinegar and let soak for 2 hours. Add the mixture to water (1:4) and simmer on low until the water is reduced by half. Then add:

½ part peppermint (catalyst)
½ part chamomile (catalyst)

Remove from heat and let steep for 30 minutes. Strain and drink 1–4 cups daily.

This formula can be made as a glycerite, simmering for at least 30 minutes to help draw the minerals out of the herbs, or it can be made as a vinegar extract. It isn't an effective mineral tonic when made as a tincture.

HOREHOUND COUGH SYRUP

Make a horehound decoction using 1 ounce dried horehound or a small handful of fresh horehound leaves in 1 pint water. Simmer for 20 minutes, strain, and reduce to 1 cup. Add 2 cups honey or 1 cup honey and 1 cup dark brown raw sugar. Add the juice of 1 lime and ½ cup brandy. Store in a cool, dark place. Take 1–2 teaspoons as needed.

IMMUNE BOOSTING FORMULA

This formula is a fast-acting immune stimulant.

    4 parts echinacea (key herb)
    2 parts boneset (supporting herb)
    1 part astragalus (balancing herb)
    1 part osha (catalyst)

Prepare from individual tinctures, or macerate at 1:5 in 50% alcohol. Take 30 drops (1 milliliter) every hour during acute infection, then take 3 milliliters 3 times daily for a week following the resolution of symptoms.

IMMUNE SYRUP

The following is a tasty syrup that can be used by children or adults to strengthen the immune system. Mix together the following:

    1 part astragalus (key herb)
    1 part elder berry (key herb)
    ½ part wild cherry bark (optional, as cooling cough suppressant with aller-
        gies or fair skin)
    ½ part white pine bark (optional, warming decongestant and expectorant)
    ½ part licorice (supporting herb, soothing to mucous membranes,
        antiviral)

Make as a syrup at 1:5 with 50% honey (or other sweetener) and 50% water. This can also be made as a 1:6 glycerite or sealed simmer glycerite (60% glycerin, 40% water). If made as a syrup, store in the refrigerator after making.

INFLAMMATION FORMULA

Most structural pain is caused by inflammation. This formula addresses inflammation.

   4 parts Solomon's seal (key herb)
   2 parts boswellia (supporting herb)
   2 parts ginger (preferably fresh juice) (catalyst)
   1 part teasel (supporting herb)
   1 part black pepper (balancing herb)
   1 part arnica (catalyst and key herb) (omit in high blood pressure)

Prepare from tinctures and take 3–5 milliliters 3 times daily.

LIVER FORMULA

This is a basic liver formula. It stimulates the flow of bile and is hepatoprotective (protects the liver).

   8 parts milk thistle (key herb)
   4 parts dandelion root (key herb)
   2 parts artichoke leaf (supporting herb)
   1 part fringe tree bark (supporting herb)
   1 part red root (balancing herb)
   1 part wild yam root (balancing herb)
   1 part turmeric root (catalyst)

Prepare from individual tinctures, or macerate at 1:5 in 50% alcohol or as a 1:6 glycerite.

LYMPHATIC CLEANSING FORMULA

This formula helps with swollen lymph nodes, sore throats, frequent earaches, and chronic congestion. It shrinks swollen lymph nodes, fights infection, and promotes lymphatic drainage.

2 parts red root (key herb)
2 parts echinacea (key herb)
1 part mullein (supporting herb)
1 part lobelia (supporting herb)
½ part yarrow (supporting herb)
½ part calendula (supporting herb)

Prepare from individual tinctures, or macerate at 1:5 in 50% alcohol or as a 1:6 glycerite.

NERVE FORMULA

This is a reliable formula for stress and stress-induced tension and panic.

4 parts scullcap (fresh tincture) (key herb)
2 parts blue vervain (supporting herb)
2 parts motherwort (supporting herb)
1 part pulsatilla (catalyst)

Prepare from tinctures. Take 1 milliliter every 10 minutes for an anxiety attack or 1–3 milliliters 3–4 times daily for acute stress or to induce sleep.

PAIN FORMULA

This formula combines a central-acting analgesic with an antispasmodic and hypnotic analgesic. This doesn't address the cause of the pain, but it helps you get through it.

4 parts Corydalis yanhusuo (key herb)
1 part Jamaican dogwood (supporting herb)

Mix from tinctures and take 1–5 milliliters as needed.

PREGNANCY TEA

This is a formula for helping to maintain a healthy pregnancy and make delivery easier. It is consumed daily during pregnancy. It tones the uterus and reduces morning sickness.

2 parts red raspberry (key herb)

2 parts nettle (supporting herb)

2 parts alfalfa (balancing herb)

1 part peppermint (optional) (catalyst)

Prepare as a standard decoction and drink 1 quart daily.

SOOTHING DIURETIC

This is a formula that doesn't have the harsh stimulating effect on the kidneys that the Stimulating Diuretic formula does. It is gentler and more suitable for children. It is also more suitable for inflamed and irritated kidneys and urinary passages and helps promote lymphatic drainage. Mix together:

4 parts cleavers (key herb)

4 parts nettle leaf (key herb)

2 parts dandelion leaf (supporting herb)

2 parts red clover (supporting herb)

2 parts goldenrod (supporting herb)

1 part corn silk (supporting herb)

This formula is best made as a strong infusion, but can be made as a glycerite or syrup.

STIMULATING DIURETIC

This formula stimulates the kidneys to produce more urine to relieve water retention. It also helps fight urinary tract infections. Do not use long term.

2 parts juniper berry (key herb)

2 parts uva ursi (key herb)

1 part parsley (supporting herb)

1 part dandelion leaf (supporting herb)

1 part barberry (supporting herb)

Mix from tinctures or make as a 1:8 glycerite.

THROAT COAT

Mix together the following:

2 parts licorice (key herb)

1 part marshmallow root (supporting herb)

½ part spearmint or peppermint (optional balancing herb)

Use as a tea (infusion) or a glycerite for sore or irritated throats. It may also be useful for dry coughs.

UTI FORMULA

This formula works well for uncomplicated cystitis and is not for long-term use.

3 parts juniper berry (key herb)

1 part barberry (supporting herb)

1 part licorice (balancing herb)

Prepare from individual tinctures; or macerate at 1:5 in 50% alcohol, 10% glycerin, and 40% water; or make a 1:6 glycerite. Take 5 milliliters 3 times daily.

OTHER FORMULAS

These are formulas designed as topical preparations, salves, ear drops, and other unique preparations.

BASIC HEALING SALVE

This is a basic salve for soothing minor irritations and injuries and promoting more rapid regeneration of tissue.

2 parts comfrey leaf (key herb)

1 part calendula flower and/or yarrow flowering herb (supporting herb)

1 part plantain (supporting herb)

1 part myrrh (optional supporting herb for a more antiseptic effect)

Extract the herbs in olive oil, almond oil, or another quality fixed oil for 12–24 hours. Strain. Add 1 ounce of beeswax for each 8 ounces of oil. See directions for making salves in the "Salves, Ointments, and Balms" section of Chapter Eight.

BASIC POULTICE FORMULA

This is a base formula for making a poultice. Mix together the following:

1 part plantain powder (key herb)

1 part calendula powder (key herb)

This powder can be moistened with water or aloe vera juice and applied topically. It can also be modified as follows.

For an astringent effect to reduce the swelling of bites and stings, add:

1 part white oak bark (key herb)

For infection, add:

½ part echinacea (supporting herb)

½ part barberry (supporting herb)

½ part lobelia (catalyst)

For an increased drawing action (to pull out pus, infection, or slivers), add one of the following as an additional supporting herb:

2 parts activated charcoal or fine clay (Redmond or other bentonite clay) to the base formula. (You can also use hydrated bentonite as the liquid.)

2 parts freshly crushed lily of the valley leaves

2 parts comfrey root powder

Tincture of pine gum as the liquid

For a greater styptic action (to reduce bleeding or oozing), add the following to the base formula:

1 part yarrow (supporting herb)

GARLIC-MULLEIN EAR OIL

This oil is a very effective remedy for earache. Mullein flowers are soothing and anodyne, while the garlic fights infection.

Pick mullein flowers and pack them into a jar (do not wash them). Fill the jar with olive oil. Crush some garlic cloves and put them in a separate jar. Cover them with olive oil, too. Infuse each mixture for 2 weeks, then strain. Mix the two oils in equal parts and bottle.

St. John's wort flowers can also be added to this oil. They help increase the pain-relieving action of the ear drops.

HEMORRHOID SUPPOSITORY

This is a healing suppository for hemorrhoids. Blend the following together with enough cocoa butter to form pellets the size of the last joint of the little finger. Refrigerate to harden before using.

1 part powdered white oak bark (key herb)
1 part powered comfrey root (supporting herb)
½ part powered goldenseal (supporting herb)
½ part collinsonia (optional supporting herb)
½ part powdered lavender flowers (optional catalyst)

HERBAL EYEWASH

This blend can be used for conjunctivitis or other eye infections. Mix together:

4 parts eyebright (key herb)
2 parts bayberry root bark (supporting herb)
2 parts goldenseal (supporting herb)
2 parts red raspberry (supporting herb)
1 part capsicum (optional catalyst)

Make as an infusion and apply using an eyecup. Can also be used as eye drops (mix with Nature's Sunshine's Silver Shield or Aqua Sol Silver to preserve). Can also be used as a compress.

HERBAL SINUS SNUFF

This blend is used as snuff to clear sinus congestion and sinus infection. Mix together the following:

1 part goldenseal root powder (key herb)
1 part bayberry root bark powder (key herb)

HERBAL TOOTH POWDER

Mix together the following:

1 part white oak bark (key herb)
1 part elecampane (supporting herb)
½ part thyme (optional catalyst)
½ part myrrh powder (optional catalyst)

Sprinkle some of the powder into the palm of the hand. Dip a moistened toothbrush in the powder and brush teeth.

MEDICATED OIL

This oil combination infused with herbs is a powerful anti-inflammatory for the skin. It's appropriate for dry, cracked skin, eczema, psoriasis, and rashes.

2 parts licorice root (key herb)
1 part calendula (supporting herb)

Make a 1:4 extract with gentle heat in equal parts grape seed oil and avocado oil. Strain and add enough jojoba oil to make 25% of the final volume.

PAIN-RELIEVING LINIMENT

This liniment is very effective for spasms, inflammation, and the resulting lymphatic congestion associated with chronic structural inflammation.

4 parts lobelia (key herb)
2 parts cayenne (key herb)
1 part arnica (supporting herb)
1 part poke (supporting herb)

1 part datura seeds (optional catalyst): topical use only; poisonous when taken internally

Macerate for 2 weeks, or percolate in 91% rubbing alcohol.

Add 5 drops per ounce of camphor and wintergreen essential oils.

Warning: Datura is a very potent addition to this formula, and makes it an excellent pain reliever. However, datura is very poisonous when taken internally. KEEP OUT OF REACH OF CHILDREN. Don't apply to more than 1 square foot of skin per application. In some states, datura is illegal to grow and potentially to use. Please check your local laws before using it.

RESPIRATORY CONGESTION OIL

Mix together:

1 tablespoon fixed oil

7–8 drops of any of the following oils: eucalyptus, rosemary, thyme, pine, frankincense, and/or cajeput

Rub into back and chest. Start at the back and work between the ribs to the breastbone. Helps to relieve coughing and congestion. Can also be used on sore throats; rub gently onto the neck.

ROSE WATER LOTION

Melt the following ingredients together in a pan:

4 parts grape seed oil

1 part mango butter

1 part emulsifier (see Lotions section of Chapter Eight)

Allow to cool to room temperature. Slowly, using a blender or immersion blender, add 4 parts rose hydrosol. Add 1 drop rosemary essential oil for every 110 milliliters (4 ounces) of liquid, and add 1 milliliter vitamin E oil per 240 milliliters (8 ounces) of liquid.

SUPPOSITORY FOR VAGINAL INFECTIONS

This blend will help with vaginal infections. Blend the following together with enough cocoa butter to form pellets the size of the last joint of the little finger. Refrigerate to harden before using.

2 parts powdered goldenseal (key herb)
1 part powdered plantain (supporting herb)
1 part powdered lavender flowers (supporting herb)
1 part powdered calendula flowers (optional supporting herb)

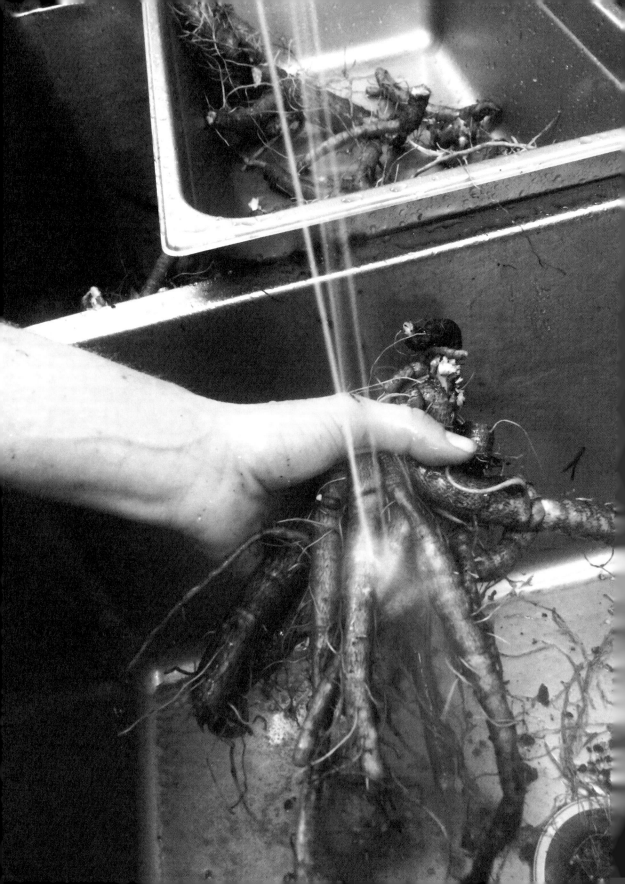

CHAPTER THIRTEEN

Single Herbs

INSTRUCTIONS FOR PREPARING AND USING SINGLE HERBS

This chapter provides you with instructions for preparing and using 235 single herbs. We've included information about each plant's energetics and properties as well as warnings. We've also listed which major bulk herb suppliers carry the herb. Directions for making preparations are starting suggestions; feel free to experiment.

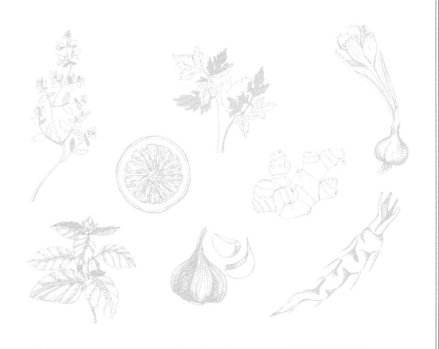

AÇAÍ

Latin name: *Euterpe oleracea*

Like other berries, açaí berries are loaded with antioxidants that help to protect cells from damage that may lead to chronic diseases such as heart disease, diabetes, and cancer. Açaí berry contains vitamin A, fiber, calcium, iron, essential fatty acids (omega-9), anthocyanins (antioxidant), and polysterols. The *Journal of Agricultural and Food Chemistry* published a 2008 study showing that the açaí berry has more antioxidants than blackberries, blueberries, strawberries, and raspberries, but fewer antioxidants than red wine and pomegranate juice.

WARNINGS: No known warnings

ENERGETICS: Cooling and nourishing

PROPERTIES: Anti-inflammatory, antioxidant, and nutritive

SOURCES: Mountain Rose Herbs, Starwest Botanicals

DOSAGE FORMS

FRESH OR DRIED BERRIES: A handful of the berries 2–3 times daily

CAPSULE: 1 500 mg capsule 1–2 times daily with food

POWDER: 1–5 grams 1–2 times daily with food

JUICE: 1–4 ounces 1–2 times daily with food

AGRIMONY

Latin name: *Agrimonia eupatoria*

Agrimony is an astringent that helps stop urinary bleeding and diarrhea. It's helpful for those with cloudy, smelly urine and for those with incontinence. It also has an energetic action on the nervous system and helps to relieve emotional tension. Its indication as a flower remedy is a good guide to its herbal use—it helps people who mask their pain behind a facade of cheerfulness. It's helpful for people who have a tense pulse and appear friendly and cheerful, but are actually very tense and stressed. It is a great urinary tract remedy and helps urinary tract infections and cystitis. It also helps constricted liver chi, a pattern in traditional Chinese medicine that is commonly seen in many Americans.

This involves an inner resistance, anger, or frustration that constricts blood flow to the liver and creates a tense, wiry pulse. Agrimony relaxes blood flow to the liver and helps a person relax and go with the flow of life.

WARNINGS: No known warnings

ENERGETICS: Drying and relaxing

SPECIFIC INDICATIONS: Rolla Thomas: Atonic conditions of the urinary apparatus, and where the urine is thick and gelatinous. Improves the tone of all mucous membranes.

PROPERTIES: Anti-inflammatory, astringent, hemostatic, and vulnerary

SOURCES: Frontier Herbs, Mountain Rose Herbs, Starwest Botanicals, Stony Mountain Botanicals

DOSAGE FORMS

STANDARD INFUSION: 4–8 ounces 1–4 times daily

TINCTURE: Fresh leaf (1:2, 95% alcohol); dried leaf (1:5, 50% alcohol); 5 drops to 3 ml (0.6 tsp.) 3 times daily

GLYCERITE: Dried leaf (1:6); ¼–1 tsp. 3 times daily

TOPICAL USE: For skin rashes, apply the salve or ointment as needed, or prepare a compress from a strong infusion or a decoction and apply several times daily.

ALFALFA

Latin name: *Medicago sativa*

Alfalfa has been called the king of herbs, and it has been used since ancient times. Roots can grow 30–60 feet deep to pick up minerals and water other plants can't reach. This makes alfalfa a rich source of vitamins, minerals, trace minerals, and other nutrients. Its trace mineral content is probably what makes it valuable for the pituitary, because trace mineral deficiencies often affect this gland. It acts as a mild alterative and blood purifier and has been used for arthritis, poor appetite, general weakness, and mineral deficiencies. Alfalfa and peppermint make a good tea for digestive troubles.

WARNINGS: Alfalfa contains canavanine, a nonprotein amino acid that induces lupus-like symptoms in monkeys. There are several reports of this in humans as well. It is contraindicated in those with lupus.

ENERGETICS: Moistening and nourishing

PROPERTIES: Anticoagulant (blood thinner), bitter, galactagogue, mineralizer, and nutritive

SOURCES: Bulk Herb Store, Frontier Herbs, Mountain Rose Herbs, San Francisco Herb Company, Starwest Botanicals, Stony Mountain Botanicals

DOSAGE FORMS

FRESH HERB: Sprouts may be added to a variety of foods and eaten daily.

SOUTHERN DECOCTION: 1 cup 1–2 times daily

TINCTURE: Alcohol is not a good solvent of minerals, so tinctures are rarely used.

BULK POWDER, CAPSULES, AND TABLETS: 1,000–4,000 mg, 2–3 times daily

GLYCERITE: Dried leaf (1:6); 2–10 ml (0.4–2 tsp.) 3 times daily

ALOE VERA

Latin name: *Aloe vera, syn. A. barbadensis*

Aloe vera juice and gel are made from the inner pulp of the aloe vera leaf. Aloe is extremely soothing to irritated skin and mucous membranes, burns, and other damaged tissues.

Whole leaf aloe vera juice builds the immune system to help fight arthritis, AIDS, cancer, and other degenerative diseases.

Aloe vera gel may be applied topically for burns and skin irritations. Apply liberally and keep the skin moist for best results. Aloe vera works best when fresh. Aloe plants are easy to grow and keep in the home for treating burns.

The outer leaf contains anthraquinone glycosides and is a strong purgative and stimulant laxative. This is filtered out when extracting the juice and gel.

WARNINGS: Some herbalists suggest that children, the elderly, and pregnant women should not drink aloe vera juice. However, this may apply only to the green outer leaf portion (which is strongly cathartic) or to aloe vera concentrates. The diluted pulp juice is a mild, harmless remedy.

ENERGETICS: Cooling and moistening

PROPERTIES: Anti-inflammatory, antiseptic, demulcent (mucilant), emollient, stimulant laxative, purgative (cathartic), soothing, and vulnerary

SPECIFIC INDICATIONS: Hot and dry conditions, sunburns, inflammatory bowel disease, gastroparesis

SOURCES: Frontier Herbs, Mountain Rose Herbs, Starwest Botanicals, Stony Mountain Botanicals

DOSAGE FORMS

FRESH: Cut fresh leaf to expose the gel. Apply gel topically.

CAPSULE (LEAF): 250–450 mg of the leaf extract daily as a laxative. Not for long-term use.

JUICE (PULP ONLY): 1–4 ounces of the juice daily

TOPICAL USE: Apply juice or gel topically as needed.

ANDROGRAPHIS

Latin name: *Andrographis paniculata*

Andrographis is a potent antiviral, antibacterial, and immune stimulator. Andrographis extracts have been shown to mildly inhibit Staphylococcus aureus, Pseudomonas aeruginosa, Proteus vulgaris, Shigella dysenteriae, and Escherichia coli. Extracts have also been shown to inhibit lipid peroxidation and inflammation. It is used in Ayurvedic medicine for diarrhea, dyspepsia, lack of bile flow, hepatitis, pneumonia, tonsillitis, colds, sinus infections, and flu; and is used by modern herbalists to treat intestinal parasites, colds, influenza, and hepatitis. In a clinical study, patients treated with andrographis for 3 months were two times less likely to catch colds than the placebo group.

WARNINGS: Not for use during pregnancy or lactation

ENERGETICS: Cooling and drying

PROPERTIES: Anti-inflammatory, antibacterial, bitter, cholagogue, febrifuge, and immune stimulant

DOSAGE FORMS

STANDARD INFUSION: ½ cup 3–4 times daily. Tastes too bad for most people to drink.

TINCTURE: Dried leaf (1:5, 50% alcohol); 1–4 ml (0.2–0.8 tsp.) 3–4 times daily

GLYCERITE: Dried leaf (1:8); 5–10 ml (1–2 tsp.) 3–4 times daily

CAPSULE: 500–1,000 mg, 3 times daily

ANGELICA

Latin name: *Angelica archangelica*

Angelica is a warming aromatic tonic useful for many ailments. Angelica helps to warm a cold, stiff, weakened body and is especially warming to the stomach, spleen, and intestines. This makes it helpful for poor digestion, colic, and intestinal cramps. It promotes perspiration, making it useful for reducing fever. It also helps recovery from colds, flu, and congestion in the lungs. Angelica is related to dong quai and has similar actions; it is a valuable remedy for women that helps to regulate menses and balance hormones. It is an uplifting remedy and can be helpful for stagnant depression. It can also be applied externally for bruises, sprains, and muscle and joint pain.

WARNINGS: Not for use during pregnancy or while nursing. Also contraindicated in heavy menstrual bleeding.

ENERGETICS: Warming and drying

PROPERTIES: Aromatic, decongestant, and digestive tonic

SPECIFIC INDICATIONS: King's American Dispensatory: Flatulent colic and heartburn, and nervous headache.

SOURCES: Frontier Herbs, Mountain Rose Herbs, San Francisco Herb Company, Starwest Botanicals, Stony Mountain Botanicals

DOSAGE FORMS

STANDARD DECOCTION: 2–4 ounces 3 times daily

TINCTURE: Fresh root (1:2, 95% alcohol); dried root (1:5, 65% alcohol); 1–3 ml (0.2–0.6 tsp.) 3 times daily

GLYCERITE: Dried root (1:5); 2–5 ml (0.4–1 tsp.) 3 times daily

CAPSULE: 1 500 mg capsule 3 times daily (doesn't work on digestion; only for pelvic circulation)

ANISE

Latin name: *Pimpinella anisum*

Anise is a soothing aromatic with properties similar to those of fennel. Tea, tincture, or oil can be used to settle the stomach and expel gas. It is useful for colic in infants and helps promote lactation for the breastfeeding mother. It is a mucolytic agent, helping to thin mucus and expel it from the lungs. It is a common ingredient in formulas for indigestion, but is not a key herb in these formulas.

WARNINGS: Anise is a traditional abortifacient. There are no reports of it being harmful when used in normal food doses, but avoid medicinal doses when pregnant except under the supervision of a well-trained herbalist.

ENERGETICS: Warming and drying

PROPERTIES: Aromatic, carminative, and galactagogue

SPECIFIC INDICATIONS: King's American Dispensatory: Flatulency, flatulent colic of infants, and to remove nausea.

SOURCES: Mountain Rose Herbs, San Francisco Herb Company, Starwest Botanicals, Stony Mountain Botanicals

DOSAGE FORMS

WEAK INFUSION: 2–8 ounces 2–3 times daily. For gastrointestinal complaints in children, give 1 ounce as needed, sweetened with maple syrup. For infants, add 1 teaspoon to their bottle, or give breastfeeding mothers strong doses.

TINCTURE: Dried (1:5, 50% alcohol and 10% glycerin); 1–3 ml (0.2–0.6 tsp.) 3 times daily

GLYCERITE: Sealed simmer dried (1:8); 2–5 ml (0.4–1 tsp.) 3 times daily

ARJUNA

Latin name: *Terminalia arjuna*

Valued as a remedy for the heart and poor circulation in Ayurvedic medicine, arjuna is used as a treatment for angina, congestive heart failure, heart problems related to smoking, and elevated blood pressure. It is used in a very similar manner as hawthorn and works well when combined with it.

WARNINGS: Not for use during pregnancy except under the supervision of a qualified health care practitioner

ENERGETICS: Cooling and slightly relaxing

PROPERTIES: Anti-arrhythmic, cardiac, hypotensive, and vasodilator

DOSAGE FORMS

TINCTURE: Dried bark (1:5, 50% alcohol); 2–4 ml (0.4–0.8 tsp.) 3 times daily

GLYCERITE: Dried bark (1:8); 5–10 ml (1–2 tsp.) 3 times daily

CAPSULE: 500–1,500 mg, 3 times daily

ARNICA

Latin name: *Arnica montana*

Arnica is used to reduce swelling, bruising, and pain from injury and trauma. It is most often used as a homeopathic preparation both internally and topically to treat swelling, bruises, and injuries. It is a good idea to keep homeopathic arnica (both tablets and topical cream) in your first aid kit.

Taken internally, arnica tincture has an even stronger anti-inflammatory action than the homeopathic preparation. In higher doses it acts as a cardiac tonic and improves the supply of blood through the coronary vessels. Arnica tincture is toxic and should be taken only under professional supervision. It should be highly diluted when used internally—just a few drops in a cup of water.

WARNINGS: Gastric irritation may develop with internal use of the herb. High doses taken internally can cause intoxication, dizziness, tremors, tachycardia, arrhythmia, and collapse. Arnica tincture should not be used during pregnancy or nursing. Homeopathic preparations do not cause these problems, but neither the herb nor the homeopathic preparation should be applied to broken skin. Arnica contains sesquiterpene lactones that can produce contact dermatitis in sensitive persons.

ENERGETICS: Warming and drying

PROPERTIES: Analgesic (anodyne), anticoagulant (blood thinner), vasodilator, and vulnerary

SPECIFIC INDICATIONS: Rolla Thomas: Tensive pain in the back as if bruised or strained; muscular pain and soreness when the limbs are moved; feeble respiration.

SOURCES: Bulk Herb Store, Frontier Herbs, Mountain Rose Herbs, Starwest Botanicals, Stony Mountain Botanicals

DOSAGE FORMS

TINCTURE: Fresh leaf or root (1:2, 70% alcohol); dried leaf (1:5, 50% alcohol); 1–5 drops in 8 ounces of water, sipped slowly, up to 3 times daily

TOPICAL USE: Apply tincture, ointment, or oil topically to unbroken skin as needed.

ARTICHOKE

Latin name: *Cynara scolymus*

This is the leaf of the globe artichoke that is eaten as a vegetable. It contains cynarin, which has proven liver protection capabilities. Artichoke leaf also contains silymarin, the active constituent of milk thistle. The leaves are used as a digestive bitter for a sluggish liver and poor digestion.

WARNINGS: People with an existing hypersensitivity to any member of the Asteraceae family should use caution.

ENERGETICS: Cooling and drying

PROPERTIES: Alterative (blood purifier), anticholesteremic, bitter, cholagogue, and digestive tonic

SOURCES: Mountain Rose Herbs, Starwest Botanicals

DOSAGE FORMS

STANDARD DECOCTION: 2–4 ounces 3 times daily

TINCTURE: Fresh leaf (1:2, 95% alcohol); dried leaf (1:5, 40% alcohol); 1–4 ml (0.2–0.8 tsp.) 3 times daily

GLYCERITE: Dried leaf (1:8); 1–5 ml (0.2–1 tsp.) 3 times daily

ASHWAGANDHA

Latin name: *Withania somnifera*

An important herb from Ayurvedic medicine, ashwagandha is a nervine and adrenal tonic that helps anxiety, depression, exhaustion, and poor muscle tone. It is adaptogenic and reduces the effects of stress while promoting energy and vitality. It is used as a supporting herb for recovery from debilitating diseases. It is effective for treating sexual dysfunction caused by stress. It is also an effective anti-inflammatory that can relieve symptoms associated with arthritis pain. Ashwagandha helps boost the conversion of T4 (the thyroid storage hormone) to T3 (the active thyroid hormone).

WARNINGS: Use cautiously during pregnancy. Contraindicated in those with sensitivity to the nightshade family.

ENERGETICS: Slightly warming

PROPERTIES: Adaptogen, anti-inflammatory, antidepressant, and nervine

SOURCES: Frontier Herbs, Mountain Rose Herbs, Starwest Botanicals, Stony Mountain Botanicals

DOSAGE FORMS

STANDARD DECOCTION: 4–8 ounces 3 times daily, or decoct in coconut milk with vanilla and honey

TINCTURE: Dried root (1:5, 70% alcohol); 1–10 ml (0.2–2 tsp.) 3 times daily

CAPSULE: 2–6 capsules (1,000–3,000 mg) 3 times daily

ASTRAGALUS

Latin name: *Astragalus membranaceus*

Astragalus is an adaptogenic and tonic herb used in traditional Chinese medicine to boost energy and strengthen immunity. Research suggests that the polysaccharides and saponins in astragalus may be helpful to those with heart disease, improving heart function and providing relief from symptoms. Astragalus appears to restore immune function in people whose immune systems have been weakened by chemotherapy or chronic illness. It has antibacterial and antiviral properties, making it useful as a topical treatment for healing wounds. It can be helpful in preventing and treating common colds and respiratory infections. Astragalus may also have benefits in treating allergic asthma.

WARNINGS: No known warnings

ENERGETICS: Slightly warming and moistening

PROPERTIES: Adaptogen, anti-inflammatory, antiviral, diuretic, hypotensive, and immune amphoteric

SOURCES: Bulk Herb Store, Mountain Rose Herbs, San Francisco Herb Company, Starwest Botanicals, Stony Mountain Botanicals

DOSAGE FORMS

STANDARD DECOCTION: 1–3 cups daily

TINCTURE: Dried root (1:5, 40% alcohol); 2–4 ml (0.4–0.8 tsp.) 3 times daily. The tincture is not as effective as other forms of administration.

GLYCERITE: Dried root (1:8); 10–20 ml (2–4 tsp.) 3 times daily

SYRUP: Dried root (1:8, 50% honey); 2–3 tsp. 3 times daily

CAPSULE OR POWDER: 1,000–3,000 mg, 3 times daily

ATRACTYLODES

Latin name: *Atractylodes ovata, A. macrocephala*

This Chinese herb is used in digestive and urinary combinations. It may also be helpful for treating fungal and bacterial infections.

WARNINGS: Contraindicated with high fever, excessive sweating, severe inflammation, and dehydration

ENERGETICS: Warming and drying

PROPERTIES: Anti-inflammatory, carminative, digestive tonic, and diuretic

DOSAGE FORMS

WEAK INFUSION: 4 ounces 3 times daily

POWDER: 500–1,000 mg, 3 times daily

BACOPA (WATER HYSSOP)

Latin name: *Bacopa monnieri*

Used in Ayurveda to treat nervous disorders such as anxiety, seizures, and poor memory, bacopa has become a popular herb for aiding brain function in Western herbalism. In a recent clinical trial of ninety-eight healthy people over age fifty-five, bacopa significantly improved memory acquisition and retention.

WARNINGS: Not for use with hyperthyroidism

ENERGETICS: Cooling

PROPERTIES: Anti-inflammatory, antioxidant, cerebral tonic, and nervine

DOSAGE FORMS

WEAK INFUSION: 1 cup up to 3 times daily

TINCTURE: Dried leaf (1:5, 50% alcohol); 1–3 ml (0.2–0.6 tsp.) 3 times daily

CAPSULE: 400–500 mg of a standardized extract 2 times daily

BARBERRY

Latin name: *Berberis vulgaris or B. aristata*

One of the best bitter liver tonics, barberry contains berberine, an antimicrobial and antifungal compound. Barberry has been shown to increase bile production and is one of the most useful cholagogues. Barberry also contains a compound called 5'-MHC, which helps keep bacteria from developing resistance to antibiotics, making it useful for many infections. Barberry is a common ingredient in blood purifying formulas.

WARNINGS: Not for use during pregnancy or when emaciated

ENERGETICS: Cooling and drying

PROPERTIES: Alterative (blood purifier), antiseptic, aperient, bitter, and cholagogue

SPECIFIC INDICATIONS: Fyfe: Chronic blood dyscrasia (imbalance), with scaly skin eruptions and impaired nutrition and waste.

SOURCES: Frontier Herbs, Mountain Rose Herbs, Starwest Botanicals, Stony Mountain Botanicals

DOSAGE FORMS

STANDARD DECOCTION: 4 ounces 3 times daily

TINCTURE: Fresh root (1:2, 95% alcohol); dried root (1:5, 50% alcohol); 1–4 ml (0.2–0.8 tsp.) 4 times daily

GLYCERITE: Dried root (1:5); 1–5 ml (0.2–1 tsp.) 3–4 times daily

CAPSULE: 500–1,500 mg, 3 times daily

TOPICAL USE: Use a compress of the decoction for bacterial infections. For fungal infections, apply a salve to the skin 3 times daily. Barberry will stain whatever it comes in contact with, including skin.

BAYBERRY

Latin name: *Myrica cerifera*

Bayberry is a strong astringent with a mild stimulant action. It is a good astringent for the gastrointestinal tract. It inhibits or slows bleeding, arrests diarrhea, and loosens phlegm to aid the discharge of mucus from the sinuses and gastrointestinal tract.

WARNINGS: Use with caution during pregnancy.

ENERGETICS: Slightly warming, drying, and constricting

PROPERTIES: Astringent, expectorant, hemostatic, styptic, and vulnerary

SOURCES: Mountain Rose Herbs, Starwest Botanicals

DOSAGE FORMS

STANDARD INFUSION: 1 cup 3 times daily

TINCTURE: Dried root bark (1:5, 50% alcohol, 10% glycerin); 0.25–2 ml (0.05–0.4 tsp.) as needed in warm water. Take frequently for colds and flu.

GLYCERITE: Dried root bark (1:5); 1–3 ml (0.2–0.6 tsp.) 3–4 times daily

CAPSULE: 1–3 capsules (500–1,500 mg) up to 3 times daily

POWDER: Very small doses (100 mg or less) used as a snuff can help dry up runny noses and help with nasal polyps.

TOPICAL: Powder, tincture, or glycerite can be applied topically as an astringent.

BEE POLLEN

Bee pollen contains every known nutrient in trace amounts. It is highly energizing and used to increase stamina and endurance. It supports the glands and aids the immune system. Bee pollen has been used to overcome allergies to pollen. It is best to get bee pollen from local beekeepers and start with a small amount (just a few grains). Gradually increase the dose over a period of several weeks to develop a tolerance to pollen and improve immune function.

WARNINGS: A few allergic reactions have been reported from the use of bee pollen. Symptoms of allergy include itching, dizziness, and difficulty swallowing. If you have allergies, be sure to start with a few grains.

ENERGETICS: Neutral and nourishing

PROPERTIES: Nutritive and metabolic stimulant

SOURCES: Mountain Rose Herbs, San Francisco Herb Company, Starwest Botanicals, Stony Mountain Botanicals

DOSAGE FORMS

POWDER: Bee pollen granules are gathered from the bees' legs as they reenter the hive, and are sold as granules or are ground into powder. For general health purposes, take 1–2 heaping teaspoons of the raw granules daily. Mix them in juice, a smoothie, yogurt, applesauce, or cereal, or simply chew and swallow.

CAPSULES: 2–4 capsules (1,000–2,000 mg) up to 4 times daily.

BILBERRY

Latin name: *Vaccinium myrtillus*

Bilberries have been shown to improve night vision and help heal eye irritations. They contain anthocyanidins, which protect collagen structures in the eyes, thereby preventing and treating macular degeneration and retinopathy. Bilberries tone blood vessels and improve circulation. Studies suggest that the antioxidants in bilberries can protect against diseases of the circulatory system. Blueberry is a cousin of bilberry and can be used interchangeably. Blueberries and bilberries can improve atherosclerosis and varicose veins.

WARNINGS: None known for the fruit; long-term use of the leaves can potentially cause gastric irritation and kidney damage, but they have a history of safe use.

ENERGETICS: Cooling, slightly drying, and nourishing

PROPERTIES: Nutritive and vascular tonic

SOURCES: Bulk Herb Store, Frontier Herbs, Mountain Rose Herbs, Starwest Botanicals

DOSAGE FORMS

FRESH HERB: The fresh berries can be eaten daily.

POWDER: 2–5 grams 3 times daily

SOLID EXTRACT: Fresh berries can be cooked down and preserved with glycerin to make a solids extract. Take 1 teaspoon 2 times daily.

SYRUP: Juice berries, warm, and mix with an equal part honey. Refrigerate or can.

BITTER MELON

Latin name: *Momordica charantia*

Bitter melon has long been used in Ayurvedic medicine to treat type 2 diabetes. It protects the pancreas, improves insulin resistance, and lowers blood lipids. Compounds in the plant inhibit *Helicobacter pylori,* which is useful in cases of gastric ulcers. Bitter melon may be helpful for parasites, intestinal worms, and stomach pain or colic accompanied by constipation.

WARNINGS: May cause diarrhea, stomachache, and bloating. Do not take with diabetes medications without professional supervision.

ENERGETICS: Cooling and drying

PROPERTIES: Anthelminthic, antibacterial, anticancer, antidiabetic, antioxidant, antiviral, and bitter

SOURCES: Mountain Rose Herbs, Starwest Botanicals

DOSAGE FORMS

CULINARY: Eaten in traditional Asian cuisine. For most Americans this isn't a pleasant-tasting food.

TINCTURE: Dried fruit (1:5, 50% alcohol); 2–4 ml (0.4–0.8 tsp.) up to 4 times daily

CAPSULE: 1–3 capsules (500–1,500 mg) up to 3 times daily

JUICE EXTRACT: 2 ounces daily

BLACK COHOSH

Latin name: *Cimicifuga racemosa; Actaea racemosa*

Black cohosh is typically used for its estrogenic effects, but its role as a source of natural estrogens is questionable. It does seem to help with menopausal symptoms. Black cohosh is antispasmodic and mildly analgesic. It is a good remedy for venomous bites and stings. Black cohosh can help lower blood pressure, reduce joint inflammation, and enhance circulation. It helps improve dark, gloomy depression, and relieves dark, twisted emotional congestion.

WARNINGS: Black cohosh stimulates uterine contractions. It is contraindicated in early pregnancy but can be used (especially as part of a formula) during the last weeks of pregnancy or during labor.

In large doses, black cohosh can cause headaches, dizziness, irritation of the central nervous system, nausea, and vomiting. If headache or dizziness occurs, reduce dose or discontinue use. When black cohosh is used in a formula, it is unlikely to cause any of these effects, because the dose is too low. Black cohosh headaches can often be remedied with a strong cup of green tea.

ENERGETICS: Cooling and relaxing

PROPERTIES: Analgesic (anodyne), anti-arrhythmic, antidepressant, antirheumatic, antispasmodic, antivenomous, emmenagogue, and hypotensive

SPECIFIC INDICATIONS: Rolla Thomas: Muscular pains; uterine pain with tenderness; false pains; irregular pains; rheumatism of the uterus; dysmenorrhea. An antirheumatic when the pulse is open, the pain paroxysmal, the skin not dry and constricted.

SOURCES: Frontier Herbs, Mountain Rose Herbs, Starwest Botanicals, Stony Mountain Botanicals

DOSAGE FORMS

STANDARD DECOCTION: 2–4 ounces up to 3 times daily

TINCTURE: Fresh root (1:2, 80% alcohol); dried root (1:5, 80% alcohol); 3–30 drops (0.1–1 ml) 3 times daily; fresh root tincture is vastly superior to dried root.

GLYCERITE: Dried root (1:5); 6 drops to 1 ml (0.2 tsp.) 3 times daily

CAPSULE: ½–1 capsule (250–500 mg) 2–3 times daily. Difficult to effectively regulate dosage with capsules.

BLACK HAW

Latin name: *Viburnum prunifolium*

Black haw is an antispasmodic used to relieve painful menstruation and low back pain. It is similar in action to cramp bark, though it's not considered as strong. Black haw may be added to formulas for high blood pressure.

WARNINGS: Contraindicated during pregnancy, except in cases of threatened miscarriage or in the last 5 weeks. Large doses can be hypotensive.

ENERGETICS: Neutral, drying, relaxing

PROPERTIES: Antispasmodic

SPECIFIC INDICATIONS: Rolla Thomas: This has been regarded as especially the remedy to arrest abortion or miscarriage, and it may be used for the same indications as the other species. Felter: Uterine irritability and hyperesthesia. Uterine colic with severe lumbar and pelvic cramps.

SOURCES: Mountain Rose Herbs, Starwest Botanicals, Stony Mountain Botanicals

DOSAGE FORMS

DECOCTION: 1–2 tsp. dried bark in 8 ounces water, decoct 15–20 minutes, then steep for 30 minutes; 2–3 cups daily

STANDARD DECOCTION: 4–8 ounces 3 times daily

TINCTURE: Fresh root (1:2, 40–50% alcohol); dried root (1:5, 40–50% alcohol); 1–4 ml (0.2–0.8 tsp.) 3 times daily

CAPSULE: 2–3 capsules (1,000–1,500 mg) 3 times daily

BLACK PEPPER

Latin name: *Piper nigrum*

Pepper is the world's most traded spice and has been used since ancient times for culinary and medicinal purposes. It stimulates digestion and intestinal mobility to ease gas and bloating. It increases the activity of transport proteins at the tight gap junctions in the gut, which helps larger compounds like curcumin and berberine absorb better.

WARNINGS: Large doses can cause gastrointestinal irritation in some people.

ENERGETICS: Warming and slightly drying

PROPERTIES: Antiseptic, carminative, and circulatory stimulant

SOURCES: Bulk Herb Store, San Francisco Herb Company, Stony Mountain Botanicals

DOSAGE FORMS

CULINARY: As a spice, sprinkle on meals as desired.

TINCTURE: Dried fruit (1:5, 50% alcohol); 1–2 ml (0.2–0.4 tsp.) 3 times daily

CAPSULE: 1 capsule (500 mg) 3 times daily, or 10 mg piperine extract 3 times daily

BLACK WALNUT

Latin name: *Juglans nigra*

Black walnut hulls are a locally acting antifungal and antimicrobial, excellent for gut infections, gastric candida overgrowth, and general dysbiosis. It's a traditional remedy for hypothyroidism, probably acting on autoimmunity through gut bacteria regulation. Externally, it can be applied to athlete's foot, ringworm, boils, and infected wounds. It builds tooth enamel when used as a tooth powder.

Black walnut leaf is less antimicrobial and more astringent and carminative than the hulls.

WARNINGS: Not recommended during pregnancy

ENERGETICS: Slightly warming; drying and slightly constricting

PROPERTIES: Antifungal, antiparasitic, bitter, and vermifuge

SPECIFIC INDICATIONS: Felter: Gastrointestinal irritation with acid eructations and flatulence. Tenesmus with burning, fetid alvine discharges. Chronic vesicular skin disease with free discharge.

SOURCES: Bulk Herb Store, Mountain Rose Herbs, Starwest Botanicals, Stony Mountain Botanicals

DOSAGE FORMS

TINCTURE: Fresh hulls (1:2, 95% alcohol); dried hulls (1:5, 50% alcohol); 5 drops to 3 ml (0.6 tsp.) 3 times daily

GLYCERITE: Dried hulls (1:6); 1–5 ml (0.2–1 tsp.) 3 times daily

CAPSULE OR BULK POWDER: 1,000–2,000 mg, 3 times daily

BLACKBERRY

Latin name: *Rubus fruticosus*

Blackberry root bark is a powerful astringent and an excellent remedy for childhood diarrhea. It can be used topically as an astringent for injuries.

WARNINGS: No known warnings

ENERGETICS: Drying and constricting

PROPERTIES: Antidiarrheal, antifungal, antiseptic, and astringent

SOURCES: Starwest Botanicals

DOSAGE FORMS

STANDARD DECOCTION: 4 ounces up to 4 times daily

TINCTURE: Fresh root (1:2, 80% alcohol, 10% glycerin); dried root (1:5, 50% alcohol); 1–3 ml (0.2–0.6 tsp.) up to 4 times daily

POWDER: 1,000–2,000 mg in applesauce as needed

BLADDERWRACK

Latin name: *Fucus vesiculosus*

Bladderwrack is a seaweed. It contains iodine, alginic acid, and fucoidan. Iodine is an essential mineral for the thyroid, uterus, breasts, and prostate. Alginic acid is a special type of fiber that can help acid reflux and acts as a mild appetite suppressant. Fucoidan is a compound shown to reduce inflammation and improve arthritis, diabetes, and other inflammatory conditions. Fucoidan is known to have a variety of antitumor and antiangiogenic properties.

WARNINGS: Not for use with hyperthyroidism or Graves' disease. Use cautiously with Hashimoto's thyroiditis and during pregnancy.

ENERGETICS: Cooling, moistening, and nourishing

PROPERTIES: Anti-inflammatory, antirheumatic, and nutritive

SOURCES: Stony Mountain Botanicals

DOSAGE FORMS

TINCTURE: Dried seaweed (1:3, 45% alcohol); 1–3 ml (0.2–0.6 tsp.) up to 4 times daily

CAPSULE OR POWDER: 1,000–2,000 mg, 2 times daily

BLESSED THISTLE

Latin name: *Cnicus benedictus*

Blessed thistle is a bitter herb with high mineral content and properties similar to those of milk thistle. It is used to strengthen the liver and digestive system, and it is used by nursing mothers to enrich and increase breast milk. The dried leaf is generally used.

WARNINGS: Not recommended during pregnancy

ENERGETICS: Cooling and drying

PROPERTIES: Alterative (blood purifier), bitter, cholagogue, galactagogue, and hepatic

SOURCES: Bulk Herb Store, Frontier Herbs, Mountain Rose Herbs, San Francisco Herb Company, Starwest Botanicals, Stony Mountain Botanicals

DOSAGE FORMS

STANDARD INFUSION: 1 cup 3 times daily

TINCTURE: Dried leaf (1:5, 45% alcohol); 1–2 ml (0.2–0.4 tsp.) up to 3 times daily

GLYCERITE: Dried leaf (1:5); 2–5 ml (0.4–1 tsp.) 3 times daily

CAPSULE: 1,000–1,500 mg, 3 times daily

BLOODROOT

Latin name: *Sanguinaria canadensis*

Bloodroot is an antimicrobial expectorant for chronic lung infections. It is a very powerful lymph-moving herb, normally used as part of a formula for chronically swollen lymph nodes. Externally it is used for fungal infections, eczema, skin disorders, skin cancers, ringworm, scabies, warts, and venereal sores.

WARNINGS: Used internally in very small doses. Large doses can cause nausea, vomiting, headaches, and respiratory failure. Do not use during pregnancy. For use under professional supervision only.

ENERGETICS: Drying and cooling

PROPERTIES: Antifungal, antiseptic, bitter, and lymphatic

SPECIFIC INDICATIONS: Fyfe: Burning, itching of throat; air passages hot, dry, and swollen. Sense of constriction in throat, difficult deglutition. Bronchial irritation with increased secretion. Uneasiness and burning in stomach.

SOURCES: Frontier Herbs, Mountain Rose Herbs, Starwest Botanicals, Stony Mountain Botanicals

DOSAGE FORMS

TINCTURE: Dried root (1:10, 60% alcohol); 1–5 drops up to 3 times daily. Larger doses can be heating and irritating. Start small and don't exceed 20 drops daily.

OIL AND SALVE: Dried root (1:4); make into salve, and apply as needed.

BLUE COHOSH

Latin name: *Caulophyllum thalictroides*

Herbalists use the herb in small doses over a period of time to induce delayed labor. This also works for inducing delayed menstruation. Taken during labor, blue cohosh strengthens contractions and eases the pain of childbirth. Its tonic action stimulates and relaxes the uterus at the same time, making it helpful for relieving painful menstrual symptoms such as cramps and breast pain. It can also be used to help ovarian pain.

WARNINGS: Because it stimulates uterine contractions, it should be avoided by pregnant women or women who are trying to become pregnant. It should also be avoided during heavy menstrual bleeding. It can be used by women after their due date to induce labor, but professional supervision is advised. Blue cohosh is mildly toxic in large doses.

ENERGETICS: Cooling, drying, and relaxing

PROPERTIES: Antispasmodic, emmenagogue, and oxytocic

SPECIFIC INDICATIONS: Felter: Uterine heaviness and sense of soreness in legs, with pelvic congestion. Sluggish labor pains.

SOURCES: Frontier Herbs, Mountain Rose Herbs, Starwest Botanicals, Stony Mountain Botanicals

DOSAGE FORMS

STANDARD DECOCTION: ½–1 cup 3 times daily

TINCTURE: Dried root (1:5, 60% alcohol); 0.5–2 ml (0.1–0.4 tsp.) up to 4 times daily

CAPSULE: 500 mg, 2 times daily

BLUE FLAG

Latin name: *Iris versicolor*

This powerful liver cleansing herb is best used in small doses or as part of a combination. It is considered helpful for chronic skin diseases and gallbladder problems involving a lack of bile flow. It helps with hypoglycemia associated with migraines, sugar cravings, and red-colored skin.

WARNINGS: The fresh root is too strong for internal use and can be toxic. Only the dried herb should be used. Large doses of the dried herb can cause nausea, vomiting, intestinal pain, and diarrhea. Not for use during pregnancy or lactation.

ENERGETICS: Cooling and drying

PROPERTIES: Bitter, cholagogue, emetic, and lymphatic

SPECIFIC INDICATIONS: Felter: Enlarged, soft, yielding lymphatic tissue. Gastrointestinal irritation, burning in the epigastrium, acid eructations.

SOURCES: Mountain Rose Herbs, Starwest Botanicals

DOSAGE FORMS

STANDARD INFUSION: 1 ounce 2–3 times daily

TINCTURE: Dried root (1:5, 50% alcohol); 1–10 drops 2 times daily

BLUE VERVAIN

Latin name: *Verbena hastata (blue vervain), V. officinalis (vervain)*

Blue vervain can be used internally to relax the nerves and combat anxiety. It is very helpful for nervous exhaustion from long-term stress or fanatical, hard-driving personalities and for people who suffer from neck and shoulder pain who feel like they're tied up in knots. It's helpful for women who get angry and tense just before their period, and for anger in general. It can alleviate some types of headaches, including migraines associated with PMS.

Detail-oriented people who suffer from surface and peripheral nervous system problems and have neuralgias and skin problems may also benefit from blue vervain. It is helpful for many spasmodic nervous disorders, including tics, palsy, and Tourette's syndrome. It can be helpful for mild pain and colds, flu, and respiratory congestion.

WARNINGS: Extremely large doses may cause nausea and vomiting. Large doses may stimulate a miscarriage in pregnant women, although in normal doses blue vervain was used traditionally to protect against miscarriage.

ENERGETICS: Slightly cooling, drying, and relaxing

PROPERTIES: Bitter, diaphoretic, diuretic, expectorant, hypotensive, nervine, and relaxant

SOURCES: Mountain Rose Herbs, Starwest Botanicals, Stony Mountain Botanicals

DOSAGE FORMS

WEAK INFUSION: For nervine properties, 1 cup up to 3 times daily

SOUTHERN DECOCTION: Use leaf or root for a strong lymphatic and diaphoretic remedy, 1 cup as needed.

TINCTURE: Fresh leaf and flowers (1:2, 60% alcohol); dried leaf and flowers (1:5, 40% alcohol); 5–10 drops. If no results are seen, increase to 1–2 ml (0.2–0.4 tsp.) up to 4 times daily.

GLYCERITE: Dried leaf and flowers (1:6); 1–5 ml (0.2–1 tsp.) as needed 3–4 times daily

BONESET

Latin name: *Eupatorium perfoliatum*

Boneset is an aromatic and bitter herb traditionally used for colds, fevers, and flu. Studies show that compounds in boneset stimulate white blood cell action. It is very helpful for flu accompanied by aches in the muscles. Taken as a warm tea, it helps to promote perspiration and acts as an emetic. Taken as a cold tea (a standard infusion that has been left to cool), it acts as a bitter tonic and mild laxative to strengthen and tone the bowels. It helps to relieve vomiting and bloating when combined with mint, and when combined with ginger and anise it aids coughs.

WARNINGS: Use cautiously during pregnancy. Long-term use is not recommended.

ENERGETICS: Cooling, drying, and slightly relaxing

PROPERTIES: Bitter, diaphoretic, and emetic

SPECIFIC INDICATIONS: Felter: Large, full pulse, current showing small waves, skin hot and full, with tendency to moisture. Deep-seated aching in bones with general body aches. Hoarseness, cough, soreness of chest. Urine turbid and high.

SOURCES: Mountain Rose Herbs, Starwest Botanicals

DOSAGE FORMS

STANDARD INFUSION: 4–8 ounces, hot, 3–5 times daily

TINCTURE: Fresh leaf and flowers (1:2, 95% alcohol); dried leaf and flowers (1:5, 35% alcohol); 1–4 ml (0.2–0.8 tsp.) 3 times daily

GLYCERITE: Dried leaf and flowers (1:6); 3–5 ml (0.6–1 tsp.) 3–4 times daily

BORAGE

Latin name: *Borago officinalis*

Borage seed oil is high in GLA, a type of polyunsaturated fatty acid, and is used internally for inflammation, skin conditions, and arthritis. Borage leaf supports adrenal function and lifts sadness and depression. Used as a flower essence, it promotes cheerful courage when facing adversity.

WARNINGS: None for the oil, but the herb itself contains pyrrolizidine alkaloids and should be used with caution. Borage herb is contraindicated in pregnancy.

ENERGETICS: Cooling, moistening, and nourishing

PROPERTIES: Adrenal tonic, anti-inflammatory, antidepressant, decongestant, and expectorant

SOURCES: Mountain Rose Herbs, Starwest Botanicals

DOSAGE FORMS

WEAK INFUSION: 1 cup up to 3 times daily

TINCTURE: Dried leaf and flowers (1:5, 50% alcohol); 6–12 drops 3 times daily

GLYCERITE: Dried leaf and flowers (1:6); 6–12 drops 3 times daily

BORAGE OIL: 3–4 300 mg capsules daily

BOSWELLIA

Latin name: *Boswellia serrata; also called frankincense*

Boswellia resin has been used in traditional Ayurvedic medicine as a remedy for arthritis, pulmonary diseases, ringworm, and diarrhea. The active constituent in boswellia is boswellic acids, which appear to have anti-inflammatory and anti-arthritic actions. Research studies have shown that boswellia may be helpful in treating osteoarthritis, rheumatoid arthritis, bursitis, tendonitis, Crohn's disease, and ulcerative colitis.

WARNINGS: No known warnings

ENERGETICS: Warming and drying

PROPERTIES: Analgesic (anodyne), anti-inflammatory, and expectorant

SOURCES: Mountain Rose Herbs, Stony Mountain Botanicals

DOSAGE FORMS

TINCTURE: Dried resin (1:5, 90% alcohol); 1–4 ml (0.2–0.8 tsp.) 3 times daily

CAPSULE: 400–1,000 mg, 3 times daily. This is one of the times a standardized extract works well. Standardization to 50%–65% boswellic acids is common.

ESSENTIAL OIL: Apply topically as needed.

OTHER: Frankincense tears can be burned on a charcoal disc and inhaled.

BRIGHAM TEA

Latin name: *Ephedra viridis*

Brigham tea is a southwestern herb related to Chinese ephedra (which is now illegal to sell in the United States). It is a milder stimulant and decongestant than its Chinese cousin.

WARNINGS: No known warnings

ENERGETICS: Warming, drying, and slightly constricting

PROPERTIES: Metabolic stimulant

DOSAGE FORMS

STANDARD INFUSION: 1–2 cups daily

TINCTURE: Dried plant (1:5, 50% alcohol); 5 drops to 8 ml (1.6 tsp.) 2–3 times daily

OTHER: Michael Moore says that the dark brown resinous scales that settle into the collection bags or cleaning area are one-third tannin and make an excellent topical hemostatic.

BUCHU

Latin name: *Barosma betulina*

A strong diuretic native to Africa, buchu is used primarily for problems with the urinary tract. It can also be helpful for the prostate.

WARNINGS: Contraindicated with dryness. Not recommended for children under two years of age. Not to be used with acute inflammation of the urinary tract.

ENERGETICS: Warming and drying

PROPERTIES: Antiseptic, carminative, and diuretic

SPECIFIC INDICATIONS: Felter: Acid urine, with constant desire to urinate; vesico-renal irritation, with copious mucus or mucopurulent discharges.

SOURCES: Mountain Rose Herbs, Starwest Botanicals

DOSAGE FORMS

STANDARD INFUSION: 1 cup 3 times daily

TINCTURE: Dried root (1:5, 80% alcohol); 1–2 ml (0.2–0.4 tsp.) up to 3 times daily

CAPSULE: 500–1,000 mg, 3 times daily

BUCKTHORN

Latin name: *Rhamnus frangula*

A bitter laxative with properties similar to those of cascara sagrada but not as harsh, buckthorn is most often used to relieve constipation. Buckthorn bark should be dried for a year before use.

WARNINGS: Not recommended for use during pregnancy or by persons who are weak. Avoid prolonged use.

ENERGETICS: Cooling and drying

PROPERTIES: Anthelminthic, bitter, and stimulant laxative

SOURCES: Frontier Herbs, Mountain Rose Herbs, Starwest Botanicals, Stony Mountain Botanicals

DOSAGE FORMS

STANDARD DECOCTION: 2–8 ounces in the morning or evening. Takes about 12 hours to work.

TINCTURE: Dried bark (1:5, 50% alcohol); 0.5–2 ml (0.1–0.4 tsp.) night and morning

CAPSULES: 500–1,000 mg, at bedtime

BUGLEWEED

Latin name: *Lycopus virginicus*

Bugleweed inhibits peripheral iodine metabolism and helps to reduce an overactive thyroid. It is used with lemon balm and motherwort for Graves' disease. It also influences the lungs and heart and can be beneficial for a rapid or irregular heartbeat, especially when it coincides with sleep difficulties.

WARNINGS: Bugleweed should not be used in cases of underactive thyroid (hypothyroidism). It should not be taken during pregnancy or with excessive menstrual bleeding.

ENERGETICS: Cooling and drying

PROPERTIES: Antithyrotropic and cardiac

SPECIFIC INDICATIONS: Rolla Thomas: Chronic cough with frequent pulse and high range of temperature; hemorrhage with frequent pulse; albuminuria with frequent pulse; Bright's disease.

SOURCES: Mountain Rose Herbs, Starwest Botanicals

DOSAGE FORMS

WEAK INFUSION: 1 cup 3 times daily

TINCTURE: Fresh leaves (1:2, 95% alcohol); dried leaves (1:5, 55% alcohol); 1–2 ml (0.2–0.4 tsp.) up to 3 times daily

CAPSULE: 500–600 mg, 2 times daily

BUPLEURUM

Latin name: *Bupleurum chinense, syn. B. scorzoneraefolium*

A bitter and aromatic Chinese herb, bupleurum is an ingredient in many Chinese formulas for liver, blood, and skin conditions. Bupleurum contains saikosides, which strengthen liver function while protecting the liver from toxins. It has an anti-inflammatory effect and can reduce the risk of liver cancer in people with cirrhosis.

WARNINGS: No known warnings

ENERGETICS: Cooling and drying

PROPERTIES: Alterative (blood purifier), antidepressant, and carminative

SOURCES: Mountain Rose Herbs, Starwest Botanicals

DOSAGE FORMS

STANDARD DECOCTION: 2–4 ounces 2–4 times daily

TINCTURE: Dried bark (1:5, 50% alcohol); 1–2 ml (0.2–0.4 tsp.) up to 3 times daily

GLYCERITE: Dried bark (1:8); 1–5 ml (0.2–1 tsp.) 3 times daily

BURDOCK

Latin name: *Arctium lappa*

Burdock is a bitter herb used for skin conditions and general liver problems. Burdock stimulates bile function and strengthens the liver. It helps with indigestion and clearing up acne and other skin irritations. Burdock leaves may be applied as a poultice to infected sores. A strong decoction of the root can be used in baths for itching. Burdock helps to stabilize mast cells, which reduces allergic reactions.

WARNINGS: No known warnings.

ENERGETICS: Cooling, moistening, and nourishing

PROPERTIES: Alterative (blood purifier), anticancer, bitter, cholagogue, diuretic, hepatic, lymphatic, and mast cell stabilizer

SOURCES: Bulk Herb Store, Frontier Herbs, Mountain Rose Herbs, San Francisco Herb Company, Starwest Botanicals, Stony Mountain Botanicals

DOSAGE FORMS

STANDARD DECOCTION: ½–1 cup 2–3 times daily

TINCTURE: Fresh root or seeds (1:2, 95% alcohol); dried root or seeds (1:5, 50% alcohol); 1–5 ml (0.2–1 tsp.) 3 times daily; roots for chronic issues, seeds for acute

GLYCERITE: Dried root (1:5); 2–10 ml (0.4–2 tsp.) 3 times daily

CAPSULE: 1,000–3,000 mg, 1–2 times daily

BUTCHER'S BROOM

Latin name: *Ruscus aculeatus*

Butcher's broom is a tonic for the vascular system, helping to prevent blood clots and to tone arteries and veins. It is particularly helpful for phlebitis, varicose veins, hemorrhoids, and bruises.

WARNINGS: No known warnings

ENERGETICS: Cooling, drying, and slightly constricting

PROPERTIES: Vascular tonic

SOURCES: Bulk Herb Store, Mountain Rose Herbs, Starwest Botanicals, Stony Mountain Botanicals

DOSAGE FORMS

STANDARD DECOCTION: 2–4 ounces up to 3 times daily

TINCTURE: Dried herb (1:5, 60% alcohol); 1 ml (0.2 tsp.) 1–3 times daily

CAPSULE: 300–1,000 mg up to 3 times daily

TOPICAL USE: Apply as a fomentation or compress.

BUTTERBUR ROOT

Latin name: *Petasites hybridus*

This herb was tested on hay fever (allergic rhinitis) symptoms and found to be as effective as many OTC and prescription drugs. Butterbur has also been shown to reduce the frequency, intensity, and duration of migraines. It is a useful remedy for cramps and asthma.

WARNINGS: The plant contains pyrrolizidine alkaloids, which can be toxic to the liver. Some commercial extracts claim to remove the PAs, but the jury is still out. To be safe, limit use to 6 weeks a year.

ENERGETICS: Cooling and drying

PROPERTIES: Analgesic (anodyne), anti-allergenic, antitussive, and expectorant

SOURCES: Mountain Rose Herbs, Starwest Botanicals

DOSAGE FORMS

There is no commercially available source of bulk butterbur that is PA-free. Until there is, we recommend you stick to the standardized PA-free products.

CAPSULE: 1–2 50 mg capsules standardized to 7.5 mg petasin up to 2 times daily

BUTTERNUT BARK

Latin name: *Juglans cinerea*

Butternut bark is a laxative and mild alternative to cascara sagrada and buckthorn. As with cascara and buckthorn, the bark should be dried for a year before use. The laxative effects are dependent on gut bacteria and take effect 6–8 hours after ingestion. A dose in the evening normally produces defecation upon arising in the morning. The unripe nut is used to kill intestinal worms.

WARNINGS: Avoid using during pregnancy and lactation.

ENERGETICS: Cooling and drying

PROPERTIES: Bitter, stimulant laxative, and vermifuge

SPECIFIC INDICATIONS: Rolla Thomas: In large doses it is an excellent laxative; in small doses it relieves irritation of the stomach and intestines, and promotes digestion. It may be thought of as a remedy in chronic eczema.

SOURCES: Starwest Botanicals

DOSAGE FORMS

STANDARD DECOCTION: 1–4 ounces 3 times daily

TINCTURE: Dried bark (1:5, 40% alcohol); 5 drops to 1 ml (0.2 tsp.) 1–3 times daily

GLYCERITE: Dried bark (1:8, 60% glycerin); 2–5 ml (0.4–1 tsp.) up to 3 times daily

CALENDULA

Latin name: *Calendula officinalis*

Calendula is commonly used topically to speed tissue healing after injuries, burns, and bruises. It is a useful remedy for dry skin, eczema, and hemorrhoids and can ease pain in minor injuries when applied topically. Calendula is a wonderful remedy for gastrointestinal inflammation and is almost a specific for Crohn's disease, colitis, and gastritis.

WARNINGS: Internal use is contraindicated in pregnancy. Topical use is completely safe.

ENERGETICS: Cooling, drying, and constricting

PROPERTIES: Astringent and vulnerary

SPECIFIC INDICATIONS: Rolla Thomas: In enfeebled conditions of the capillary blood vessels. An excellent application to ulcers and wounds.

SOURCES: Bulk Herb Store, Frontier Herbs, Mountain Rose Herbs, San Francisco Herb Company, Starwest Botanicals, Stony Mountain Botanicals

DOSAGE FORMS

STANDARD INFUSION: 4–8 ounces up to 3 times daily, or use as a compress as needed.

TINCTURE: Fresh plant (1:2, 95% alcohol); dried plant (1:5, 70% alcohol); 1–3 ml (0.2–0.6 tsp.) up to 3 times daily

GLYCERITE: Dried plant (1:8); 5–10 ml (1–2 tsp.) up to 3 times daily

TOPICAL USE: Apply tincture, oil, salve, or liniment as needed.

CALIFORNIA POPPY

Latin name: *Eschscholzia californica*

California poppy is in the same family as the opium poppy and has mild sedative and analgesic properties, but is not narcotic. It helps to normalize nervous system function to ease nervous tension, anxiety, insomnia, and pain (internal and external). It has an affinity for GABA receptors in the brain, calming the mind without depressing the central nervous system.

WARNINGS: Not for use during pregnancy except under the supervision of a professional

ENERGETICS: Cooling and relaxing

PROPERTIES: Analgesic (anodyne), sedative, and soporific (hypnotic)

SOURCES: Mountain Rose Herbs, San Francisco Herb Company, Starwest Botanicals, Stony Mountain Botanicals

DOSAGE FORMS

STANDARD INFUSION: 2–4 ounces at night to promote restful sleep

TINCTURE: Fresh plant (1:2, 95% alcohol); dried plant (1:5, 60% alcohol); 0.5–2 ml (0.1–0.4 tsp.) in 2 ounces of water or chamomile tea as needed

CAMPHOR

Latin name: *Cinnamomum camphora*

Camphor is a local anesthetic, numbing the nerve endings where it is applied. It helps open congested air passages when inhaled. Camphor is toxic internally; internal use should be reserved for professionals only.

WARNINGS: Use only as part of a topical analgesic formula. Don't use topically in children under two years of age or in pregnancy. The herb itself is for professional use only.

ENERGETICS: Warming and relaxing

PROPERTIES: Anti-inflammatory, antiseptic, antispasmodic, and expectorant

DOSAGE FORMS

TINCTURE: Dried leaf (1:10, 95% alcohol); 1–10 drops in simple syrup no more than 2 times daily

TOPICAL USE: Apply tincture or liniment as needed.

ESSENTIAL OIL: Put 5 drops in a pot of water, bring to a low simmer, and inhale the steam.

CAPSICUM (CAYENNE)

Latin name: *Capsicum frutescens or C. annuum*

Capsicum is a major stimulant for the circulatory system. It increases circulation to every area of the body it comes in contact with, internally or externally.

Capsicum also strengthens the heartbeat. Capsicum is useful for shock, heart attack, and trauma. Because adequate blood supply is necessary for all tissues to heal, capsicum has earned a reputation in the West as a kind of cure-all. It is analgesic: the capsaicin in capsicum depletes substance P and thereby partially blocks pain receptors. A small part of capsicum is commonly added to formulas made in the Thomsonian and Physiomedicalism systems as an accelerant.

WARNINGS: Due to its irritating nature, some people have a hard time taking capsicum. Large doses can be irritating to the stomach and cause painful bowel eliminations. Although capsicum stops bleeding and has been used to heal ulcers, this herb can cause pain when used for these purposes; hence, it should be used with caution. It is best to start with extremely small doses to build up tolerance. When applied locally, capsicum causes burning sensations in sensitive areas such as genitals, sinuses, and eyes. It is not recommended for people with hemorrhoids or anal fissures. Topical use may exacerbate coughs caused by ACE inhibitors.

ENERGETICS: Warming and drying

PROPERTIES: Analgesic (anodyne), carminative, counterirritant, diaphoretic, hemostatic, circulatory stimulant, and styptic

SPECIFIC INDICATIONS: Felter: Marked depression with feeble pulse and scanty secretions. Tongue dry and harsh, salivary secretions suppressed.

SOURCES: Bulk Herb Store, Mountain Rose Herbs, San Francisco Herb Company, Starwest Botanicals, Stony Mountain Botanicals

DOSAGE FORMS

TINCTURE: Fresh fruit (1:2, 95% alcohol); dried fruit (1:5, 60% alcohol); 5 drops to 1 ml (0.2 tsp.) in water, or, as a less irritating alternative, milk or coconut milk

GLYCERITE: Dried fruit (1:5); 1–5 drops diluted in water or alternative

CAPSULE AND POWDER: 500–1,500 mg up to 3 times daily, preferably with food to buffer the irritating effects

TOPICAL USE: Apply tincture, oil, salve, or liniment as needed.

CARDAMOM

Latin name: *Eletteria cardamomum*

An aromatic spice, cardamom acts as a carminative and digestive aid. It has a reputation as an aphrodisiac and has been used in India for respiratory and kidney ailments. It can add a nice flavor to formulas.

WARNINGS: No known warnings

ENERGETICS: Warming and slightly drying

PROPERTIES: Aromatic and carminative

SOURCES: Bulk Herb Store, Mountain Rose Herbs, San Francisco Herb Company, Stony Mountain Botanicals

DOSAGE FORMS

DRIED SEED: Chew a few seeds as needed.

STANDARD INFUSION: 1 cup of the crushed seed tea 3 times daily

TINCTURE: Dried seeds (1:5, 50% alcohol); 10 drops to 3 ml (0.6 tsp.) up to 3 times daily

CASCARA SAGRADA

Latin name: *Rhamnus purshiana*

A bitter purgative, cascara sagrada increases bile flow and stimulates peristalsis of the colon. The name cascara sagrada means holy or sacred bark. It is known for its effectiveness in relieving constipation and for colon cleansing. The bark should be dried for 1 year before use. The correct dose is the smallest dose necessary to create soft stool.

WARNINGS: Not recommended for use during pregnancy or in those with inflammatory bowel disorders, abdominal pain, or obstruction. Avoid prolonged use. If a person appears dependent on this or other stimulant laxatives or if cramps or griping become a problem, use nervines for the dependency and bowel spasms, and use magnesium to counteract spasms. In case of diarrhea caused by excessive use, use charcoal or mucilaginous herbs. Long-term use will darken the tissue color of the bowel and create laxative dependency. Triphala is helpful for people who have become dependent on laxatives.

ENERGETICS: Cooling and drying

PROPERTIES: Bitter, cholagogue, stimulant laxative, and purgative (cathartic)

SPECIFIC INDICATIONS: Felter: Constipation due to neglect, or to nervous or muscular atony of the bowels.

SOURCES: Frontier Herbs, Mountain Rose Herbs, San Francisco Herb Company, Starwest Botanicals, Stony Mountain Botanicals

DOSAGE FORMS

STANDARD DECOCTION: 2–4 ounces at bedtime, but the taste is very unpleasant.

TINCTURE: Aged dried bark (1:5, 40% alcohol); 1–2 ml (0.2–0.4 tsp.) in a little water just before bedtime

CAPSULE: 500–1,000 mg, morning and/or evening

CAT'S CLAW (UÑA DE GATO, GAMBIER)

Latin name: *Uncaria tomentosa*

Cat's claw is one of the very best remedies for normalizing the function of the gastrointestinal tract. It is often helpful for ulcers, gastritis, Crohn's disease, and irritable bowel syndrome. Aside from inflammation of the bowel and intestines, it can also address inflammation of the joints and muscles. Cat's claw has a broad-spectrum mild antimicrobial action and also balances immune function. Cat's claw seems to have antiviral and antimutagenic properties, making it a good complementary treatment for a variety of degenerative diseases and helping to strengthen the immune system against the effects of chemotherapy.

WARNINGS: Avoid during pregnancy and while trying to get pregnant.

ENERGETICS: Cooling and slightly constricting

PROPERTIES: Anti-inflammatory, antimicrobial, antimutagenic, and antioxidant

SOURCES: Bulk Herb Store, Frontier Herbs, Mountain Rose Herbs, Starwest Botanicals, Stony Mountain Botanicals

DOSAGE FORMS

STANDARD DECOCTION: 6–12 ounces 3 times daily

TINCTURE: Dried bark (1:5, 60% alcohol); 3–5 ml (0.6–1 tsp.) up to 3 times daily

CAPSULE OR POWDER: 2,000–7,000 mg, 3 times daily

CATNIP

Latin name: *Nepeta cataria*

A mild aromatic herb that is soothing and settling to the stomach and nerves, catnip is helpful for colds, chills, congestion, sore throats, and indigestion. It is excellent for colic in infants when combined with fennel. It helps produce perspiration without increasing body heat. Catnip can also be used for nervousness or stress and at bedtime as a sleep aid. It is one of the best remedies for stress-induced IBS. The fresh leaf tincture is a strong gastrointestinal antispasmodic, but the dried leaf loses most of this property.

WARNINGS: Excellent herb for children and babies and generally mild and extremely safe, but in extremely large doses it can cause vomiting. Avoid during pregnancy.

ENERGETICS: Cooling and drying

PROPERTIES: Aromatic, carminative, diaphoretic, nervine, and sedative

SPECIFIC INDICATIONS: Rolla Thomas: Pain in abdomen, flexing of the thighs upon the abdomen, writhing of the patient, persistent crying.

SOURCES: Bulk Herb Store, Frontier Herbs, Mountain Rose Herbs, San Francisco Herb Company, Stony Mountain Botanicals

DOSAGE FORMS

STANDARD INFUSION: 2–6 ounces up to 3 times daily

TINCTURE: Fresh leaf (1:2, 95% alcohol); dried leaf (1:5, 50% alcohol); 1–5 ml (0.4–1 tsp.) up to 3 times daily

GLYCERITE: Fresh leaf (1:5, 90% glycerin sealed simmer method; puree leaf and glycerin in blender before extracting); dried leaf (1:8), 1–2 tsp. up to 3 times daily

CELANDINE

Latin name: *Ranunculus ficaria*

A bitter herb with a strong affinity for the liver and gallbladder, celandine is usually used in combination with other herbs to stimulate bile flow. The juice of celandine has traditionally been used for warts, corns, and ringworm.

WARNINGS: Contraindicated with liver disease, emaciation, or weak digestion. Not for long-term use. Not for use during pregnancy or while breastfeeding.

ENERGETICS: Cooling and drying

PROPERTIES: Bitter and cholagogue

SPECIFIC INDICATIONS: Felter: Full, pale, sallow tongue and membranes; skin sallow, sometimes greenish. Hepatic congestion with light, pasty stools; fullness in right hypochondrium, with tensive throbbing to the right shoulder.

SOURCES: Mountain Rose Herbs, Starwest Botanicals

DOSAGE FORMS

STANDARD DECOCTION: 4 ounces 3 times daily

TINCTURE: Fresh leaf (1:2, 95% alcohol); dried leaf (1:5, 50% alcohol); 10 drops to 2 ml (0.4 tsp.) up to 3 times daily

CELERY SEED

Latin name: *Apium graveolens*

The seeds of celery are used for treating rheumatic conditions and gout. They help the kidneys dispose of urine and other unwanted waste products. They are useful in arthritis, helping to detoxify the body and improve the circulation of blood to muscles and joints. Celery seeds are effective in treating cystitis; they help disinfect the bladder and urinary tubules. Celery stalks are good medicine for urinary problems and for rheumatism and gout.

WARNINGS: Avoid if there is a history of kidney inflammation. Use cautiously during pregnancy and while lactating.

ENERGETICS: Warming and drying

PROPERTIES: Antirheumatic and diuretic

SOURCES: Mountain Rose Herbs, San Francisco Herb Company, Stony Mountain Botanicals

DOSAGE FORMS

STANDARD INFUSION: 4–8 ounces up to 3 times daily (seeds)

TINCTURE: Dried seeds (1:5, 50% alcohol, 10% glycerin); 10 drops to 2 ml (0.4 tsp.) up to 3 times daily

GLYCERITE: Dried seeds (1:5); 1–5 ml (0.2–1 tsp.) up to 3 times daily

CAPSULE: 500–1,500 mg up to 3 times daily

CHAMOMILE (ENGLISH AND ROMAN)

Latin name: *Chamomilla recutita, Matricaria recutita*

Chamomile is a mild sedative and a good gastric anti-inflammatory. It calms the nerves, settles the stomach, and helps to expel gas. This is an excellent nervine agent, especially for children. Use it homeopathically or make it into a tea and sweeten for colic, hyperactivity, teething, fussiness, fever, or irritability in infants and children.

Chamomile is useful for colds and flu in children when combined with elder flower, peppermint, and yarrow. (It contains an anti-inflammatory volatile oil similar to the oil in yarrow.) Use it in combination with other nervines and anti-inflammatory agents for pain, swelling, and infection. It can be applied topically for inflammation.

WARNINGS: Allergic reactions to chamomile are not common, but are more common than with many other herbs.

ENERGETICS: Cooling and relaxing

PROPERTIES: Antispasmodic, aromatic, carminative, diaphoretic, digestive tonic, and nervine

SPECIFIC INDICATIONS: Matthew Wood: Whiny, fussy babies of any age.

SOURCES: Bulk Herb Store, Frontier Herbs, Mountain Rose Herbs, San Francisco Herb Company, Starwest Botanicals, Stony Mountain Botanicals

DOSAGE FORMS

COLD INFUSION: 2–8 ounces up to 3 times daily

TINCTURE: Dried flowers (1:2, 55% alcohol); 1–5 ml (0.2–1 tsp.) 1–4 times daily

GLYCERITE: Dried flowers (1:6); 1–5 ml (0.2–1 tsp.) 1–4 times daily

CHAPARRAL

Latin name: *Larrea tridentata*

A very bitter, acrid herb, chaparral has long been used as a cancer remedy and blood purifier. It contains an antioxidant substance known as NDGA. Chaparral cleanses and tones the liver, blood, and lymphatics, making it useful for parasites, bacterial infection, viruses, heavy metal toxicity, drug withdrawal, and radiation.

WARNINGS: Potentially hepatotoxic, although the evidence is circumstantial and may be due to taking the plant in capsules instead of its traditional form as a tea. Nevertheless, it is contraindicated in kidney disease, liver disease, and when pregnant. It has a strong action on the kidneys and should be taken with ample amounts of water to protect the kidneys.

ENERGETICS: Cooling and drying

PROPERTIES: Alterative (blood purifier), anthelminthic, antibacterial, anticancer, antioxidant, antiparasitic, antiseptic, and bitter

SOURCES: Frontier Herbs, Mountain Rose Herbs, San Francisco Herb Company, Starwest Botanicals, Stony Mountain Botanicals

DOSAGE FORMS

STANDARD DECOCTION: 2–4 ounces internally (if you can manage the taste)

TINCTURE: Dried leaf (1:5, 75% alcohol); 1–2 ml (0.2–0.4 tsp.) up to 3 times daily

OIL AND SALVE: Can be extracted in oil (1:8) to make an oil or salve for topical use

TOPICAL USE: Apply a compress of the decoction or the tincture, oil, salve, or liniment as needed.

CHASTETREE (VITEX)

Latin name: *Vitex agnus-castus*

Chastetree helps to regulate female hormones, making it useful for PMS and menopause. It is a good remedy to balance reproductive hormones in teenagers and adults. It is generally a better remedy for women than men because it inhibits androgens (male sex hormones). It may take 3–6 months of use to see optimal results.

WARNINGS: Chastetree might reduce the effectiveness of hormonal birth control.

ENERGETICS: Warming and drying

PROPERTIES: Hormonal balancing, anaphrodisiac

SOURCES: Bulk Herb Store, Frontier Herbs, Mountain Rose Herbs, Starwest Botanicals, Stony Mountain Botanicals

DOSAGE FORMS

TINCTURE: Dried berries (1:5, 45% alcohol); 1–3 ml (0.2–0.6 tsp.) 3 times daily

CAPSULE OR POWDER: 1,000–2,000 mg, 3 times daily

CHICKWEED

Latin name: *Stellaria media*

Chickweed is a mucilaginous herb thought to break down fats and fatty tumors in the body. It acts as a mild appetite suppressant and weight loss aid when taken 1 hour before mealtimes. It can be used in poultices for skin irritations, and the tea can be used as an eyewash for soothing irritated eyes. Applied topically, it is helpful for relieving itchy skin.

WARNINGS: No known warnings

ENERGETICS: Cooling and balancing

PROPERTIES: Demulcent (mucilant), emollient, and nutritive

SOURCES: Frontier Herbs, Mountain Rose Herbs, San Francisco Herb Company, Stony Mountain Botanicals

DOSAGE FORMS

STANDARD INFUSION: 6–12 ounces up to 3 times daily

TINCTURE: Fresh leaf (1:2, 95% alcohol); recently dried leaf (1:5, 50% alcohol); 2–5 ml (0.4–1 tsp.) as needed

CAPSULE OR POWDER: 1,000–2,000 mg, 2–3 times daily

TOPICAL USE: Apply a compress, oil, or salve as needed.

CILANTRO (CORIANDER)

Latin name: *Coriandrum sativum*

A widely popular culinary herb, cilantro is used by herbalists to detoxify the body. Dr. Yoshiaki Omura, director of medical research at the Heart Disease Research Foundation in New York, did early research that suggested cilantro could reduce heavy metals when taken 4 times daily for 2 weeks. Later studies showed no increase in lead excretion in children taking cilantro. More studies should be done. Until they are, cilantro shouldn't be counted on to reduce heavy metals in the body. Coriander seeds come from the cilantro plant and are used as a carminative and digestive aid.

WARNINGS: No known warnings

ENERGETICS: Cooling and drying

PROPERTIES: Carminative, chelating, and condiment

SOURCES: Mountain Rose Herbs, San Francisco Herb Company

DOSAGE FORMS

STANDARD INFUSION: 2–8 ounces up to 3 times daily

TINCTURE: Fresh leaf (1:2, 95% alcohol); dried leaf (1:5, 50% alcohol); 10 drops to 3 ml (0.6 tsp.) up to 3 times daily

GLYCERITE: Dried seeds (1:5, sealed simmer method); 1–5 ml (0.2–1 tsp.) up to 3 times daily

CINNAMON

Latin name: *Cinnamomum verum, syn. C. zeylanicum*

Cinnamon is a spicy aromatic herb used in traditional Chinese medicine as a warming stimulant. It is useful as a digestive and circulatory stimulant. Modern research has shown that cinnamon increases the capability of beta cells in the pancreas to produce insulin, reducing blood glucose levels in diabetics. Cinnamon also has astringent properties and can help control heavy menstrual flows and postpartum bleeding. Cinnamon is a strong antimicrobial and is helpful for certain types of dysbiosis. Cinnamon essential oil (Cassia variety) has powerful antibacterial and antifungal properties.

WARNINGS: Large amounts of cinnamon oil ingested internally can cause kidney damage or coma. Cinnamon oil and bark are not recommended during pregnancy except as a seasoning in food. It is a good idea to avoid cinnamon while breastfeeding. Taking more than 2 grams of cinnamon bark daily can cause gastrointestinal irritation.

ENERGETICS: Warming, drying, and constricting

PROPERTIES: Antidiabetic, antiseptic, aromatic, astringent, and carminative

SPECIFIC INDICATIONS: Felter: Passive hemorrhage. Gastric irritation with flatulence.

SOURCES: Bulk Herb Store, Mountain Rose Herbs, San Francisco Herb Company

DOSAGE FORMS

TEA: Compound Cinnamon Tea: ¼ tsp. ground ginger, ¼ tsp. ground cinnamon, and 1 tsp. lemon juice in 8 ounces hot water; 4–8 ounces up to 3 times daily

TINCTURE: Dried bark (1:5, 60% alcohol, 5% glycerin); 30–60 drops up to 3 times daily

GLYCERITE: Dried bark (1:5, sealed simmer method); 3–10 drops up to 3 times daily

CAPSULE OR POWDER: 500–2,000 mg up to 3 times daily. Mix powder with food; do not try to take it straight.

SPIRIT OF CINNAMON: 10 ml of essential oil in 100 ml of 40% alcohol; 1 tsp. in 4 ounces of sweetened water every 5, 10, or 30 minutes for postpartum hemorrhage. Don't use at this dosage for more than a day.

ESSENTIAL OIL: Avoid internal use, as cinnamon essential oil is very irritating. For topical use, dilute 1 drop in 50–60 drops of fixed vegetable oil. Test on a small patch of skin before applying.

CLEAVERS (BEDSTRAW)

Latin name: *Galium aparine*

Cleavers, also known as bedstraw, is used to promote urination and to stimulate the lymphatic system. It can be used externally as a poultice for skin inflammation and swollen lymph nodes.

WARNINGS: No known warnings

ENERGETICS: Cooling and drying

PROPERTIES: Diuretic, kidney tonic, and lymphatic

SOURCES: Frontier Herbs, Mountain Rose Herbs, Starwest Botanicals

DOSAGE FORMS

FRESH PLANT JUICE: 2–5 ml up to 3 times daily

STANDARD INFUSION: 4–8 ounces up to 3 times daily

TINCTURE: Fresh herb (1:2, 95% alcohol); 5–10 ml (1–2 tsp.) 3 times daily

CLOVE

Latin name: *Eugenia caryophyllata, syn. Syzygium aromaticum*

A spicy aromatic often used in combination with other herbs, cloves are valuable in liniments, gargles, and digestive formulas. Powdered cloves have been used to expel parasites. Clove essential oil applied topically has a numbing effect on the nerves. It can be mixed with olive oil and applied to the gums for teething babies or toothache.

WARNINGS: Clove can be irritating in large quantities. Clove oil should not be used internally without professional supervision. Use caution in pregnancy. Dilute essential oil for topical use.

ENERGETICS: Warming and drying

PROPERTIES: Analgesic (anodyne), antiseptic, aromatic, carminative, counterirritant, circulatory stimulant, and vermifuge

SOURCES: Bulk Herb Store, Mountain Rose Herbs, San Francisco Herb Company, Stony Mountain Botanicals

DOSAGE FORMS

STANDARD INFUSION: 1 ounce up to 3 times daily

TINCTURE: Dried buds (1:5, 50% alcohol, 10% glycerin); 5–25 drops up to 3 times daily

GLYCERITE: Dried buds (1:5, sealed simmer method); 2–10 drops up to 3 times daily

TOPICAL USE: Apply diluted essential oil (1:20) as needed

CODONOPSIS

Latin name: *Codonopsis pilosula*

Codonopsis is used in place of ginseng as a milder and safer general tonic for both men and women. It balances adrenal cortex activity (balancing cortisol) and improves immune function. It is used in Fu Zheng therapies to prevent side effects from chemotherapy or radiation, and it increases hemoglobin levels and red blood cells. Codonopsis stimulates appetite and strengthens the immune system.

WARNINGS: No known warnings

ENERGETICS: Neutral, moistening, and nourishing

PROPERTIES: Adaptogen, lung tonic, and tonic

SOURCES: Mountain Rose Herbs

DOSAGE FORMS

STANDARD DECOCTION: 4–12 ounces up to 3 times daily

CAPSULE OR POWDER: 1,000–3,000 mg, 2–3 times daily

BULK HERB: Commonly cooked in broth with medicinal mushrooms and astragalus

COLLINSONIA (STONEROOT)

Latin name: *Collinsonia canadensis*

Collinsonia is an excellent astringent for rectal problems such as anal fistulas and hemorrhoids. It can be taken orally and applied topically. It is also used for sore throats and laryngitis, being a specific remedy for speakers and singers who develop throat irritation. It can be used topically for poison oak and ivy and for injuries.

WARNINGS: No known warnings

ENERGETICS: Cooling and constricting

PROPERTIES: Astringent and vascular tonic

SPECIFIC INDICATIONS: Felter: Atony of venous circulation, irritation and constriction of mucous membrane of larynx, hoarseness. Gastrointestinal irritation with sluggish portal circulation. Rolla Thomas: In chronic laryngeal irritation or inflammation, with sense of tickling in larynx, and cough arising from use of the voice.

SOURCES: Starwest Botanicals

DOSAGE FORMS

STANDARD DECOCTION: 1–4 ounces up to 3 times daily

TINCTURE: Fresh leaf (1:2, 95% alcohol); dried leaf (1:5, 60% alcohol; not as effective); 1–2 ml (0.2–0.4 tsp.) up to 3 times daily

COLTSFOOT

Latin name: *Tussilago farfara*

Coltsfoot is a great remedy for debilitated individuals with chronic respiratory conditions. It is indicated for asthma and emphysema; the active constituents can decrease the time for bronchial cilia to recover after damage from smoking. Extracts of the plant have been shown to increase immune resistance and act as a natural antihistamine.

WARNINGS: Not for use during pregnancy and lactation. Contains pyrrolizidine alkaloids; may be toxic in higher doses. Use only as directed and for no longer than 6 weeks a year.

ENERGETICS: Cooling and moistening

PROPERTIES: Antitussive and expectorant

SOURCES: Frontier Herbs, Mountain Rose Herbs, Starwest Botanicals

DOSAGE FORMS

STANDARD INFUSION: 4 ounces up to 3 times daily

COMFREY

Latin name: *Symphytum officinale*

Comfrey is a mucilaginous herb with a slight astringent quality. It has been used for generations to aid in the healing of injuries. Not only does it contain important minerals needed in the healing process, but it also contains allantoin, a substance that stimulates cell growth. Comfrey is primarily used externally in compresses, poultices, and salves. It has been used internally, but most herbalists no longer use it this way because of concerns about hepatic toxicity.

WARNINGS: Completely safe for topical use. It contains pyrrolizidine alkaloids, which are believed to cause liver problems when taken internally. Many people have used comfrey internally with no reported ill effects, and it is probably safe to use internally for short periods. It should be avoided during pregnancy, lactation, when cancer or tumors are present, or when there is a history of liver problems.

ENERGETICS: Cooling, moistening, and slightly constricting

PROPERTIES: Emollient and vulnerary

SOURCES: Bulk Herb Store, Frontier Herbs, Mountain Rose Herbs, San Francisco Herb Company, Starwest Botanicals

DOSAGE FORMS

STANDARD INFUSION: 4–8 ounces up to 3 times daily for no more than 6 weeks a year. We recommend the internal use of comfrey only for broken bones that don't seem to be healing together naturally or with the assistance of safer herbs.

TOPICAL USE: Apply fresh or dried leaf as a poultice; a standard infusion as a compress or soak; or the oil or salve as needed

CORDYCEPS

Latin name: *Cordyceps sinensis, C. militaris*

Cordyceps entered Western medicine after the Chinese government demonstrated its efficacy at the 2008 Olympic games in Beijing, where the Chinese athletes set new world records in nearly every competition they entered. The spectacular performance of the athletes stimulated a burst of pharmacological and clinical research into its health benefits. Cordyceps is an adaptogen and general health tonic. It benefits the lungs, kidneys, adrenal glands, and cardiovascular system. Wildcrafted cordyceps is very difficult to find; when available, be sure it has been tested for heavy metals. Cultured Cs-4 strain powder works well and is easier to find.

WARNINGS: No known warnings

ENERGETICS: Balancing and slightly warming

PROPERTIES: Adaptogen, anti-inflammatory, anticancer, anticholesteremic, antioxidant, immune amphoteric, and tonic

SOURCES: Mountain Rose Herbs

DOSAGE FORMS

POWDER: 5–10 grams daily

TINCTURE: Dried mushrooms (1:4, 25% alcohol); 2–4 ml (0.4–0.8 tsp.) 3 times daily

CAPSULE OR POWDER: 1,000–2,000 mg, 2–3 times daily

CORN SILK

Latin name: *Zea mays*

A mild and soothing diuretic agent, corn silk is useful for kidney inflammation and relieving discomfort associated with urinary tract conditions such as inflamed bladder and painful urination.

WARNINGS: No known warnings

ENERGETICS: Cooling and slightly drying

PROPERTIES: Demulcent (mucilant), diuretic, and soothing

SOURCES: Bulk Herb Store, Frontier Herbs, Starwest Botanicals

DOSAGE FORMS

STANDARD INFUSION: 4–6 ounces up to 3 times daily

TINCTURE: Fresh corn silk (1:2, 95% alcohol); dried corn silk (1:5, 25% alcohol); 3–5 ml (0.6–1 tsp.) in water up to 3 times daily

CAPSULE: 1,000–3,000 mg up to 3 times daily

CORYDALIS

Latin name: *Corydalis yanhusuo*

Corydalis is a natural pain reliever. It contains an alkaloid called THP that acts similarly to opium poppy but is much milder. It is a central nervous system depressant and appropriate for pain from any cause. It has traditionally been used for pain associated with rheumatism, arthritis, or menstruation. It can also be used as an aid for sleep and anxiety.

WARNINGS: Not for use during pregnancy

ENERGETICS: Warming and relaxing

PROPERTIES: Analgesic (anodyne), sedative, and soporific (hypnotic)

DOSAGE FORMS

STANDARD DECOCTION: Tastes vile, but is effective. 3–8 ounces as needed

TINCTURE: Dried rhizome (1:3, 50% alcohol); 1–5 ml (0.2–1 tsp.) as needed

STANDARDIZED EXTRACT: THP 100–200 mg daily

CAPSULE OR POWDER: A tea powder concentrate works best; 1,000–2,000 mg, 2–3 times daily

COTTON ROOT

Latin name: *Gossypium herbaceum*

Cotton root is used for menstrual cramping with scanty bleeding. It can also be used to induce labor and to aid contractions during labor.

WARNINGS: Avoid during pregnancy, as the plant is an abortifacient that causes uterine contractions.

ENERGETICS: Warming and moistening

PROPERTIES: Abortifacient and emmenagogue

SPECIFIC INDICATIONS: Felter: Tardy menstruation with backache and dragging pelvic pain; fullness and weight in the bladder, with difficult micturition; sexual lassitude with anemia; hysteria, with pelvic atony and anemia.

DOSAGE FORMS

TINCTURE: Freshly dried root (1:4, 50% alcohol); 2–4 ml (0.4–0.8 tsp.) 1–3 times daily

STANDARD DECOCTION: 1–2 ounces 3 times daily

CRAMP BARK

Latin name: *Viburnum opulus*

As its name implies, cramp bark is used to relax muscle spasms. It is commonly used for women as a uterine tonic, because it both relaxes and tones the uterus. It has been used to ease menstrual cramps and prevent miscarriage, but may also be helpful for angina, backache, and other problems involving tension.

WARNINGS: Don't take with low blood pressure.

ENERGETICS: Relaxing

PROPERTIES: Anti-abortive and antispasmodic

SOURCES: Frontier Herbs, Mountain Rose Herbs, Starwest Botanicals, Stony Mountain Botanicals

DOSAGE FORMS

STANDARD DECOCTION: 3–4 ounces 3 times daily

TINCTURE: Dried bark (1:5, 50% alcohol); 1–5 ml (0.2–1 tsp.) 1–4 times daily

CRANBERRY

Latin name: *Vaccinium macrocarpon*

Cranberries contain antioxidants that mitigate the damaging effects of free radicals in the body. They also contain two compounds that prevent the adherence of E. coli to the bladder: mannose and proanthocyanidins. Cranberries are an effective preventative for urinary tract infections, and they also help treat H. pylori and gastric E. coli infections. They are high in vitamin C and have been used to prevent scurvy in sailors. Commercially prepared cranberry juice can be used; it works better if it has no added sugar.

WARNINGS: No known warnings

ENERGETICS: Cooling and slightly drying

PROPERTIES: Antibacterial, antioxidant, and nutritive

SOURCES: Mountain Rose Herbs

DOSAGE FORMS

FRESH: Whole cranberries. Eat 1.5 ounces daily.

JUICE: 3–8 ounces daily of unsweetened juice

CAPSULE OR POWDER: 1,000–3,000 mg, 2–3 times daily

CULVER'S ROOT

Latin name: *Leptandra virginica*

A bitter tonic used to cleanse the liver and colon, Culver's root is a strong cholagogue (an agent that stimulates bile flow). It is best used for short periods or in combination with other herbs.

WARNINGS: Contraindicated with emaciation, weak digestion, and pregnancy. High doses can cause diarrhea, vomiting, abdominal pain, vertigo, and other undesirable effects.

ENERGETICS: Slightly cooling and drying

PROPERTIES: Bitter and cholagogue

DOSAGE FORMS

TINCTURE: Dried root (1:5, 65% alcohol); 10–30 drops 3 times daily

DAMIANA

Latin name: *Turnera diffusa, syn. T. diffusa var. aphrodisiaca*

Damiana is most commonly used to increase libido, but it is really a tonic for stress and low energy; in other words, it works best when low sex drive is due to fatigue and stress. It also has antidepressant effects.

WARNINGS: Safe herb, but should avoid during pregnancy.

ENERGETICS: Warming

PROPERTIES: Antidepressant, aphrodisiac, nervine, and metabolic stimulant

SOURCES: Frontier Herbs, Mountain Rose Herbs, San Francisco Herb Company, Starwest Botanicals, Stony Mountain Botanicals

DOSAGE FORMS

WEAK INFUSION: 1 cup up to 3 times daily

TINCTURE: Fresh leaf (1:2, 95% alcohol); dried leaf (1:5, 60% alcohol); 1–2 ml (0.2–0.4 tsp.) up to 4 times daily

GLYCERITE: Dried leaf (1:6); 1–3 ml (0.2–0.6 tsp.) up to 4 times daily

CAPSULE OR POWDER: 1,000–2,000 mg, 2–3 times daily

DANDELION

Latin name: *Taraxacum officinale*

This common lawn and garden weed has a beneficial effect on the digestive system, the urinary system, and the pancreas. The root is primarily used to stimulate bile flow and aid the liver, whereas the leaf is more often employed as a diuretic to aid kidney function. It acts on the microflora of the gut and helps stimulate digestive secretions. Dandelion leaf is often combined in equal parts with nettle leaf as a potassium-sparing diuretic. Dandelion flower wine makes a nice digestive tonic.

WARNINGS: No known warnings

ENERGETICS: Cooling and drying

PROPERTIES: Alterative (blood purifier), bitter, cholagogue, digestive tonic, diuretic, hepatoprotective

SOURCES: Bulk Herb Store, Frontier Herbs, Mountain Rose Herbs, San Francisco Herb Company, Starwest Botanicals, Stony Mountain Botanicals

DOSAGE FORMS

FRESH: Eat young spring leaves raw.

STANDARD INFUSION: Leaf: 4–8 ounces 3 times daily

STANDARD DECOCTION: Root: 2–4 ounces 3 times daily

TINCTURE: Fresh leaf (1:2, 95% alcohol); dried leaf (1:5, 30% alcohol); 2–5 ml (0.4–1 tsp.) 3 times daily; fresh root (1:2, 30% alcohol) 4–5 ml (0.8–1 tsp.) 3 times daily

GLYCERITE: Dried root (1:5); 1–3 ml (0.2–0.6 tsp.) 3 times daily

DEVIL'S CLAW

Latin name: *Harpagophytum procumbens*

Used by indigenous people for thousands of years to treat pain, stomach disorders, and fever, devil's claw is used as an anti-inflammatory in modern herbalism to treat problems like arthritis and low back pain. It increases mobility in the joints and is a common ingredient in formulas for inflammation and arthritis.

WARNINGS: Contraindicated in gastric and duodenal ulcers

ENERGETICS: Cooling and drying

PROPERTIES: Analgesic (anodyne), anti-inflammatory, and bitter

SOURCES: Mountain Rose Herbs, Starwest Botanicals

DOSAGE FORMS

TINCTURE: Dried root (1:5, 25% alcohol); 1–2 ml (0.2–0.4 tsp.) 3 times daily

CAPSULE OR POWDER: 500–1,000 mg, 2–3 times daily

DEVIL'S CLUB

Latin name: *Oplopanax horridus*

Pacific Northwest Indians used devil's club for a myriad of conditions, much the same as ginseng is used in traditional Chinese medicine. Although it has numerous potential benefits, devil's club is most often used to help regulate blood sugar. It also helps adrenal burnout, especially in people who have dry mucous membranes.

WARNINGS: If collecting devil's club in the wild, be careful to avoid the prickles, which may cause painful wounds.

ENERGETICS: Cooling and moistening

PROPERTIES: Adaptogen, adrenal tonic, alterative (blood purifier), antidiabetic, and tonic

SOURCES: Starwest Botanicals

DOSAGE FORMS

TINCTURE: Fresh root bark (1:2, 60% alcohol); dried root bark (1:5, 60% alcohol); ½–2 ml (0.1–0.4 tsp.) 3 times daily

DONG QUAI

Latin name: *Angelica sinensis*

Dong quai has been used extensively in Asia for improving the general health of women. It is a blood tonic and helps to rebuild the blood from the monthly blood loss women experience in menstruation during their childbearing years. It also eases pain and congestion associated with periods. It stimulates blood flow to the pelvic floor, which helps relieve a variety of reproductive issues.

WARNINGS: Not recommended during pregnancy or with excessive menstrual flow

ENERGETICS: Warming, moistening, and nourishing

PROPERTIES: Anticoagulant, blood building, and emmenagogue

SOURCES: Frontier Herbs, Mountain Rose Herbs, Starwest Botanicals

DOSAGE FORMS

STANDARD DECOCTION: 2–4 ounces 3 times daily

TINCTURE: Dried root (1:5, 40% alcohol); 2–4 ml (0.4–0.8 tsp.) 3 times daily

GLYCERITE: Dried root (1:5); 2.5–10 ml (0.5–2 tsp.) 3 times daily

CAPSULE: 500 mg, 3–6 times daily

DULSE

Latin name: *Palmaria palmata*

Dulse is a seaweed. It is a nourishing food containing numerous trace minerals as well as iodine. It can be used in baths and other topical preparations to promote healthy skin.

WARNINGS: No known warnings

ENERGETICS: Cooling, moistening, and nourishing

PROPERTIES: Emollient, mineralizer, and nutritive

SOURCES: Starwest Botanicals, Stony Mountain Botanicals

DOSAGE FORMS

POWDER: Add dried dulse as you would salt to food. It has a pleasant, salty taste.

CAPSULE: 1,000–10,000 mg daily, divided into 2–3 doses

GLYCERITE: Dried seaweed (1:6); 2–5 ml (0.4–1 tsp.) daily

ECHINACEA

Latin name: *Echinacea angustifolia*

There are several species of echinacea used. We prefer Echinacea angustifolia, or a combination of E. angustifolia and E. purpurea. E. pallida lacks the alkamides that contribute to E. angustifolia's and E. purpurea's action. E. angustifolia is superior to E. purpurea for topical application to wounds, bites, and stings. Echinacea aids the process of antibody formation and stimulates the production of white blood cells. It helps to strengthen and clear lymph nodes. It inhibits hyaluronidase (an enzyme produced by bacteria that breaks down compounds that bind cells together), thus inhibiting the spread of infection. Echinacea also helps the body fight viral infections. Echinacea is a wonderful herb to use topically for infections. It is often used to treat colds and flu, but is actually not the best herb for this purpose. Due to its popularity, echinacea is probably overused for many applications when other herbs would be just as effective.

WARNINGS: Echinacea is nontoxic and mostly harmless. Use very cautiously if you have an autoimmune disorder. High-quality preparations of echinacea can cause excessive salivation and a scratchy, tingling sensation in the throat.

ENERGETICS: Cooling and drying

PROPERTIES: Alterative (blood purifier), antiseptic, antivenomous, antiviral, immune stimulant, and lymphatic

SPECIFIC INDICATIONS: Felter: Systemic sepsis, tendency to boils and to formation of semiactive multiple cellular abscesses, with adynamia and asthenia. Foul discharges with emaciation. Dirty brownish or bluish tongue, with sordes. Skin and mucous membranes dull bluish or purplish in color.

SOURCES: Bulk Herb Store, Frontier Herbs, Mountain Rose Herbs, San Francisco Herb Company, Starwest Botanicals, Stony Mountain Botanicals

DOSAGE FORMS

STANDARD DECOCTION: 2–4 ounces 3 times daily

TINCTURE: Fresh root for E. angustifolia, fresh herb for E. purpurea (1:2, 95% alcohol); dried root for E. angustifolia, dried herb for E. purpurea (1:5, 60% alcohol); 1–5 ml (0.2–1 tsp.) 3–6 times daily

GLYCERITE: Dried root or herb (1:5); 2–8 ml (0.4–1.6 tsp.)

CAPSULE: 400–1,200 mg, 3–4 times daily

TOPICAL USE: A standard decoction or tincture can be used as a wash or compress.

ELDER

Latin name: *Sambucus canadensis, S. nigra*

Elder is a very versatile herb with many useful parts. Elder flowers are an excellent remedy for acute ailments. They help to promote perspiration and reduce inflammation. Research suggests they may have anti-inflammatory, antiviral, and anticancer properties, as well as the ability to shorten the duration and severity of flu symptoms. They work especially well in combination with yarrow and peppermint. They can also be used topically in skin lotions.

The fruits (elder berries) have a mild laxative and decongestant action, and they inhibit the spread of many viral infections. The bark, although not commonly used now, was traditionally used as a laxative and to soothe mucous membranes.

WARNINGS: All parts of the fresh plant are mildly toxic and can cause nausea and diarrhea. Even dried, the stems, bark, and root contain enough residual compounds to induce nausea. The flowers should be dried before using. The berries should be used dried, or boil fresh berries for 3 minutes before preserving.

ENERGETICS: Cooling and drying

PROPERTIES: Anti-inflammatory, antiviral, decongestant, diaphoretic, febrifuge, and nutritive

SOURCES: Bulk Herb Store, Frontier Herbs, Mountain Rose Herbs, San Francisco Herb Company, Starwest Botanicals, Stony Mountain Botanicals

DOSAGE FORMS

STANDARD INFUSION: Flowers: 4–8 ounces served hot as a diaphoretic up to 3 times daily

TINCTURE: Dried flowers (1:5, 60% alcohol); 1–3 ml (0.2–0.6 tsp.) 2–4 times daily

GLYCERITE: Dried flowers (1:6, sealed simmer method); dried berries (1:5, sealed simmer method); 5–10 ml (1–2 tsp.) 4 times daily

SYRUP: Cook fresh or dried berries with a little water until soft, then press through a jelly bag. Measure juice, add an equal amount of honey, bring to a boil, remove from heat, and refrigerate or can; 1–2 teaspoons 4 times daily

TOPICAL USE: Use salve made from flowers as needed.

ELECAMPANE

Latin name: *Inula helenium*

Elecampane is an outstanding remedy for clearing phlegm and mucus from the lungs, urinary system, and digestive system. Elecampane is specific for chronic irritation and infection of the respiratory system. It is a great ingredient in glycerites and syrups for cough. It contains inulin, which feeds friendly bacteria in the colon.

WARNINGS: No known warnings

ENERGETICS: Warming and drying

PROPERTIES: Antiseptic, bitter, diaphoretic, and expectorant

SOURCES: Frontier Herbs, Mountain Rose Herbs, Starwest Botanicals, Stony Mountain Botanicals

DOSAGE FORMS

TINCTURE: Fresh root (1:2, 75% alcohol); dried leaf (1:5, 60% alcohol); 1–2 ml (0.2–0.4 tsp.) 2–4 times daily
Glycerite: Dried root (1:8); 5 ml (1 tsp.) 3 times daily

ELEUTHERO

Latin name: *Eleutherococcus senticosus*

Eleuthero has had more than three thousand studies performed on it, more than any other herb in the world. It was the first plant identified as an adaptogen by Russian scientists. Not only does it help the body cope better with stress, but it also increases endurance and stimulates the brain to improve concentration. Soviet researchers found that eleuthero improved athletic performance, aided cosmonauts in preventing space sickness, caused secretaries to make fewer mistakes, and helped workers have fewer sick days. In other words, eleuthero enhances endurance, immunity, brain function, and general good health. Eleuthero is one of the more stimulating adaptogens and should be used short term, or in lower doses, to prevent overstimulation and insomnia.

WARNINGS: Insomnia and agitation can occur at higher doses or in sensitive people.

ENERGETICS: Balancing and slightly warming

PROPERTIES: Adaptogen, antirheumatic, hypotensive, and immune amphoteric

SOURCES: Bulk Herb Store, Frontier Herbs, Mountain Rose Herbs, Starwest Botanicals

DOSAGE FORMS

TINCTURE: Dried root concentrate (2:1, 30% alcohol), 10 drops to 5 ml (1 tsp.) up to 3 times daily for short term; dried root (1:4, 30% alcohol), 1–3 ml (0.2–0.6 tsp.) daily, normally as part of a formula

GLYCERITE: Dried root (1:5); 5–10 ml (1–2 tsp.) 2–3 times daily

CAPSULE: 500–1,000 mg, 2–3 times daily

ERIGERON (FLEABANE)

Latin name: *Erigeron canadensis*

Erigeron is extremely useful for stopping capillary bleeding. It also helps to halt excessive urination and watery secretions from the gastrointestinal tract.

WARNINGS: No known warnings

ENERGETICS: Warming and constricting

PROPERTIES: Antidiarrheal, antidiuretic, circulatory stimulant, and styptic

SPECIFIC INDICATIONS: King: Free discharge from mucous membranes. Passive capillary hemorrhage. Choleraic discharges, sudden, gushing, and watery, attended by cramping and distress.

DOSAGE FORMS

TINCTURE: Dried leaf (1:5, 60% alcohol); 5 drops to 2 ml (0.4 tsp.) up to 3 times daily

EUCALYPTUS

Latin name: *Eucalyptus globulus*

The leaves of eucalyptus are an underutilized expectorant, helpful for damp coughs, lingering bronchitis, damp asthma, and some cases of COPD. The oil can be diffused and inhaled, and also applied topically as an analgesic in arthritis.

WARNINGS: Eucalyptus leaf is safe for internal use in adults, and in small doses as part of a formula for children. Use the essential oil with caution in children under the age of four, because of possible neurotoxicity.

ENERGETICS: Warming and drying

PROPERTIES: Antibacterial, antimicrobial, and expectorant

SPECIFIC INDICATIONS: Rolla Thomas: Sensations of coldness and weight in bowels; cold extremities; cold perspiration; perspiration during chills.

SOURCES: Bulk Herb Store, Frontier Herbs, Mountain Rose Herbs, San Francisco Herb Company, Starwest Botanicals, Stony Mountain Botanicals

DOSAGE FORMS

STANDARD INFUSION: 1–2 ounces up to 3 times daily

TINCTURE: Fresh leaf (1:2, 80% alcohol, 10% glycerin); dried leaf (1:5, 60% alcohol, 10% glycerin); 1–2 ml (0.2–0.4 tsp.) up to 3 times daily

ESSENTIAL OIL: Best inhaled with steam. Can be diluted in a fixed oil and rubbed on the chest.

EYEBRIGHT

Latin name: *Euphrasia officinalis*

Eyebright is commonly used to treat eye infections and strengthen the eyes. Although it is commonly taken internally for these conditions, it works best when used as an eyewash. The best use of eyebright is as an internal remedy for upper respiratory congestion with acute irritation of the sinuses and eyes with thin, watery mucus and itching eyes and ears, such as rhinitis or the early stages of a cold. A tincture made from the fresh plant will open the Eustachian tubes in children, allowing the inner ear to drain and thus preventing earaches. The dried leaf is almost entirely ineffective for allergies and Eustachian tube issues.

WARNINGS: Eyebright tinctures used as eye drops can cause increased eye pressure, redness, watering, and swelling; when using eyebright topically, use the tea.

ENERGETICS: Cooling, drying, and slightly constricting

PROPERTIES: Anti-allergenic, anti-inflammatory, astringent, and ophthalmicum

SPECIFIC INDICATIONS: Ellingwood: Acute irritating inflammation of mucous membranes of eyes and upper respiratory passages, with acrid, watery discharges.

SOURCES: Frontier Herbs, Starwest Botanicals

DOSAGE FORMS

TINCTURE: Fresh leaf (1:2, 60% alcohol); 1–4 ml (0.2–0.8 tsp.) 1–4 times daily

TOPICAL USE: Prepare a compress or fomentation from a standard infusion of the dried leaf. Apply as needed.

FALSE UNICORN (HELONIAS)

Latin name: *Chamaelirium luteum, syn. Helonias dioica*

False unicorn appears to have a progesterone-enhancing effect. It is used as a female tonic to balance excess estrogen and has been used to help prevent miscarriage. Traditionally it was used for painful ovulation, vaginal discharge, and lack of menstruation.

WARNINGS: Not recommended with emaciation or inflammation

ENERGETICS: Cooling and moistening

PROPERTIES: Anti-abortive, emmenagogue, and uterine tonic

SOURCES: Starwest Botanicals

DOSAGE FORMS

STANDARD DECOCTION: 1–2 ounces up to 3 times daily

TINCTURE: Dried root (1:5, 50% alcohol); 1–4 ml (0.2–0.8 tsp.) 3 times daily

FENNEL

Latin name: *Foeniculum vulgare*

Fennel is a wonderful carminative, commonly used in combination with catnip for colic. Catnip combined with fennel is an excellent remedy for colic, indigestion, and diarrhea in infants and young children as well as adults. Like most carminatives, fennel stimulates digestion and reduces intestinal gas. It also helps to sweeten and increase breast milk. Crush seeds to release oils before using.

WARNINGS: Use cautiously during pregnancy.

ENERGETICS: Warming and drying

PROPERTIES: Aromatic, carminative, condiment, and galactagogue

SOURCES: Bulk Herb Store, Mountain Rose Herbs, San Francisco Herb Company, Stony Mountain Botanicals

DOSAGE FORMS

WEAK INFUSION: 4–6 ounces up to 3 times daily

TINCTURE: Dried seeds (1:3, 60% alcohol, 10% glycerin); 20–40 drops 3 times daily

GLYCERITE: Dried seeds (1:8, sealed simmer method); 3–10 ml (0.6–2 tsp.) as needed

FENUGREEK

Latin name: *Trigonella foenum-graecum*

Fenugreek encourages weight gain and is helpful for strengthening the body during convalescence. It helps to balance blood sugar and therefore may be helpful for diabetes. Fenugreek also helps to enrich breast milk in nursing mothers. It is a soothing remedy for ulcers, burns, abscesses, and other injuries. Used with thyme, it helps decongest the sinuses.

WARNINGS: Not recommended for use during pregnancy

ENERGETICS: Warming and drying

PROPERTIES: Antidiabetic, decongestant, and galactagogue

SOURCES: Bulk Herb Store, Mountain Rose Herbs, San Francisco Herb Company, Stony Mountain Botanicals

DOSAGE FORMS

WEAK DECOCTION: 4–8 ounces 3 times daily. To make a more pleasant-tasting drink, add 1 teaspoon anise seed.

TINCTURE: Dried seeds (1:3, 70% alcohol, 10% glycerin); 1–3 ml (0.2–0.6 tsp.) 3 times daily

TOPICAL USE: Pulverize seeds for use as a poultice.

FEVERFEW

Latin name: *Tanacetum parthenium*

Feverfew is a popular natural remedy for migraine headaches. It does not work very well once the migraine has started, but when taken regularly it helps to prevent migraines and lessen their severity. Its name comes from its traditional use as a remedy for fevers. It is an effective small intestinal anti-inflammatory that combines well with chamomile and calendula for gastritis and leaky gut.

WARNINGS: Not for use during pregnancy. If mouth soreness or ulcerations develop, reduce dosage or discontinue use. It does not work on migraine headaches caused by weakness or deficiency (for example, anemia).

ENERGETICS: Cooling and drying

PROPERTIES: Analgesic (anodyne), anthelminthic, anti-inflammatory, and nervine

SOURCES: Bulk Herb Store, Frontier Herbs, Mountain Rose Herbs, Starwest Botanicals, Stony Mountain Botanicals

STANDARD INFUSION: 1–4 ounces 3 times daily

TINCTURE: Fresh leaf (1:2, 95% alcohol); dried leaf (1:5, 60% alcohol); 2–5 ml (0.4–1 tsp.) 2 times daily

FLAXSEED

Latin name: *Linum usitatissimum*

Freshly ground flaxseed's ability to heal an inflamed gut is amazing. It is a stool softener and bulk laxative for chronic constipation. Flax lignans are phytoestrogens and may be helpful in preventing estrogen-dependent cancers.

WARNINGS: Flaxseeds oxidize very rapidly after being ground. Grinding your own fresh flaxseeds as needed is best.

ENERGETICS: Cooling, moistening, and nourishing

PROPERTIES: Bulk laxative and phytoestrogen

SOURCES: Bulk Herb Store, Mountain Rose Herbs, San Francisco Herb Company, Starwest Botanicals, Stony Mountain Botanicals

DOSAGE FORMS

POWDER: Grind whole flaxseeds in a coffee grinder and use fresh (flaxseed begins to oxidize within 20 minutes of grinding). Sprinkle on food or mix in liquid. Start with 1 teaspoon, and gradually work your way up to a dose of 2–3 tablespoons 2 times daily.

FRINGE TREE

Latin name: *Chionanthus virginicus*

A bitter tonic with blood purifying, laxative, and mild diuretic actions, fringe tree is a very effective gallbladder remedy. It stimulates bile flow and helps relieve intestinal gas, bloating, and a stuffy feeling under the right rib cage. It is one of the best herbs for gallstones, especially when combined with other cholagogues like wild yam, turmeric, dandelion, and barberry.

WARNINGS: Should not be used in bile duct obstruction or pregnancy

ENERGETICS: Cooling and drying

PROPERTIES: Cholagogue

SPECIFIC INDICATIONS: Felter: Jaundice of skin and conjunctiva. Hepatic tenderness upon deep pressure, light, clay-colored stools, high-colored urine.

SOURCES: Mountain Rose Herbs

DOSAGE FORMS

STANDARD DECOCTION: 2–4 ounces 3 times daily

TINCTURE: Dried root (1:5, 65% alcohol); 10 drops to 2 ml (0.4 tsp.) 3 times daily

GARLIC

Latin name: *Allium sativum*

Garlic is a strong aromatic herb that acts as an expectorant to expel phlegm from the lungs, and as a circulatory tonic to lower high blood pressure. It combines well with other herbs for treating certain bacterial and fungal infections. For hypertension, it must be taken daily for at least 3–6 months to see full results. The fresh bulb has the best anti-hypertensive and antimicrobial properties.

WARNINGS: Not for feeble, emaciated, or wasting conditions. Gastric irritation is possible; take with or after meals to lessen this effect.

ENERGETICS: Warming and drying

PROPERTIES: Anthelminthic, antibacterial, anticoagulant (blood thinner), antifungal, antiseptic, aromatic, decongestant, expectorant, and circulatory stimulant

SOURCES: Bulk Herb Store, Mountain Rose Herbs, San Francisco Herb Company, Stony Mountain Botanicals

DOSAGE FORMS

FRESH HERB: Finely mince 1 clove and take 3 times daily. If the taste is objectionable, add an equal amount of honey.

CAPSULE: Aged garlic capsules can slightly lower blood pressure, but are totally ineffective as an expectorant or antimicrobial.

GENTIAN

Latin name: *Gentiana lutea*

This intensely bitter herb is commonly used to stimulate digestive system function. It is often combined with other bitters and carminatives for this purpose. It is best taken in liquid form prior to meals.

WARNINGS: Not for use during pregnancy or acute gastrointestinal inflammation

ENERGETICS: Cooling and drying

PROPERTIES: Alterative (blood purifier), antacid, bitter, and digestive tonic

SOURCES: Frontier Herbs, Mountain Rose Herbs, Starwest Botanicals, Stony Mountain Botanicals

DOSAGE FORMS

TINCTURE: Dried root (1:5, 30% alcohol); 10 drops to 2 ml (0.4 tsp.) 3 times daily, 15–30 minutes before a meal

GHOST PIPE (INDIAN PIPE)

Latin name: *Monotropa uniflora*

Ghost pipe is used primarily to help ease pain. It does not numb pain, but rather takes the pain, whether physical or emotional, outside of the mind so that you remain aware of the pain but no longer feel it. It can be helpful for panic attacks from emotional pain and bad trips from LSD. Ghost pipe is difficult to find and is impossible to grow because it parasitizes fungal mycorrhiza and has never been cultivated. Reserve its use for pain that doesn't respond to anything else.

WARNINGS: Consumption of large doses can bring deep sleep and ultra-vivid dreams.

ENERGETICS: Relaxing and cooling

PROPERTIES: Antispasmodic, nervine, and sedative

DOSAGE FORMS

TINCTURE: Fresh aboveground parts (1:2, 95% alcohol); 3 drops. If nothing happens after 10 minutes, gradually increase dose to 30 drops. Repeat effective dose every 2–4 hours as needed.

GINGER

Latin name: *Zingiber officinale*

A pungent aromatic, ginger is used to relieve nausea, vomiting, and motion sickness. Take capsules or the extract before traveling, to prevent motion sickness. It stimulates digestive secretions when taken with or after meals. Research indicates that ginger root enhances immune function, promotes the secretion of bile and gastric fluids, and increases blood circulation by inhibiting platelet aggregation. It is a potent anti-inflammatory, and studies show it is as effective as ibuprofen for reducing the pain and inflammation associated with arthritis. Fresh ginger is also a potent antiviral and antibacterial, helpful for treating influenza, the common cold, and both bacterial and viral gastroenteritis.

WARNINGS: Some authors caution against use during pregnancy, but no adverse effects have been reported by women using ginger for morning sickness.

ENERGETICS: Warming and drying

PROPERTIES: Analgesic (anodyne), anti-emetic (antinauseous), aromatic, carminative, counterirritant, diaphoretic, digestive tonic, and circulatory stimulant

DOSAGE FORMS

FRESH JUICE: Juice fresh and use 4 ounces, mixed with equal parts hot water, 3 times daily. Add honey and lemon or lime to taste. You can freeze the fresh juice in ice cube trays for later use, or preserve by adding enough alcohol to bring the total alcohol content above 20% (25 ml of 95% alcohol and 75 ml fresh ginger juice).

TINCTURE: Preserve the fresh juice with 25% alcohol, 1–5 ml (0.2–1 tsp.) up to 8 times daily; dried root (1:5, 60% alcohol), 0.8–1.5 ml (0.1–0.3 tsp.) in water 3 times daily

GLYCERITE: Dried root (1:5, sealed simmer method), 1–3 ml (0.2–0.6 tsp.) in water as needed; preserve fresh juice with 50% glycerin, measure the total amount of liquid, and add 20% brandy or rum, ½–1 tsp. with water as needed

CAPSULES: 500–1,000 mg, as needed, up to 8 daily

POWDER: Taken as a food, ginger promotes digestive and general health.

GINKGO

Latin name: *Ginkgo biloba*

Extensive research has been conducted in Europe using concentrated extracts of the flavonoids in this herb. Ginkgo is best used as a standardized extract. It is commonly used to enhance memory and brain function. It improves blood flow to the brain and acts as an antioxidant to protect brain cells from damage. It also improves peripheral circulation and may be beneficial in diabetic retinopathy, tinnitus, vertigo, and dizziness. Best results are obtained when the herb is used consistently for 2–3 months. Ginkgo is an excellent remedy to take to slow the aging process and protect the nervous and cardiovascular systems.

WARNINGS: Use with caution when taking blood thinners. Safety during pregnancy hasn't been established.

ENERGETICS: Slightly cooling

PROPERTIES: Anticoagulant (blood thinner), antioxidant, cerebral tonic, hypotensive, and vasodilator

SOURCES: Bulk Herb Store, Frontier Herbs, Mountain Rose Herbs, San Francisco Herb Company, Starwest Botanicals, Stony Mountain Botanicals

DOSAGE FORMS

STANDARDIZED EXTRACT: Concentration and standardization are required for therapeutic activity. There is no demonstrated therapeutic activity to the crude, powdered, tinctured, infused, or decocted leaf—only adverse allergic reactions to ginkgolic acid. The usual daily dose is 120 mg of a 50:1 ginkgo standardized extract, equivalent to 27–30 mg ginkgo flavone glycosides and about 10 mg terpenoids.

GINSENG (AMERICAN)

Latin name: *Panax quinquefolius*

American ginseng is used as a tonic for strengthening the overall system, improving stamina and resistance to disease. It helps counteract the effects of aging and improves overall health when taken in very small doses. American ginseng is less stimulating than Asian (Korean) ginseng. It helps regulate blood sugar, improves digestion, helps the body cope better with stress, and strengthens adrenal and general glandular function. Ginseng works best in small doses.

WARNINGS: Not toxic, but should not be taken by persons with high blood pressure, fevers, acute inflammation, or acute diseases like colds and flu. Regular large doses can cause insomnia and nervous overstimulation.

ENERGETICS: Cooling and moistening

PROPERTIES: Adaptogen, adrenal tonic, antidiabetic, hypertensive, and tonic

SPECIFIC INDICATIONS: Rolla Thomas: Nervous dyspepsia; sensation of dullness in head, with inability to control the voluntary muscles.

SOURCES: Mountain Rose Herbs, Stony Mountain Botanicals

DOSAGE FORMS

STANDARD DECOCTION: For weakened people, 2–10 grams daily as a decoction can be used for 2–3 days to speed up recovery from acute illness. Don't give this dose if there are any heat signs.

TINCTURE: Dried root (1:4, 30% alcohol); 2–5 drops 1–3 times daily for long-term use

GLYCERITE: Dried root (1:5); 3–7 drops 1–3 times daily for long-term use

CAPSULE: One capsule is a large dose for most people. 100 mg 1–2 times daily is normally all that is needed as a long-term tonic.

GINSENG (ASIAN, KOREAN)

Latin name: *Panax ginseng*

Ginseng is one of the most highly prized herbs in the world. Asian or Korean ginseng has been shown to increase energy, help fight fatigue, and increase physical stamina and agility. It may even enhance the body's ability to recover from physical injuries. Small doses of ginseng are used to slow aging, reduce stress, balance mood, and enhance a person's general health. Ginseng may lower the risk of cancer and build up a weakened immune system. Asian ginseng is more warming than American ginseng and is well suited to older men and women who tend to be cold, pale, and easily fatigued. Red ginseng, which is steamed before drying, is more warming in energy, whereas white ginseng, which is just peeled and dried, is more neutral in energy.

WARNINGS: Has no toxic effects but is contraindicated with signs of heat, in acute diseases, high fevers, or inflammation

ENERGETICS: Warming and moistening

PROPERTIES: Adaptogen, hypertensive, immune stimulant, and tonic

SOURCES: Mountain Rose Herbs, Starwest Botanicals, Stony Mountain Botanicals

DOSAGE FORMS

STANDARD DECOCTION: 2–4 ounces 2 times daily

TINCTURE: Dried root (1:4, 30% alcohol); 1–2 ml (0.2–0.4 tsp.) 1–3 times daily

GLYCERITE: Dried root (1:5); 1–3 ml (0.2–0.6 tsp.) 1–3 times daily

CAPSULE: 500 mg, 1–2 times daily

GOLDENROD

Latin name: *Solidago virgaurea, S. canadensis, and other species*

Goldenrod is very soothing and healing. It is a useful diuretic for urinary tract problems, obstructions, kidney stones, and inflammation. It is helpful for hay fever and allergies to cats. It can be helpful for upper respiratory infections and yeast infections like thrush. Topically, it is a good anti-inflammatory for sore muscles.

WARNINGS: Not for use with edema from kidney failure

ENERGETICS: Warming and drying

PROPERTIES: Anti-inflammatory, antiseptic, diuretic, and kidney tonic

SOURCES: Mountain Rose Herbs, Starwest Botanicals

DOSAGE FORMS

STANDARD INFUSION: 4–8 ounces 3 times daily

TINCTURE: Fresh flowers (1:2, 95% alcohol); dried flowers (1:5, 50% alcohol); 2–4 ml (0.4–0.8 tsp.) 1–4 times daily

GLYCERITE: Dried flowers (1:8); 2.5–10 ml (0.5–2 tsp.) 2–4 times daily

TOPICAL USE: Dried flowers (1:4, oil or salve); apply 2–3 times daily.

GOLDENSEAL

Latin name: *Hydrastis canadensis*

Goldenseal is a locally acting antibiotic, meaning it has to come in contact with the infected tissue, and a mild immune stimulant, useful in urinary and digestive tract infections. It is very drying to the mucous membranes and particularly helpful after the acute infection has passed and there is lingering stagnation in the respiratory, digestive, or urinary mucous membranes. Goldenseal lowers blood sugar and, like most bitters, stimulates digestion. It is a specific remedy for diarrhea caused by giardia. It may be used as a wash for sore red eyes and as a topical application for canker sores.

Goldenseal is overharvested, and other herbs should be used as substitutes when possible. Coptis root, Oregon grape, and barberry all contain the alkaloid berberine, and have similar antimicrobial properties as goldenseal.

WARNINGS: Goldenseal is safe when used at the recommended dosages and times, but should not be used as a single herb for longer than 2 weeks. It is contraindicated in dry conditions. When used for long periods, it can cause malabsorption of B vitamins, resulting in fatigue and listlessness. Goldenseal should be used under professional supervision during pregnancy.

ENERGETICS: Cooling, drying, and slightly constricting

PROPERTIES: Alterative (blood purifier), antibacterial, antiseptic, and digestive tonic

SPECIFIC INDICATIONS: Felter: Relaxed mucous membranes, with feeble circulation, and profuse mucus flow of thick, tenacious, yellowish or greenish-yellow character. Gastric irritability and anorexia.

SOURCES: Frontier Herbs, Mountain Rose Herbs, San Francisco Herb Company, Starwest Botanicals, Stony Mountain Botanicals

DOSAGE FORMS

STANDARD DECOCTION: 2–4 ounces 3 times daily

TINCTURE: Dried root (1:5, 60% alcohol); 10 drops to 2 ml (0.4 tsp.) 2–4 times daily

GLYCERITE: Dried root (1:8); 2.5–10 ml (0.5–2 tsp.) 2–4 times daily

CAPSULE: 500–2,000 mg, 2–3 times daily

POWDER: Use the dry powered herb as a snuff; works well with bayberry; can also be applied topically for skin ulcerations or used as an ingredient in poultices.

GOTU KOLA

Latin name: *Centella asiatica, syn. Hydrocotyle asiatica*

Gotu kola has a reputation for improving memory and brain function. It is balancing to the adrenals. Gotu kola is used in India for skin diseases and wasting diseases such as leprosy. It is a wonderful topical remedy for wound healing and scar prevention.

WARNINGS: Overdose may cause dizziness. Use caution with blood thinning medications. It appears safe during pregnancy and lactation in animal studies, and no human adverse events have been reported, but some sources suggest caution.

ENERGETICS: Cooling and drying

PROPERTIES: Adaptogen and cerebral tonic

SOURCES: Frontier Herbs, Mountain Rose Herbs, San Francisco Herb Company, Starwest Botanicals, Stony Mountain Botanicals

DOSAGE FORMS

STANDARD INFUSION: 4–8 ounces 3 times daily

TINCTURE: Fresh plant (1:2, 95% alcohol); dried plant (1:5, 40% alcohol); 1–4 ml (0.2–0.8 tsp.) 3 times daily

CAPSULE: 500–1,000 mg, 3 times daily

GRAVEL ROOT

Latin name: *Eupatorium purpureum*

Gravel root is a diuretic that helps to remove urinary stones and flush the urinary passages. It is used for kidney infections, prostatitis, pelvic inflammatory disease, gout, and diabetes.

WARNINGS: Contains pyrrolizidine alkaloids. Not recommended for long-term use or for pregnant or nursing women.

ENERGETICS: Cooling and drying

PROPERTIES: Diuretic and lithotriptic

SPECIFIC INDICATIONS: Fyfe: Functional derangements of urinary organs, scanty, burning urination.

SOURCES: Frontier Herbs, Mountain Rose Herbs, Starwest Botanicals, Stony Mountain Botanicals

DOSAGE FORMS

STANDARD DECOCTION: 4–8 ounces 3 times daily

Tincture: Dried root (1:5, 60% alcohol); 1–3 ml (0.2–0.6 tsp.) 2–4 times daily

Glycerite: Dried root (1:8); 5–15 ml (1–3 tsp.) 2–4 times daily

GRINDELIA (GUMWEED)

Latin name: *Grindelia spp.*

This resinous expectorant and decongestant is very good at breaking up hardened mucus in the respiratory tract. It eases breathing in bronchitis and asthma. Its antispasmodic action opens the smaller passages in the lungs and can make breathing easier. It can be combined with plantain to pull thick mucus out of the lungs. It can also be applied topically as a salve to heal skin afflictions like poison ivy and rashes and is helpful for insect bites.

WARNINGS: Can be toxic in large doses. Not for long-term use or for use by people suffering from kidney or heart disease.

ENERGETICS: Warming, drying, and constricting

PROPERTIES: Antiseptic, astringent, decongestant, and expectorant

SPECIFIC INDICATIONS: Rolla Thomas: Asthma; labored respiration with dusky flushing of face; old atonic ulcers; tissues full.

SOURCES: Starwest Botanicals

DOSAGE FORMS

TINCTURE: Dried leaf (1:5, 70% alcohol); fresh unopened flower buds (1:2, 95% alcohol); 1–3 ml (0.2–0.6 tsp.) 2–4 times daily. 5 drops every 15–30 minutes during coughing fits.

OIL: Dried leaves and unopened flower buds (1:4); can be made into a salve

GUARANA

Latin name: *Paullinia cupana, P. sorbilis*

Guarana contains caffeine, but it may be a better stimulant than coffee, as it is released more slowly into the body to provide a more sustained energy release.

WARNINGS: Avoid taking guarana if combined with ephedrine, or if you have high blood pressure, heart disease, or sensitivity to caffeine. May cause irregular heartbeat, anxiety, jitteriness, and insomnia in susceptible persons.

ENERGETICS: Warming and drying

PROPERTIES: Diuretic and metabolic stimulant

SOURCES: Frontier Herbs, Starwest Botanicals, Stony Mountain Botanicals

DOSAGE FORMS

STANDARDIZED EXTRACT: 150 mg dry extract standardized to 11%–13% alkaloid concentration once daily

CAPSULES: 500 mg, 1–2 times daily

GUGGUL

Latin name: *Commiphora mukul*

Research has shown that guggul may be able to lower both cholesterol and triglycerides. It inhibits platelet aggregation and can help prevent and possibly reverse arterial plaque. It is mildly stimulating to the thyroid and may be helpful for weight loss.

WARNINGS: Because it thins the blood, it should not be used in persons who bleed easily or during pregnancy. Avoid with hyperthyroid disorders.

ENERGETICS: Warming and drying

PROPERTIES: Anti-inflammatory, antibacterial, anticholesteremic, and antirheumatic

SOURCES: Mountain Rose Herbs

DOSAGE FORMS

TINCTURE: Dried resin (1:3, 95% alcohol); 1–3 ml (0.2–0.6 tsp.) 2–4 times daily

CAPSULE: 75 mg standardized guggulsterones daily

GYMNEMA

Latin name: *Gymnema sylvestre*

Ayurvedic practitioners have used gymnema to treat type 2 diabetes for at least two thousand years. When it comes in contact with the tongue, gymnema makes it impossible to taste sugar. It is believed that it not only blocks sweet receptors on the tongue, but also slows absorption of sugar in the digestive tract. Peer-reviewed studies now support the use of gymnema as a treatment for high blood sugar.

WARNINGS: Gymnema is generally regarded as safe.

ENERGETICS: Cooling and drying

PROPERTIES: Antidiabetic

SOURCES: Mountain Rose Herbs, Starwest Botanicals

DOSAGE FORMS

TINCTURE: Dried leaf (1:5, 30% alcohol); 1–3 ml (0.2–0.6 tsp.) 2–4 times daily. Use smaller, more frequent doses to reduce cravings for sweets and to control the appetite.

GLYCERITE: Dried leaf (1:8); 2.5–10 ml (0.5–2 tsp.) 2–4 times daily

CAPSULE: 1,000–2,000 mg, 3 times daily

HAWTHORN

Latin name: *Crataegus oxyacantha, C. monogyna*

Studies around the world have confirmed that hawthorn berries improve the tone of the heart muscle, improve oxygen uptake by the heart, improve circulation in the heart, energize the heart cells, and dilate blood vessels in the extremities to reduce strain on the heart. Thus, hawthorn berries are an excellent herbal food for building up the heart muscle. Hawthorn needs to be taken on a regular basis for best results. Generally, it improves cardiac function in heart disorders with or without chest pain. Besides benefiting the heart, hawthorn helps reduce stress and improves digestion.

WARNINGS: Completely safe for long-term use

ENERGETICS: Cooling and moistening

PROPERTIES: Anti-arrhythmic, antiseptic, cardiac, hypertensive, and hypotensive

SPECIFIC INDICATIONS: Fyfe: Cardiac weakness and palpitation, irregular, intermittent pulse, with increased rate, dyspnea, and nervous depression.

SOURCES: Bulk Herb Store, Frontier Herbs, Mountain Rose Herbs, San Francisco Herb Company, Starwest Botanicals, Stony Mountain Botanicals

DOSAGE FORMS

STANDARD DECOCTION: 4–8 ounces 3 times daily

TINCTURE: Dried leaf and flowers (1:5, 45% alcohol); 1–5 ml (0.2–1 tsp.) 2–4 times daily

FLUID EXTRACT: Dried berries and flowers (1:1, 50% alcohol); 1–2 ml (0.2–0.4 tsp.) 2–4 times daily

GLYCERITE: Dried flowers and berries (1:8); 5–20 ml (1–4 tsp.) 2–4 times daily

SOLID EXTRACT: 0.5–1 tsp. up to 3 times daily

CAPSULE: 1,000–2,000 mg, 3 times daily

HE SHOU WU (HO SHOU WU, FO-TI)

Latin name: *Polygonum multiflorum*

This herb is considered an anti-aging tonic and is believed to help prevent (and possibly reverse) the graying of hair when taken regularly. It helps to balance blood sugar levels and improve thyroid function.

WARNINGS: Not for persons with diarrhea, weak digestion, or heavy mucus congestion. There is some concern over potential liver toxicity when used in large amounts.

ENERGETICS: Neutral and moistening

PROPERTIES: Anticholesteremic, blood building, glandular, and tonic

SOURCES: Frontier Herbs, Mountain Rose Herbs, Starwest Botanicals, Stony Mountain Botanicals

DOSAGE FORMS

STANDARD DECOCTION: 4–8 ounces 3 times daily

TINCTURE: Dried root (1:5, 60% alcohol); 1–5 ml (0.2–1 tsp.) 2–4 times daily

CAPSULE: 1,000 mg, 3 times daily

HOLY BASIL

Latin name: *Ocimum sanctum*

Holy basil is heavily used in Ayurvedic medicine. In Western herbalism it is considered an adaptogen and general tonic. It protects the heart from stress, lowers blood pressure and cholesterol levels, and stabilizes blood sugar levels. It reduces feelings of stress and reduces excessive immune responses in conditions like hay fever (allergic rhinitis) and asthma. At the same time, it enhances digestion, cerebral circulation, memory, concentration, and mental acuity. Avicenna considered all basils to be heart exhilarants, useful for increasing joy and happiness.

WARNINGS: No known warnings

ENERGETICS: Cooling and drying

PROPERTIES: Adaptogen, antibacterial, antiviral, carminative, hypotensive, and immune amphoteric

SOURCES: Bulk Herb Store, Frontier Herbs, Mountain Rose Herbs, Starwest Botanicals, Stony Mountain Botanicals

DOSAGE FORMS

STANDARD INFUSION: 4–8 ounces 3 times daily

TINCTURE: Dried leaf (1:5, 60% alcohol); 2–4 ml (0.4–0.8 tsp.) 3 times daily

HOPS

Latin name: *Humulus lupulus*

Hops is a powerful nervine and sleep aid, and can be combined with other carminatives for settling a nervous, acidic stomach. It is estrogenic and is used to increase sex drive in women and reduce it in men. Hops is indicated for a hot digestive system or irritated nervous system. It works best on hot, damp people who are often overweight and red-faced with fiery personalities and have poor digestion and insomnia.

WARNINGS: Hops is contraindicated in clinical depression, estrogen dominance, or with allergies to hops. Hops is not the best choice for young children, but are all right as part of a formula. Use with caution during pregnancy due to its estrogenic effects.

ENERGETICS: Cooling and relaxing

PROPERTIES: Analgesic (anodyne), anaphrodisiac, antacid, anthelminthic, antispasmodic, nervine, phytoestrogen, sedative, and soporific (hypnotic)

SPECIFIC INDICATIONS: Felter: Nervousness, irritability, insomnia. Acid eructations. Vesical irritation.

SOURCES: Bulk Herb Store, Mountain Rose Herbs, Starwest Botanicals, Stony Mountain Botanicals

STANDARD INFUSION: 4–8 ounces up to 3 times daily

TINCTURE: Dried leaf (1:5, 75% alcohol); 1–3 ml (0.2–0.6 tsp.) 3 times daily

CAPSULE: 1,000–2,000 mg, 3 times daily

HOREHOUND

Latin name: *Marrubium vulgare*

Horehound has traditionally been used to make cough drops or cough syrup. Horehound drops can still be found in some stores. It increases the secretion of thinner mucus to break up congestion. It is a great remedy for coughing, wheezing, and difficulty breathing. It stimulates digestion and has a mild cardiac effect.

WARNINGS: Use with caution during pregnancy.

ENERGETICS: Cooling and drying

PROPERTIES: Anti-arrhythmic, bitter, cardiac, decongestant, and expectorant

SOURCES: Frontier Herbs, Mountain Rose Herbs, Starwest Botanicals, Stony Mountain Botanicals

DOSAGE FORMS

STANDARD INFUSION: 4–8 ounces 3 times daily. Mix with honey or lemon to make it more palatable.

TINCTURE: Dried leaf (1:5, 60% alcohol); 0.5–3 ml (0.1–0.6 tsp.) 3 times daily

HORNY GOAT WEED (EPIMEDIUM)

Latin name: *Epimedium grandiflorum*

Horny goat weed has been traditionally used in treating sexual dysfunction, fatigue, and arthritis. The herb's active constituent, icariin, has been shown in animal studies to help the body form and maintain an erection. Horny goat weed also stimulates the production of osteoblasts, which are specialized cells involved in building bone mass. The flavonoids in horny goat weed are believed to stimulate the nerves, improving the sensation of touch.

WARNINGS: High doses of horny goat weed may result in breathing trouble, dizziness, vomiting, thirst, and dry mouth.

ENERGETICS: Warming, drying, and slightly relaxing

PROPERTIES: Aphrodisiac and vasodilator

SOURCES: Mountain Rose Herbs, Starwest Botanicals, Stony Mountain Botanicals

DOSAGE FORMS

CAPSULE: 1,000–2,000 mg, 3 times daily

HORSE CHESTNUT

Latin name: *Aesculus hippocastanum*

Horse chestnut is a specific tonic for the vascular system. It improves the tone of veins, helping to control varicose veins, bruises, and hemorrhoids. It can be taken internally or applied topically.

WARNINGS: There is some toxicity to the horse chestnut plant, but standardized extracts of the seeds are safe when used as directed. Avoid with children, during pregnancy, and with nursing mothers. Use cautiously when taking blood thinning medications.

ENERGETICS: Cooling, drying, and slightly constricting

PROPERTIES: Astringent and vascular tonic

SPECIFIC INDICATIONS: Rolla Thomas: A stimulant to the nervous system, and useful in difficult breathing of asthma when not of a paroxysmal character; also a good remedy in hemorrhoids.

SOURCES: Mountain Rose Herbs, Starwest Botanicals, Stony Mountain Botanicals

DOSAGE FORMS

TINCTURE: Dried seeds (1:5, 40% alcohol); 1–2 ml (0.2–0.4 tsp.) 1–3 times daily. The seed tincture is a toxic botanical and should be used only under professional supervision.

STANDARDIZED EXTRACT: 2–4 capsules or tablets daily (or as recommended on the product label)

OIL: Dried seeds (1:4); apply 1–2 times daily.

HORSERADISH

Latin name: *Armoracia rusticana*

Horseradish helps stimulate the digestion as well as metabolism of protein. It can be used for colds, flu, and other acute ailments and may be helpful for allergies, hay fever, and congestion in the lungs.

WARNINGS: Large amounts can cause gastrointestinal upset.

ENERGETICS: Warming and drying

PROPERTIES: Carminative, decongestant, and expectorant

SOURCES: Mountain Rose Herbs

DOSAGE FORMS

FRESH HERB: Peel and grate fresh roots. Horseradish loses potency when dried. Mix with vinegar (prepare this in a well-ventilated area), and refrigerate as a condiment.

TINCTURE: Fresh root (1:2, 95% alcohol); 1–3 ml (0.2–0.6 tsp.) 2–4 times daily

GLYCERITE: Fresh root (1:4, 100% glycerin sealed simmer method); 2.5–10 ml (0.5–2 tsp.) 2–4 times daily

HORSETAIL

Latin name: *Equisetum arvense*

Horsetail is rich in the mineral silica, which is used along with calcium to form bones, nails, hair, and skin. Silica adds elasticity to tissues, making them strong but not brittle. It is astringent and is useful for internal bleeding, such as blood in the urine. It has a mild diuretic effect.

WARNINGS: Excessive consumption may lead to a thiamine deficiency. The powdered herb is not recommended for children, but the tea is okay.

ENERGETICS: Cooling, drying, and slightly constricting

PROPERTIES: Diuretic, hemostatic, kidney tonic, mineralizer, and vulnerary

SPECIFIC INDICATIONS: Rolla Thomas: A mild diuretic, invaluable in gravel and irritation of the urinary organs, with dysuria and pain after urinating; also in suppression of urine and dropsical affections.

SOURCES: Bulk Herb Store, Frontier Herbs, Mountain Rose Herbs, San Francisco Herb Company, Starwest Botanicals, Stony Mountain Botanicals

DOSAGE FORMS

STANDARD INFUSION: 4–8 ounces 3 times daily

TINCTURE: Dried herb (1:5, 35% alcohol); 1–2 ml (0.2–0.4 tsp.) 3 times daily

HYDRANGEA

Latin name: *Hydrangea arborescens*

Hydrangea is used as a diuretic and urinary anodyne. It is useful to help rid the body of kidney stones. It can also be helpful for back pain and arthritis.

WARNINGS: Not recommended for long-term use

ENERGETICS: Cooling and drying

PROPERTIES: Analgesic (anodyne), diuretic, and lithotriptic

SPECIFIC INDICATIONS: Felter: Vesical and urethral irritation with dull aching in back; urine tinged with blood.

SOURCES: Frontier Herbs, Mountain Rose Herbs, Starwest Botanicals, Stony Mountain Botanicals

DOSAGE FORMS

TINCTURE: Dried root (1:3, 60% alcohol); 1–4 ml (0.2–0.8 tsp.) 3 times daily

STANDARD DECOCTION: 2–4 ounces 3 times daily

CAPSULE: 1,000–2,000 mg, 3 times daily

POWDER: 2 grams in 3 ounces of hot lemon water every 20 minutes for acute kidney stones

HYSSOP

Latin name: *Hyssopus officinalis*

Hyssop is considered a cure-all for respiratory ailments. It helps clear thick and congested phlegm from the lungs to restore free breathing. Hyssop has antiseptic properties that are helpful in the treatment of cuts and abrasions and can also be used to provide immediate relief from insect bites.

WARNINGS: The essential oil of hyssop is toxic. The herb is generally recognized as safe when used as directed, but should be avoided during pregnancy.

ENERGETICS: Warming and drying

PROPERTIES: Antiseptic, antiviral, carminative, decongestant, emmenagogue, and expectorant

SOURCES: Frontier Herbs, Mountain Rose Herbs, San Francisco Herb Company, Starwest Botanicals, Stony Mountain Botanicals

DOSAGE FORMS

STANDARD INFUSION: 4–8 ounces 3 times daily

TINCTURE: Dried leaf (1:5, 60% alcohol); 1–3 ml (0.2–0.6 tsp.) 2–4 times daily

IRISH MOSS

Latin name: *Chondrus crispus*

Irish moss is a seaweed rich in iodine and trace minerals and a source of protein, amino acids, and manganese. It soothes dry and irritated tissues and is helpful for chronic, dry lung conditions and sore throats. Irish moss arrests diarrhea, but it may also act as a mild laxative in conditions involving dry, hard stools. It contains a mucilage (carrageenan) that is widely used as a stabilizer in dairy products and cosmetics.

WARNINGS: No known warnings

ENERGETICS: Cooling, moistening, and nourishing

PROPERTIES: Anti-inflammatory, emollient, bulk laxative, mucilaginous (mucilant), and nutritive

SOURCES: Frontier Herbs, Starwest Botanicals, Stony Mountain Botanicals

DOSAGE FORMS

POWDER OR CAPSULES: 1,000–5,000 mg up to 3 times daily

ISATIS

Latin name: *Isatis tinctoria*

Isatis is a potent antiviral, used for infections involving fever and inflammation. It is extremely cooling; if taken for extended periods, it can make a person feel as if they have an ice cube in their stomach and can cause uncontrolled shivering. For this reason it is normally taken only for short periods or combined with ginger.

WARNINGS: Isatis is contraindicated for cold, chronic conditions and is not recommended for long-term use.

ENERGETICS: Very cooling

PROPERTIES: Antiviral and refrigerant

DOSAGE FORMS

TINCTURE: Dried root (1:5, 75% alcohol); 1–3 ml (0.2–0.6 tsp.) 3 times daily

JAMAICAN DOGWOOD

Latin name: *Piscidia erythrina, P. piscipula*

A mild narcotic and anodyne herb, Jamaican dogwood is a relatively potent sedative known as a remedy for migraine headaches, neuralgia, and the treatment of insomnia caused by pain, nervous tension, and stress. The bark is anti-inflammatory and antispasmodic and can be used for painful menstrual periods. It is used in combination with other herbs to treat the musculoskeletal pain of arthritis and rheumatism. Jamaican dogwood mixes well with Corydalis yanhusuo for pain relief.

WARNINGS: Use with caution with hypotension and in children or pregnant women. May potentiate sedative medications.

ENERGETICS: Cooling and relaxing

PROPERTIES: Analgesic (anodyne), antispasmodic, narcotic, sedative, and soporific (hypnotic)

SPECIFIC INDICATIONS: Amidon: Insomnia and nervous unrest, spasm, pain, nervous irritability; neuralgias of trigeminal and cervical plexuses.

SOURCES: Mountain Rose Herbs, Starwest Botanicals

DOSAGE FORMS

TINCTURE: Dried bark (1:5, 80% alcohol); 10 drops to 3 ml (0.6 tsp.) every 4 hours. Do not exceed recommended dose.

GLYCERITE: Dried bark (1:8); 5–10 ml (0.5–1 tsp.) every 4 hours

JAMBUL

Latin name: *Syzygium cumini*

Jambul helps to maintain blood sugar levels and has been studied for use with type 2 diabetes. The seeds regulate the conversion of starch into sugar, checking the production of glucose. The fruit reduces sugar in the urine and abates thirst. It is helpful for bile insufficiency, gallbladder troubles, and hepatitis.

WARNINGS: No known warnings

ENERGETICS: Cooling and constricting

PROPERTIES: Antidiabetic, antidiarrheal, astringent, and bitter

DOSAGE FORMS

TINCTURE: Dried leaf (1:5, 60% alcohol); 1–4 ml (0.2–0.8 tsp.) 3 times daily

CAPSULE OR POWDER: 3,000–10,000 mg (3–10 grams) daily

JUNIPER BERRY

Latin name: *Juniperus spp.*

Juniper berry strongly stimulates kidney function and has antiseptic properties. It is commonly used for edema and other urinary problems. It also stimulates digestion. One species of juniper (*J. monosperma*) is sometimes called cedar berries and is used in formulas to reduce blood sugar. Juniper berries must be cured (dried) for 1 year before use.

WARNINGS: The volatile oils in juniper can be irritating to the kidneys and the nervous system with long-term use. Not recommended when kidneys are inflamed or in cases of nephritis and nephrosis. Not recommended for use in pregnancy.

ENERGETICS: Warming and drying

PROPERTIES: Antifungal, antiseptic, aromatic, carminative, and diuretic

SOURCES: Frontier Herbs, Mountain Rose Herbs, San Francisco Herb Company, Starwest Botanicals, Stony Mountain Botanicals

DOSAGE FORMS

STANDARD INFUSION: Powder berries before adding boiling water; 4–8 ounces 1–4 times daily

TINCTURE: Dried berries (1:5, 65% alcohol, 10% glycerin); 1–2 ml (0.2–0.4 tsp.) 2–4 times daily

GLYCERITE: Dried berries (1:8); 10–20 ml (1–2 tsp.) 3–4 times daily

CAPSULES: 1,000–2,000 mg, 3 times daily

KAVA-KAVA

Latin name: *Piper methysticum*

Kava-kava has long been used to treat stress, anxiety, and insomnia. It is used in Polynesian religious ceremonies to reduce anxiety and relax muscles while maintaining mental alertness. It also elevates mood. Kava-kava is a diuretic and reduces the pain of urinary tract infections and interstitial cystitis.

WARNINGS: Large doses over a long period of time may cause liver problems and skin eruptions. Do not drive or operate heavy machinery under the influence of large doses of kava-kava, as it can impair motor function. If you have liver health problems or drink alcohol regularly, you should avoid kava-kava.

ENERGETICS: Relaxing, drying, and warming

PROPERTIES: Acrid, analgesic (anodyne), anesthetic, antispasmodic, diuretic, and sedative

SPECIFIC INDICATIONS: Felter: Irritation, inflammation, atony of urinary passages, painful micturition, scanty and irregular. Pale edematous tissues.

SOURCES: Mountain Rose Herbs, Starwest Botanicals, Stony Mountain Botanicals

DOSAGE FORMS

STANDARD INFUSION: 4–8 ounces as needed

TINCTURE: Fresh root (1:2, 95% alcohol); dried root (1:5, 65% alcohol); 1–5 ml (0.2–1 tsp.) as needed

CAPSULE: 500–1,000 mg, as needed; if standardized product, use 100–200 mg of kava lactones daily.

KELP

Latin name: *Laminaria spp.*

Kelp is a large, fast-growing seaweed rich in iodine, minerals, trace minerals, vitamins, and chlorophyll. Kelp is sometimes considered a super-food because of the many nutrients it contains.

WARNINGS: Avoid with hyperthyroid disorders. Use cautiously in Hashimoto's thyroiditis and selenium deficiencies.

ENERGETICS: Cooling, moistening, and nourishing

PROPERTIES: Emollient and nutritive

SOURCES: Bulk Herb Store, San Francisco Herb Company, Starwest Botanicals, Stony Mountain Botanicals

DOSAGE FORMS

DRIED OR POWDERED: 2–5 grams daily; can be sprinkled on food

POWDER OR CAPSULES: 1,000–5,000 mg up to 3 times daily

KHELLA

Latin name: *Ammi visnaga*

Khella is a vasodilator and calcium channel blocker used to treat cardiovascular problems. Its antispasmodic properties make it helpful for asthma and cramps. It may also be helpful for passing stones from the gallbladder and kidneys.

WARNINGS: Not for use during pregnancy

ENERGETICS: Warming and relaxing

PROPERTIES: Anti-arrhythmic, antispasmodic, bronchial dilator, cardiac, hypotensive, and vasodilator

DOSAGE FORMS

TINCTURE: Dried seeds (1:5, 65% alcohol); 1–3 ml (0.2–0.6 tsp.) 3 times daily

KUDZU

Latin name: *Pueraria lobata, P. thunbergiana*

Kudzu has a history of use in traditional Chinese medicine for counteracting the effects of alcohol. Extracts of the flower are used for treating alcoholism and relieving hangover. The roots are used for neutralizing poisons and viral infections. The roots are also used to treat venous problems and the headache, dizziness, and numbness caused by high blood pressure. Kudzu is helpful for leaky gut syndrome, muscle aches, and neck and upper back pain. It is also used for diarrhea, dysentery, and increasing blood flow in patients with arteriosclerosis.

WARNINGS: No known warnings

ENERGETICS: Cooling and constricting

PROPERTIES: Astringent, demulcent (mucilant), and tonic

SOURCES: Mountain Rose Herbs, Starwest Botanicals

DOSAGE FORMS

TINCTURE: Dried root (1:5, 50% alcohol); 1–4 ml (0.2–0.8 tsp.) 3 times daily

POWDER OR CAPSULES: 1,000–3,000 mg up to 3 times daily

LADY'S MANTLE

Latin name: *Alchemilla vulgaris*

Lady's mantle is used as a tonic for the uterus and as a remedy for vaginal discharge and heavy menstrual bleeding, internally or externally. It is a styptic and can also be used for other types of bleeding. It has a diuretic effect and eases edema.

WARNINGS: Avoid during pregnancy.

ENERGETICS: Drying and constricting

PROPERTIES: Antidiarrheal, astringent, uterine tonic, and vulnerary

SOURCES: Mountain Rose Herbs, Starwest Botanicals, Stony Mountain Botanicals

DOSAGE FORMS

STANDARD INFUSION: 4–8 ounces 3 times daily

TINCTURE: Fresh root (1:2, 75% alcohol); dried leaf (1:5, 50% alcohol); 5 drops to 3 ml (0.6 tsp.) 3 times daily

LAVENDER

Latin name: *Lavandula officinalis, syn. L. angustifolia*

Lavender is a relaxing nervine that eases tension and anxiety. It is a specific for high-strung, nervous, self-absorbed people who need to relax. It lifts mood and is mildly antidepressant. Lavender has a mild analgesic effect and can ease headaches and migraines when taken soon after onset. The essential oil of lavender is antifungal and is a great remedy for burns.

WARNINGS: No known warnings

ENERGETICS: Relaxing and slightly warming

PROPERTIES: Analgesic (anodyne), antifungal, aromatic, and relaxant

SOURCES: Bulk Herb Store, Frontier Herbs, Mountain Rose Herbs, San Francisco Herb Company, Starwest Botanicals, Stony Mountain Botanicals

DOSAGE FORMS

STANDARD INFUSION: 4–8 ounces 1–4 times daily

TINCTURE: Dried flower and leaf (1:5, 75% alcohol, 10% glycerin); 1–3 ml (0.2–0.6 tsp.) 3 times daily

ESSENTIAL OIL: Use in baths with Epsom salts for stress, nervousness, depression, and anxiety. Blend in fixed oil for massage to relieve stress. Apply neat for burns and skin irritation.

LEMON

Latin name: *Citrus limon*

Lemon juice is used to help fight colds and flu. It has a cooling effect on the body and helps with calcium deposits, gallstones, and kidney stones.

WARNINGS: No known warnings

ENERGETICS: Cooling

PROPERTIES: Antiseptic, febrifuge, lithotriptic, nutritive, and refrigerant

SOURCES: Bulk Herb Store, Mountain Rose Herbs, San Francisco Herb Company, Starwest Botanicals, Stony Mountain Botanicals

DOSAGE FORMS

FRESH SQUEEZED JUICE: 1 ounce diluted in water as needed

TINCTURE: Fresh peel (1:3, 95% alcohol); 1–5 ml (0.2–1 tsp.) 1–3 times daily

GLYCERITE: Dried peel (1:6, sealed simmer method); 2–10 ml (0.4–2 tsp.) 1–3 times daily

ESSENTIAL OIL: Apply topically. Internally dilute 1 drop in a cup of water and sip once daily. Do not use lemon oil internally for more than 7 days.

LEMON BALM

Latin name: *Melissa officinalis*

Lemon balm is an aromatic with a lemony scent and a mild astringent action. It is useful for many acute ailments such as colds, digestive upset, and flu. It is used in combination with bugleweed to calm an overactive thyroid. It is helpful for nervousness that affects the heart and digestion. Lemon balm is a locally acting antiviral, used in topical applications for cold sores and shingles. It helps to ease sadness and depression, calm mania and hysteria, enhance sleep, and aid memory and concentration.

WARNINGS: No known warnings

ENERGETICS: Cooling and slightly relaxing

PROPERTIES: Antidepressant, antiseptic, antithyrotropic, antiviral, aromatic, carminative, diaphoretic, and nervine

SOURCES: Bulk Herb Store, Frontier Herbs, Mountain Rose Herbs, San Francisco Herb Company, Starwest Botanicals, Stony Mountain Botanicals

DOSAGE FORMS

WEAK INFUSION: Hot infusion, steeped 30 minutes; 8 ounces 1–4 times daily

COLD INFUSION: Steep 4–8 hours; 4–8 ounces 1–4 times daily

TINCTURE: Fresh leaf (1:2, 85% alcohol, 10% glycerin); dried leaf (1:5, 65% alcohol, 10% glycerin); 2–5 ml (0.4–1 tsp.) 3 times daily

GLYCERITE: Fresh leaf (1:6, 80% glycerin sealed simmer method); dried leaf (1:6); 2.5–10 ml (0.5–2 tsp.) 3 times daily

LICORICE

Latin name: *Glycyrrhiza glabra*

Licorice is a strong mucosal anti-inflammatory that can be used for gastric, esophageal, urinary, and respiratory inflammation. It eases dry coughs and sore throats when used as a tea or syrup. Licorice root helps to stabilize blood sugar levels and is useful in treating both hypoglycemia and diabetes. It is used in many traditional Chinese medicine formulations as a small part of the formula.

WARNINGS: Although licorice is a safe herb, some cautions are necessary when taking large doses for long periods of time. Licorice should be avoided in cases of high blood pressure or when taking digitalis. It causes retention of water and sodium and excretion of potassium, which can cause edema (water retention), high blood pressure, heart palpitations, or a slowing of the heartbeat. Vertigo (dizziness) and headaches are early symptoms of overuse of licorice. Taking a potassium supplement with licorice can help counteract some of these effects. These side effects are much more likely to occur when using licorice extracts or licorice-derived drugs than when taking whole licorice root. Deglycyrrhizinated licorice (DGL) is free of adverse effects. Use in pregnancy only under the supervision of a qualified herbalist or practitioner. Small quantities as part of a formula are okay during pregnancy.

ENERGETICS: Cooling and moistening

PROPERTIES: Adaptogen, anti-inflammatory, antitussive, demulcent (mucilant), and hypertensive

SOURCES: Bulk Herb Store, Frontier Herbs, Mountain Rose Herbs, San Francisco Herb Company, Starwest Botanicals, Stony Mountain Botanicals

DOSAGE FORMS

WEAK DECOCTION: 4–6 ounces 3 times daily

TINCTURE: Dried root (1:5, 40% alcohol); 1–5 ml (0.2–1 tsp.) 1–4 times daily

GLYCERITE: Dried root (1:5); 2.5–10 ml (0.5–2 tsp.) 1–4 times daily

CAPSULE: 500–1,000 mg up to 4 times daily

LILY OF THE VALLEY

Latin name: *Convallaria majalis*

Lily of the valley contains cardiac glycosides that affect the heart like digitalis but are less toxic. Lily of the valley normalizes heart action and increases blood pressure in hypotensive people. The crushed leaves of the fresh plant can be applied topically for drawing out infection and slivers.

WARNINGS: This toxic botanical is for professional use only. A toxic dose may cause nausea, vomiting, cardiac arrhythmias, hypertension, restlessness, trembling, confusion, weakness, depression, circulatory collapse, and death. Use formulas containing lily of the valley under professional supervision.

ENERGETICS: Warming

PROPERTIES: Cardiac, diuretic, and drawing

SPECIFIC INDICATIONS: Rolla Thomas: Painful cardiac affections, with difficulty breathing, excited heart action, palpitation, and dropsy.

SOURCES: Starwest Botanicals

DOSAGE FORMS

TINCTURE: Fresh root (1:2, 95% alcohol); freshly dried root (1:5, 65% alcohol); 5–20 drops up to 3 times daily

LINDEN

Latin name: *Tilia spp.*

Linden is a soothing nervine that relaxes tension and reduces blood pressure. It can be helpful for headaches. It is a very pleasant-tasting herbal tea and is a valuable but underused remedy.

WARNINGS: No known warnings

ENERGETICS: Cooling, drying, and relaxing

PROPERTIES: Antispasmodic, hypotensive, nervine, and relaxant

SOURCES: Frontier Herbs, Mountain Rose Herbs, Starwest Botanicals, Stony Mountain Botanicals

DOSAGE FORMS

STANDARD INFUSION: 8 ounces 1–4 times daily

TINCTURE: Dried leaf (1:5, 40% alcohol); 1–5 ml (0.2–1 tsp.) 2–4 times daily

LOBELIA

Latin name: *Lobelia inflata*

Lobelia is a powerful antispasmodic herb. It dilates the bronchial passages to ease asthma attacks and eases pain caused by tension. It helps to clear lymphatic congestion and can be applied topically to insect bites and stings.

WARNINGS: The FDA considers lobelia to be poisonous, and many sources claim it will cause convulsions, coma, and death. These are potential effects of its principal alkaloid lobeline, but there is no record of the whole herb causing these problems in anyone. Lobelia is an emetic and makes you throw up if you take too much. Lobelia can produce severe symptoms (nausea, profuse sweating, vomiting, and deep relaxation), but these symptoms typically pass quickly and the person feels better afterward. However, because of these effects, lobelia is not recommended for weak, debilitated persons or persons who are deeply relaxed. Lobelia is not recommended for long-term use and should be used cautiously during pregnancy. To avoid unpleasant effects such as nausea and vomiting, use small, repeated doses instead of large, infrequent doses, or use it as part of a formula.

ENERGETICS: Relaxing, slightly warming, and slightly drying

PROPERTIES: Acrid, anti-arrhythmic, antispasmodic, antitussive, bronchial dilator, emetic, expectorant, hypotensive, nervine, and vasodilator

SPECIFIC INDICATIONS: Rolla Thomas: Sense of fullness and oppression in precordial region; oppression of chest and difficult respiration; sharp, lancinating pain starting in heart and radiating to left shoulder and arm; mucus rattling in throat; full, oppressed pulse, weak pulse—stimulant doses, 10–20 drops at a single dose in angina pectoris; 10 drops in 4 ounces water in ordinary disease; combined with lavender for asthenic bronchitis of the child.

SOURCES: Bulk Herb Store, Mountain Rose Herbs, Starwest Botanicals, Stony Mountain Botanicals

DOSAGE FORMS

STRONG INFUSION: A strong infusion was traditionally used for emetic purposes, 2 ounces every few minutes.

TINCTURE: Fresh flowers and seeds (1:2, 95% alcohol); dried flowers and seeds (1:5, 65% alcohol, 5% vinegar); 5–20 drops as needed

GLYCERITE: Dried herb (1:6); 10–30 drops as needed

CAPSULE: ¼–1 capsule (100–400 mg) per dose. Hard to dose in capsule form, as 1 capsule is a fairly large dose.

TOPICAL USE: The tincture may be applied topically. An oil or salve preparation should use 95% alcohol as an intermediate solvent.

LOMATIUM

Latin name: *Lomatium dissectum*

Lomatium is a powerful antiviral and antiseptic and is useful for a wide variety of viral conditions. It is also beneficial for respiratory problems. Applied topically, it can ease pain and promote healing of wounds, sprains, cuts, and other injuries.

WARNINGS: Not for use during pregnancy. Discontinue if rash develops.

ENERGETICS: Cooling

PROPERTIES: Antiseptic and antiviral

SOURCES: Starwest Botanicals

DOSAGE FORMS

TINCTURE: Fresh root (1:2, 95% alcohol); dried root (1:5, 70% alcohol); 10–20 drops 3 times daily

MACA

Latin name: *Lepidium meyenii*

Maca is a rejuvenating tonic for reproductive health in both men and women. Scientific studies have shown that maca can be helpful for erectile dysfunction in men and for increasing sexual desire in women. Maca has adaptogenic and tonic properties.

WARNINGS: Maca can mildly inhibit thyroid function if there is a concurrent iodine deficiency.

ENERGETICS: Warming and nourishing

PROPERTIES: Testosterone-enhancing and tonic

SOURCES: Mountain Rose Herbs, Starwest Botanicals

DOSAGE FORMS

BULK POWDER: 1–4 tablespoons (5–20 grams) daily

MAITAKE

Latin name: *Grifola frondosa*

A powerful immune-enhancing mushroom, maitake is used to regulate the immune system. The beta glucans in maitake mushrooms activate and increase production of immune system cells such as macrophages, T-cells, natural killer cells, and neutrophils. These cells help the immune system to fight illness more quickly and efficiently. Maitake may help with diabetes, blood pressure, and cholesterol management.

WARNINGS: No known warnings

ENERGETICS: Drying and nourishing

PROPERTIES: Anticancer, antifungal, antiviral, hepatoprotective, immune amphoteric, and tonic

SOURCES: Mountain Rose Herbs, Starwest Botanicals

DOSAGE FORMS

FRESH: Dust fresh mushrooms with flour and pan-fry in butter and olive oil.

BULK DRIED: Put into soups and stews for a meaty, chicken-like flavor.

STANDARD DECOCTION: 4–8 ounces 1–4 times daily

MARSHMALLOW

Latin name: *Althaea officinalis*

Marshmallow is a mucilaginous herb that aids the bowels, mucous membranes, lungs, and kidneys. It soothes inflamed and irritated tissues and reduces swelling. Marshmallow is used in combination with other kidney herbs to soothe burning urination and inflamed kidneys and to ease the passing of kidney stones. It can ease respiratory congestion and dry coughs. It enriches breast milk in nursing mothers and is a mild, nourishing food.

WARNINGS: No known warnings. A very mild and safe remedy for children, infants, and elderly persons.

ENERGETICS: Cooling and moistening

PROPERTIES: Demulcent (mucilant), diuretic, emollient, galactagogue, nutritive, and vulnerary

SOURCES: Bulk Herb Store, Frontier Herbs, Mountain Rose Herbs, San Francisco Herb Company, Starwest Botanicals, Stony Mountain Botanicals

DOSAGE FORMS

BULK POWDER: Up to 12,000 mg daily

COLD INFUSION: 2–8 ounces 1–4 times daily

TINCTURE: Dried root (1:5, 40% alcohol); 10–60 drops 1–4 times daily. Mucilage does not extract well in alcohol; the tincture is used to soften hardened lymph nodes.

POWDER OR CAPSULES: 1,000–5,000 mg up to 3 times daily

MEADOWSWEET

Latin name: *Filipendula ulmaria*

Meadowsweet contains salicin, a compound similar to aspirin, but without the negative side effects. It's useful for reducing pain and inflammation, but it takes 6–8 hours to start acting. It settles the stomach and acts as a natural antacid. It also contains silica, which aids the skin, joints, and connective tissues.

WARNINGS: Because of its salicin content, some herbalists think meadowsweet should not be given to small children suffering with fevers from colds, flu, or chicken pox. It can cause nausea or vomiting in large doses.

ENERGETICS: Cooling and drying

PROPERTIES: Analgesic (anodyne), antacid, anti-inflammatory, and stomachic

SOURCES: Frontier Herbs, Mountain Rose Herbs, Starwest Botanicals, Stony Mountain Botanicals

DOSAGE FORMS

STANDARD INFUSION: 4–8 ounces 1–4 times daily

TINCTURE: Fresh leaf (1:2, 95% alcohol); dried leaf (1:5, 50% alcohol); 1–5 ml (0.2–1 tsp.) 1–4 times daily

POWDER OR CAPSULES: 1,000–2,000 mg up to 3 times daily

MILK THISTLE

Latin name: *Carduus marianus, syn. Silybum marianum*

There is good scientific evidence that the silymarin contained in milk thistle can protect the liver from various chemicals and toxins and aid in healing liver diseases. Milk thistle can prevent liver cell death from toxins like carbon tetrachloride and even the toxic effects of amanita (death cap) mushrooms. The flavonoids in milk thistle can increase the production of glutathione, a strong antioxidant.

WARNINGS: No known warnings

ENERGETICS: Moistening and cooling

PROPERTIES: Alterative (blood purifier), cholagogue, galactagogue, and hepatoprotective

SOURCES: Bulk Herb Store, Frontier Herbs, Mountain Rose Herbs, San Francisco Herb Company, Starwest Botanicals, Stony Mountain Botanicals

DOSAGE FORMS

TINCTURE: Dried seeds (1:3, 70% alcohol); 3–8 ml (0.6–1.6 tsp.) up to 4 times daily

STANDARDIZED EXTRACT: 140–180 mg silymarin 3 times daily

MIMOSA (ALBIZIA, SILK TREE)

Latin name: *Albizia julibrissin*

Mimosa is a traditional Chinese medicinal used to calm the spirit, relieve constriction and pain, invigorate the blood, and heal bone fractures. It is used to treat bad temper, depression, insomnia, irritability, and poor memory due to suppressed emotions. Modern Western herbalists use mimosa to relieve heartache, stress, and depression. Mimosa bark is mildly uplifting and grounding; it stretches energy upward and softens the heart. The flowers, on the other hand, concentrate energy in the head, causing mild euphoria and giddiness. It is an instant dose of feel-good that insists you take a walk in nature and enjoy life.

WARNINGS: Pregnant and breastfeeding women should avoid mimosa.

ENERGETICS: Cooling, moistening, and slightly relaxing

PROPERTIES: Antidepressant, calmative, euphoretic, relaxant, and vulnerary

DOSAGE FORMS

TINCTURE: Freshly dried flowers (1:2, 50% alcohol); dried bark (1:5, 50% alcohol); 10 drops to 5 ml (1 tsp.) 1–4 times daily

MISTLETOE

Latin name: *Viscum album*

Mistletoe is a powerful nervine. It is helpful for hypertension (without fluid retention), vasoconstrictive headaches, petit mal seizures, and tinnitus. In large doses, mistletoe induces hypertension. It is oxytocic and is used during labor to strengthen and normalize uterine contractions. Mistletoe is best mixed in small amounts with other nervines to increase the potency of sedative formulas.

WARNINGS: Use of this herb requires the supervision of a skilled herbalist or a physician.

Mistletoe may act as an abortifacient, so pregnant women should not take it. There have been some reports of ingestion of mistletoe leading to adverse reactions and even death in animals and small children; it was determined that the substance ingested in these cases was probably another species of mistletoe that is not used medicinally. Adults need not fear poisoning unless large amounts are ingested.

When mixed with prescription medicines that have a monoamine oxidase inhibitor (MAOI), mistletoe may cause a sudden drop in blood pressure. Mistletoe should not be taken with prescription blood pressure medications.

ENERGETICS: Relaxing

PROPERTIES: Cardiac, hypotensive, nervine, and sedative

SOURCES: Frontier Herbs, Mountain Rose Herbs, Stony Mountain Botanicals

DOSAGE FORMS

TINCTURE: Dried leaf (1:5, 50% alcohol); 15–30 drops 3 times daily

MOTHERWORT

Latin name: *Leonurus cardiaca*

Motherwort is a calming nervine used to lower blood pressure and as a remedy for heart problems that are related to the nervous system. It relieves anxiety and nervousness and contains glycosides that temporarily lower blood pressure and ease the strain on heart muscles. This also makes it useful for tachycardia, heart palpitations, and preventing heart disease. Motherwort is useful for hot flashes, menstrual cramps, scanty menstrual flow, and vaginal pain characterized by weakness, nervous irritability, and stress.

WARNINGS: Avoid during pregnancy and menstruation with excessive bleeding.

ENERGETICS: Cooling, drying, and relaxing

PROPERTIES: Anti-arrhythmic, cardiac, emmenagogue, hypotensive, sedative, and vasodilator

SOURCES: Frontier Herbs, Mountain Rose Herbs, Starwest Botanicals, Stony Mountain Botanicals

DOSAGE FORMS

STANDARD INFUSION: 2–4 ounces 1–4 times daily

TINCTURE: Fresh leaf (1:2, 95% alcohol); dried leaf (1:5, 60% alcohol); 1–4 ml (0.2–0.8 tsp.) 3 times daily

MUIRA PUAMA

Latin name: *Ptychopetalum olacoides*

Muira puama is a tonic that can help with impotency and performance anxiety in men as well as lack of desire in women. It was used by natives of the Amazon rain forest to promote sexual energy and arousal. It has a relaxing effect and eases neuromuscular pain and cramps, rheumatism, and poor circulation. It has been used for depression, nervous exhaustion, and some mild cases of paralysis.

WARNINGS: Not for use during pregnancy

ENERGETICS: Warming and relaxing

PROPERTIES: Antirheumatic, aphrodisiac, nervine, and tonic

SOURCES: Mountain Rose Herbs, Starwest Botanicals, Stony Mountain Botanicals

DOSAGE FORMS

COLD INFUSION: 3–6 ounces every morning

TINCTURE: Dried bark (1:5, 70% alcohol); 1–3 ml (0.2–0.6 tsp.) every morning

MULLEIN

Latin name: *Verbascum spp.*

Mullein leaves are most commonly used for respiratory complaints. They have a soothing, hydrating effect on the lungs and contain saponins that loosen mucus. Mullein is often used for chronic lung problems such as asthma and COPD, but is also helpful for colds and coughs, particularly dry coughs. Mullein flowers are used to make ear drops to soothe earache. Mullein root is specific for low back pain and inflammation.

WARNINGS: Mullein seeds contain the poisonous substance rotenone. Mullein leaf and flowers are generally regarded as safe.

ENERGETICS: Moistening and cooling

PROPERTIES: Demulcent (mucilant), expectorant, and lung tonic

SOURCES: Bulk Herb Store, Frontier Herbs, Mountain Rose Herbs, San Francisco Herb Company, Starwest Botanicals, Stony Mountain Botanicals

DOSAGE FORMS

STANDARD INFUSION: 4–8 ounces 2–4 times daily. Prepare leaves in this manner for lung issues.

TINCTURE: Fresh root (1:2, 95% alcohol); dried root (1:5, 65% alcohol); 10 drops to 3 ml (0.6 tsp.) 3 times daily for back issues

GLYCERITE: Dried leaf (1:8); 2.5–10 ml (0.5–2 tsp.) 3 times daily for lung issues

OIL: Fresh flowers (1:4, in olive oil); used as ear drops

MYRRH

Latin name: *Commiphora molmol, syn. C. myrrha*

Myrrh is an aromatic and bitter resin with antiseptic and disinfectant qualities. Myrrh combines well with goldenseal, echinacea, and other herbs for fighting infection. Like other antiseptic herbs, myrrh must come in contact with the bacteria to have an effect. It is especially helpful when used as a gargle, mouthwash, or liniment. Myrrh helps heal wounds, and can be blended with aloe vera gel to form a soothing topical wound protector. It is also a bitter tonic for digestion.

WARNINGS: Avoid taking internally while pregnant.

ENERGETICS: Warming and drying

PROPERTIES: Antibacterial, antiseptic, carminative, digestive tonic, and disinfectant

SPECIFIC INDICATIONS: Rolla Thomas: Increased secretion from mucous membranes, they being full and relaxed; full, oppressed pulse; imperfect circulation to surface and extremities.

SOURCES: Frontier Herbs, Mountain Rose Herbs, San Francisco Herb Company, Starwest Botanicals, Stony Mountain Botanicals

DOSAGE FORMS

TINCTURE: Resin (1:5, 95% alcohol); 5 drops to 2 ml (0.4 tsp.) 3 times daily

CAPSULE: 500 mg up to 3 times daily

NEEM

Latin name: *Azadirachta indica*

Neem is a popular remedy in India and has been called the village pharmacy tree because of its wide range of uses. It is strongly antimicrobial, antifungal, and anti-inflammatory. It's one of the best remedies for dysbiosis and gastrointestinal infections.

WARNINGS: Neem is not recommended for young children, the elderly, or the weak. Internal use should be for short periods (7–14 days) only.

ENERGETICS: Cooling and drying

PROPERTIES: Anti-inflammatory, antibacterial, and antifungal

SOURCES: Frontier Herbs, Starwest Botanicals, Stony Mountain Botanicals

DOSAGE FORMS

DRIED POWDER: 1–2 grams 2 times daily

CAPSULE: 1,000–2,000 mg, 2 times daily

TINCTURE: Dried leaf (1:5, 50% alcohol); 1–2 ml (0.2–0.4 tsp.) 2 times daily

NETTLE (STINGING)

Latin name: *Urtica dioica*

Nettles are a nourishing herbal food, rich in iron, calcium, magnesium, protein, and other nutrients. Nettles help to build healthy blood, bones, joints, and skin. Nettles are an excellent remedy for anemia, low blood pressure, and general weakness. They increase excretion of uric acid and help with rheumatism and gout. Nettles have anti-inflammatory and anti-allergenic properties, making them useful for respiratory allergies, asthma, and eruptive skin diseases. A blend of nettles, red raspberry, and alfalfa makes a great tonic tea for pregnancy.

Nettle seeds can slow, halt, or even partially reverse progressive renal failure. Studies have shown the root to improve benign prostatic hypertrophy (BPH) symptoms in 81% of men taking the herb (compared with 16% improvement in the placebo group).

WARNINGS: Nettle is extremely safe. The live plant can cause skin irritation (hence the name "stinging"), but the dried plant does not produce this effect.

ENERGETICS: Neutral and nourishing

PROPERTIES: Anti-allergenic, anti-inflammatory, antihistamine, diuretic, kidney tonic, mast cell stabilizer, mineralizer, and tonic

SPECIFIC INDICATIONS: Rolla Thomas: Chronic diarrhea or dysentery with evacuations of mucus; chronic inflammation of bladder with abundant mucus discharge.

SOURCES: Bulk Herb Store, Frontier Herbs, Mountain Rose Herbs, San Francisco Herb Company, Starwest Botanicals, Stony Mountain Botanicals

DOSAGE FORMS

STANDARD INFUSION: 8 ounces 1–4 times daily

TINCTURE (LEAF): Fresh leaf (1:2, 95% alcohol), 1–3 ml (0.2–0.6 tsp.) 3 times daily for allergies; dried leaf (1:4, 50% alcohol), 2–5 ml (0.4–1 tsp.) 3 times daily for the kidneys (tea works better)

TINCTURE (ROOT): Dried root (1:4, 50% alcohol); 1–3 ml (0.2–0.6 tsp.) 3 times daily for prostate issues

TINCTURE (SEED): Dried seed (1:4, 50% alcohol); 1–2 ml (0.2–0.4 tsp.) 3 times daily for the kidneys

GLYCERITE: Dried leaf (1:6); 10–20 ml (1–2 tsp.) 3 times daily for allergies and minerals

NIGHT BLOOMING CEREUS (CACTUS)

Latin name: *Selenicereus grandiflorus*

This species of cactus is used for all types of cardiopulmonary disorders, including angina, tachycardia, palpitations, and valvular disease. It has an effect similar to that of digitalis, but milder. It stimulates the action of the heart and has been used to aid recovery from heart attacks; night blooming cereus combines well with hawthorn and motherwort for this purpose. Cactus, rose, and mimosa combine well for people suffering from emotional heartbreak.

WARNINGS: Recommended for professional use only

ENERGETICS: Cooling

PROPERTIES: Anti-arrhythmic, cardiac, diuretic, relaxant, and sedative

SPECIFIC INDICATIONS: Felter: Impaired heart action, feeble, irregular, or tumultuous, with mental depression, apprehension, and precordial oppression.

DOSAGE FORMS

TINCTURE: Fresh stem (1:2, 95% alcohol); 1–15 drops in a little water 1–4 times daily

NOPAL (PRICKLY PEAR)

Latin name: *Opuntia streptacantha, O. ficus-indica*

Nopal is helpful for type 2 diabetes (reducing blood sugar) and has a very low glycemic index. It contains potent antioxidants to reduce inflammation, which is a primary driver of most chronic diseases. The warmed pads make wonderful poultices for infected wounds; make sure to place the goopy inside in contact with the skin. Be sure to remove the smooth, fixed spines and the small, hair-like prickles called glochids before using nopal. Nopal pads are available in many Mexican grocery stores.

WARNINGS: No known warnings

ENERGETICS: Cooling and moistening

PROPERTIES: Analgesic (anodyne), anti-inflammatory, and antidiabetic

SOURCES: Starwest Botanicals

DOSAGE FORMS

POWDER OR CAPSULES: 1,000–2,000 mg up to 3 times daily

TOPICAL USE: Remove the spines from the pads with a sharp knife or potato peeler. Remove remaining glochids by holding the pad over a flame. Cut the pad in half, apply warm, and secure in place. Change as needed. The flesh can also be dried on a fruit leather tray in a dehydrator and powdered; reconstitute with water for an instant demulcent.

OAT

Latin name: *Avena sativa*

The milky (unripe) seeds of the oat grain are used as a remedy for a depleted nervous system. Milky oats is a tonic that combines well with almost every other nervine. It works best for people with mental and physical exhaustion who are irritable and lack focus. They may also experience heart palpitations and loss of libido. Milky oats are used to support recovery from drug addiction.

Like horsetail, oat straw is rich in silica. It is used as a mineralizer and a mild nervine. Oat bran is used as a bulk laxative and an agent to help lower cholesterol.

WARNINGS: Use cautiously with gluten sensitivity or allergy.

ENERGETICS: Neutral, moistening, and nourishing

PROPERTIES: Bulk laxative, mineralizer, and nerve tonic

SPECIFIC INDICATIONS: Rolla Thomas: Sleeplessness with irritability, nervous prostration due to mental strain, headache, melancholia, and hysteria.

SOURCES: Bulk Herb Store, Frontier Herbs, Mountain Rose Herbs, San Francisco Herb Company, Starwest Botanicals, Stony Mountain Botanicals

DOSAGE FORMS

STANDARD INFUSION: 4–8 ounces 1–4 times daily

TINCTURE: Fresh seed (1:2, 95% alcohol); 10–30 drops 3–5 times daily

GLYCERITE: Dried green oat straw (1:6); 10–20 ml (1–2 tsp.) 3 times daily

OCOTILLO

Latin name: *Fouquieria splendens*

Ocotillo is a plant from the deserts of the Southwest. It is used for glandular and lymphatic inflammation. It moves fluid through the lymphatic system and acts more strongly on the lymphatic vessels in the abdomen and reproductive organs than other herbs.

WARNINGS: Not for use during pregnancy

ENERGETICS: Cooling and slightly drying

PROPERTIES: Antidiarrheal, astringent, and lymphatic

DOSAGE FORMS

TINCTURE: Fresh bark (1:2, 95% alcohol); 10–30 drops up to 4 times daily

OLIVE

Latin name: *Olea europaea*

The leaf of the olive tree is used, along with other herbs, to treat high blood pressure and angina. Olive leaf is widely recommended as a broad-spectrum antiviral and antibacterial agent, but its antimicrobial effects are mild at best and other herbs should be considered first.

Olive oil is nutritious and helps to lower cholesterol. It is often used with lemon juice as a natural therapy for gallstones. Olive oil is often used as a base for herbal salves and ointments.

WARNINGS: No known warnings

ENERGETICS: Cooling, drying, and slightly relaxing

PROPERTIES: Antiviral and hypotensive

SOURCES: Bulk Herb Store, Frontier Herbs, Mountain Rose Herbs, Starwest Botanicals, Stony Mountain Botanicals

DOSAGE FORMS

STANDARD INFUSION: 4–8 ounces 1–4 times daily

TINCTURE: Dried leaf (1:5, 60% alcohol); 2–3 ml (0.2–0.6 tsp.) 3 times daily

CAPSULE: 500–1,000 mg, 2 times daily with meals

ORANGE PEEL

Latin name: *Citrus sinensis*

Orange peel is aromatic and bitter; it stimulates appetite and digestion and is found in many respiratory formulas.

WARNINGS: Orange peel is contraindicated with fluid loss and excessive thirst. Use cautiously during pregnancy. Use only organic orange peel when making extracts.

ENERGETICS: Warming and drying

PROPERTIES: Aromatic, bitter, carminative, decongestant, and digestive tonic

SOURCES: Bulk Herb Store, Mountain Rose Herbs, San Francisco Herb Company, Starwest Botanicals, Stony Mountain Botanicals

DOSAGE FORMS

TINCTURE: Fresh peel (1:2, 95% alcohol, 10% glycerin); dried peel (1:5, 65% alcohol, 10% glycerin); 1–2 ml (0.2–0.4 tsp.) up to 3 times daily

GLYCERITE: Dried peel (1:6); 2–4 ml (0.4–0.8 tsp.) up to 3 times daily

OREGANO

Latin name: *Origanum vulgare*

Oregano is antiseptic and useful for infections of the respiratory and digestive tracts. It is a good remedy for fungal infections, coughs, tonsillitis, bronchitis, asthma, and chest congestion. The oil of oregano can be added to bath water or a steamer to clear the lungs.

WARNINGS: Oregano should be avoided in large quantities during pregnancy. Oregano essential oil is toxic to the liver and should not be used internally.

ENERGETICS: Warming and drying

PROPERTIES: Antifungal, antimicrobial, aromatic, and expectorant

SOURCES: Bulk Herb Store, Mountain Rose Herbs, San Francisco Herb Company, Stony Mountain Botanicals

DOSAGE FORMS

WEAK INFUSION: 2–4 ounces 1–4 times daily

TINCTURE: Dried leaf (1:5, 65% alcohol, 10% glycerin); 1–2 ml (0.2–0.4 tsp.) 3–4 times daily

GLYCERITE: Fresh leaf (1:8, 80% glycerin sealed simmer method); dried leaf (1:6); 1–2 ml (0.2–0.4 tsp.) 3–4 times daily

OREGON GRAPE

Latin name: *Berberis repens, B. aquifolium*

Oregon grape is often used as an alternative to goldenseal. Oregon grape has antimicrobial properties and is a good lymphatic cleansing herb. It stimulates bile flow and is used with other alteratives to help the liver. It can be used both internally and externally to relieve skin conditions such as acne, boils, and eczema, and may reduce itching.

WARNINGS: Not for use with emaciation or weak digestion. Use with caution during pregnancy.

ENERGETICS: Cooling and drying

PROPERTIES: Alterative (blood purifier), antiseptic, cholagogue, and lymphatic

SOURCES: Frontier Herbs, Mountain Rose Herbs, Starwest Botanicals, Stony Mountain Botanicals

TINCTURE: Dried root (1:5, 45% alcohol); 5 drops to 4 ml (0.8 tsp.) 3 times daily

GLYCERITE: Dried root (1:5); 2–5 ml (0.4–1 tsp.) 3 times daily

OSHA

Latin name: *Ligusticum porteri*

Osha is a great remedy for viral infections such as the common cold, flu, sore throats, and upper respiratory congestion. It stimulates the digestive and immune systems and expels mucus. It is used for settling the stomach after vomiting and can be used with eyebright to prevent and treat earaches in children.

Osha has been overharvested in the wild, and is very difficult if not impossible to cultivate. It is on the United Plant Savers at-risk list. Pine, grindelia, and ginger combined together make a nice replacement for osha. Until populations in the wild are stabilized, please limit your use of this wonderful plant.

WARNINGS: Not for use during pregnancy

ENERGETICS: Warming and drying

PROPERTIES: Antiviral, decongestant, and expectorant

SOURCES: Mountain Rose Herbs, Starwest Botanicals

DOSAGE FORMS

TINCTURE: Fresh root (1:2, 85% alcohol, 10% glycerin); dried root (1:5, 60% alcohol, 10% glycerin); 1–3 ml (0.2–0.6 tsp.) 1–4 times daily

SYRUP: Fresh root (1:2, in 100% honey); 2.5–10 ml (0.5–2 tsp.) 1–4 times daily

PAPAYA

Latin name: *Carica papaya*

Papaya fruit contains enzymes that help digest proteins. The seeds of papaya are a strong antiparasitic.

WARNINGS: No known warnings

ENERGETICS: Cooling and nourishing

PROPERTIES: Antiparasitic and digestant

SOURCES: Mountain Rose Herbs, Starwest Botanicals

DOSAGE FORMS

TINCTURE: Fresh seeds (1:2, 95% alcohol); 2–5 ml (0.4–1 tsp.) 3 times daily

PARSLEY

Latin name: *Petroselinum crispum*

Parsley is rich in sodium and potassium, which are necessary to regulate fluids in the body. It has a volatile oil that stimulates kidney function. Parsley helps to lower blood pressure and slow the pulse.

WARNINGS: Not recommended in cases involving fluid deficiency, wasting, or dryness. It is used to dry up breast milk, so it should be avoided while breastfeeding.

ENERGETICS: Slightly warming, slightly drying, and nourishing

PROPERTIES: Antigalactagogue, diuretic, and nutritive

SOURCES: Mountain Rose Herbs, San Francisco Herb Company, Starwest Botanicals, Stony Mountain Botanicals

DOSAGE FORMS

FRESH HERB: Can be eaten raw or cooked

STANDARD INFUSION: 4–8 ounces 1–4 times daily

TINCTURE: Fresh leaf (1:2, 95% alcohol); dried leaf (1:5, 65% alcohol); 2–4 ml (0.4–0.8 tsp.) 3 times daily

POWDER OR CAPSULES: 1,000–2,000 mg up to 3 times daily

PARTRIDGE BERRY

Latin name: *Mitchella repens*

Partridge berry was traditionally taken as a tea by Native American women during pregnancy. It was used to ease the difficulties of pregnancy in the later stages and to make childbirth fast and easy. Partridge berry salve, applied after breastfeeding, works wonders to heal sore nipples. Partridge berry tones the uterus, which eases painful, heavy menstruation and regulates periods of irregularity.

WARNINGS: No known warnings

ENERGETICS: Warming and drying

PROPERTIES: Emmenagogue and uterine tonic

SPECIFIC INDICATIONS: Rolla Thomas: Uneasy sensations in the pelvis, with dragging, tenderness on pressure, frequent desire to pass urine, and difficulty of evacuation.

SOURCES: Mountain Rose Herbs, Starwest Botanicals, Stony Mountain Botanicals

DOSAGE FORMS

STANDARD INFUSION: 2–4 ounces 3 times daily

TINCTURE: Fresh plant (1:2, 95% alcohol); dried herb (1:5, 50% alcohol); 2–5 ml (0.4–1 tsp.) 3 times daily

PASSIONFLOWER

Latin name: *Passiflora incarnata, P. quadrangularis*

Passionflower is a relaxing nervine, often combined with other nervines to reduce stress and tension and to aid sleep. It helps to quiet mental chatter. Passionflower is used for restless agitation and exhaustion, with or without muscular twitching and spasms.

WARNINGS: No known warnings

ENERGETICS: Cooling and relaxing

PROPERTIES: Nervine, relaxant, and sedative

SPECIFIC INDICATIONS: Rolla Thomas: Irritation of brain and nervous system; sleeplessness; in fact, wherever a harmless and certain soporific is demanded; in convulsions of childhood; nervous headache and neuralgia; infantile nervous irritation, tetanus, and in epilepsy.

SOURCES: Bulk Herb Store, Frontier Herbs, Mountain Rose Herbs, San Francisco Herb Company, Starwest Botanicals, Stony Mountain Botanicals

DOSAGE FORMS

STANDARD INFUSION: 4–8 ounces up to 4 times daily

TINCTURE: Fresh leaf (1:2, 95% alcohol); dried leaf (1:5, 50% alcohol); 2–8 ml (0.4–1.6 tsp.) up to 4 times daily

GLYCERITE: Dried leaf (1:6); 3–10 ml (0.6–2 tsp.) up to 4 times daily

FLUID EXTRACT: Dried leaf (1:1, 50% alcohol); 1–3 ml (0.2–0.6 tsp.) up to 4 times daily

PAU D'ARCO

Latin name: *Tabebuia impetiginosa, T. avellanedae, T. ipe, T. cassinoides, Tecoma ochracea*

Pau d'arco is commonly used as an anticancer and antifungal remedy. It may be helpful for fighting infections in the digestive tract, both bacterial and fungal. Its active constituents include lapachol and beta-lapachone, which have demonstrated potent antifungal properties in laboratory tests.

WARNINGS: Contraindicated for blood clotting disorders. Not for use by pregnant women. Side effects with high doses may include nausea, vomiting, intestinal discomfort, and anticoagulant effects.

ENERGETICS: Drying and slightly cooling

PROPERTIES: Alterative (blood purifier), anticancer, antifungal, antiseptic, and astringent

SOURCES: Bulk Herb Store, Frontier Herbs, Mountain Rose Herbs, San Francisco Herb Company, Starwest Botanicals, Stony Mountain Botanicals

DOSAGE FORMS

COLD INFUSION: 4–8 ounces up to 4 times daily

TINCTURE: Dried bark (1:5, 50% alcohol); 3–8 ml (0.6–1.6 tsp.) 3 times daily

FLUID EXTRACT: Dried bark (1:1, 50% alcohol); 1–2 ml (0.2–0.4 tsp.) up to 4 times daily

PENNYROYAL

Latin name: *Mentha pulegium*

Pennyroyal tea produces sweating and is useful for fevers and flu. The essential oil, well diluted, is used externally as a mosquito repellent. The herb can be used to regulate menstruation and reduce cramping.

WARNINGS: Pennyroyal may cause miscarriage; avoid during pregnancy. Pennyroyal essential oil has caused a number of deaths when ingested. It should not be used internally under any circumstances.

ENERGETICS: Warming, drying, and relaxing

PROPERTIES: Antispasmodic and diaphoretic

SOURCES: Frontier Herbs, San Francisco Herb Company, Starwest Botanicals, Stony Mountain Botanicals

DOSAGE FORMS

WEAK INFUSION: 4–8 ounces up to 4 times daily

TINCTURE: Fresh leaf (1:2, 95% alcohol); recently dried leaf (1:5, 50% alcohol); 1–2 ml (0.2–0.4 tsp.) in hot water

PEONY

Latin name: *Paeonia lactiflora*

Peony is used as a tonic for women in traditional Chinese medicine, commonly blended with rehmannia, dong quai, and osha. It is also used for abdominal pain, for amenorrhea, and to move blood. Peony builds the blood and can ease hot flashes or night sweats. It can also relieve abdominal cramps and pain.

ENERGETICS: Cooling and relaxing

PROPERTIES: Alterative (blood purifier), analgesic (anodyne), anti-inflammatory, and antispasmodic

DOSAGE FORMS

STANDARD DECOCTION: 1–4 ounces up to 4 times daily

TINCTURE: Fresh root (1:2, 95% alcohol); dried root (1:5, 60% alcohol); 10 drops to 1 ml (0.2 tsp.) up to 4 times daily

PEPPERMINT

Latin name: *Mentha × piperita*

Peppermint is a soothing aromatic with primary effects on the nervous system, stomach, and colon. It is an excellent ingredient in formulas for acute ailments. It settles the stomach, expels gas, and has a mild palliative effect on colds, fevers, and headaches.

WARNINGS: Peppermint can increase heartburn and symptoms of gastroesophageal reflux disease in some people.

ENERGETICS: Cooling and drying

PROPERTIES: Antacid, anti-emetic (antinauseous), aromatic, carminative, diaphoretic, and digestive tonic

SOURCES: Bulk Herb Store, Frontier Herbs, Mountain Rose Herbs, San Francisco Herb Company, Starwest Botanicals, Stony Mountain Botanicals

DOSAGE FORMS

STANDARD INFUSION: 4–8 ounces 1–4 times daily

TINCTURE: Dried leaf (1:5, 50% alcohol, 10% glycerin); 1–3 ml (0.2–0.6 tsp.) 3 times daily

GLYCERITE: Fresh leaf (1:8, 80% glycerin sealed simmer method); dried leaf (1:8); 10–20 ml (1–2 tsp.) 3–4 times daily

PERIWINKLE (LESSER)

Latin name: *Vinca minor*

Periwinkle increases blood flow and oxygen to the brain. It is used for migraines due to vasoconstriction. Clinical studies suggest periwinkle may be helpful in treating dementia, Alzheimer's disease, short-term memory loss caused by some medications, high blood pressure, age-related hearing loss, and vertigo, and reducing calcium buildup from dialysis. Periwinkle can also help stop internal bleeding.

WARNINGS: Do not use during pregnancy. Avoid with low blood pressure and liver and kidney diseases. Periwinkle is best used under professional supervision.

ENERGETICS: Drying and relaxing

PROPERTIES: Astringent, hypotensive, sedative, and styptic

SOURCES: Mountain Rose Herbs, Starwest Botanicals, Stony Mountain Botanicals

DOSAGE FORMS

WEAK INFUSION: 2–4 ounces up to 3 times daily

TINCTURE: Fresh leaf (1:2, 95% alcohol); dried leaf (1:5, 50% alcohol); 5 drops to 1 ml (0.2 tsp.) up to 3 times daily

PINE (WHITE)

Latin name: *Pinus strobus and other species*

Pine bark is used primarily as an expectorant for coughs. It helps discharge mucus and fight infection. It is particularly helpful in cases of chronic bronchitis, and for coaxing old, thick, green mucus up and out of the lungs and sinuses.

Pine gum is a good agent for wound healing and drawing out pus and slivers. Pine pollen also strengthens muscles and tendons and helps tissue regeneration and repair. The pollen contains testosterone and is used as a male glandular tonic.

WARNINGS: No known warnings

ENERGETICS: Warming and drying

PROPERTIES: Antiseptic, aromatic, drawing, expectorant, and testosterone-enhancing

DOSAGE FORMS

STANDARD INFUSION: Fresh or dried needles; 4–8 ounces 1–4 times daily

TINCTURE: Gum (1:2, 95% alcohol); 10 drops to 1 ml (0.2 tsp.) up to 4 times daily

GLYCERITE: Gum (1:4); dried or fresh bark (1:8); 10–20 ml (1–2 tsp.) 3–4 times daily

PIPSISSEWA

Latin name: *Chimaphila umbellata*

Antibacterial and astringent, pipsissewa is used primarily for urinary problems involving inflammation, such as cystitis, prostatitis, and urethritis. It is a great remedy for irritable bladder. It has the same urinary disinfectant compounds as uva ursi, but pipsissewa has less tannin, which makes it easier on the kidneys.

WARNINGS: No known warnings

ENERGETICS: Cooling and drying

PROPERTIES: Antiseptic and diuretic

SOURCES: Mountain Rose Herbs, Starwest Botanicals

DOSAGE FORMS

STANDARD INFUSION: 4–8 ounces 1–4 times daily

TINCTURE: Fresh leaf (1:2, 95% alcohol); dried leaf (1:5, 50% alcohol); 1–2 ml (0.2–0.4 tsp.) 3 times daily

PLANTAIN

Latin name: *Plantago major*

This common lawn and garden weed is a valuable remedy for bruises, insect bites, and injuries when applied topically. Plantain is used internally for ulcers, inflammatory bowel disorders, and coughs. It is helpful for drawing sticky phlegm out of the lungs, especially when combined with grindelia.

WARNINGS: No known warnings

ENERGETICS: Cooling, moistening, and slightly constricting

PROPERTIES: Antiseptic, antivenomous, astringent, decongestant, demulcent (mucilant), drawing, emollient, and vulnerary

SPECIFIC INDICATIONS: King: Nocturnal enuresis in children, with pale, abundant urine, irritation and relaxation of sphincter vesicae.

SOURCES: Bulk Herb Store, Mountain Rose Herbs, Starwest Botanicals, Stony Mountain Botanicals

DOSAGE FORMS

FRESH HERB: Crush fresh leaves and use as a poultice.

STANDARD INFUSION: 4–8 ounces 1–4 times daily

TINCTURE: Fresh leaf (1:2, 95% alcohol); 2–5 ml (0.4–1 tsp.) up to 4 times daily

OIL AND SALVE: Dried leaf (1:4); use oil to make a salve for topical use.

TOPICAL USE: Use the standard infusion as a compress.

PLEURISY ROOT

Latin name: *Asclepias tuberosa*

Native Americans used pleurisy root for ailments relating to the heart, bronchials, and lungs. As its name implies, it is one of the best remedies for pleurisy. It eases chest pain and is good for hot, dry conditions of the chest. Pleurisy root is an excellent diaphoretic: it relaxes the peripheral capillaries and increases perspiration.

WARNINGS: Excessive doses may cause vomiting. Not recommended for use during pregnancy.

ENERGETICS: Cooling and moistening

PROPERTIES: Anti-inflammatory, diaphoretic, diuretic, and expectorant

SPECIFIC INDICATIONS: Felter: Skin hot, but inclined to moisture, face flushed, vascular excitement of bronchial region, scanty urine; serous or synovial inflammation.

SOURCES: Mountain Rose Herbs, Starwest Botanicals

DOSAGE FORMS

COLD INFUSION: 1–4 ounces 3 times daily

TINCTURE: Dried root (1:5, 50% alcohol); 5 drops to 1 ml (0.2 tsp.) up to 4 times daily

POKE ROOT

Latin name: *Phytolacca decandra*

Poke root is a traditional antitumor remedy that is also used to clear the lymphatic system. It is antiviral and an immune stimulant. Poke root oil is used topically for swollen lymph nodes, mastitis, or breast cancer. Its use is similar to, though stronger than, that of castor oil packs. A tincture of the berries or root is used internally in small doses for severe lymphatic congestion and mastitis.

WARNINGS: The main toxic compounds in poke are the pokeweed mitogen (lectins) and the glycoside saponin, along with the alkaloid phytolaccin. The alkaloids are mucosal irritants and mitogenic, and they affect the medulla in the brain, causing paralysis, bradycardia, decreased respiration, and decreased skeletal muscle coordination. The alkaloids can build up in the body for up to 2 weeks. If any toxic effects are noticed, stop the use of this herb immediately. Toxic effects include: vomiting, diarrhea, nausea, stomach cramps, dizziness, hypotension, decreased respiration, and headaches. Avoid use for those with kidney disease. For professional use only, because of its toxicity, especially internally. Not for use during pregnancy.

ENERGETICS: Cooling

PROPERTIES: Alterative (blood purifier), anti-inflammatory, anticancer, immune stimulant, and lymphatic

SPECIFIC INDICATIONS: Fyfe: Enlargement and inflammation of glandular structures; mucous membranes pallid. Impaired glandular secretion and function.

SOURCES: Mountain Rose Herbs, Starwest Botanicals

DOSAGE FORMS

TINCTURE: Recently dried root (1:10, 45% alcohol); 1–10 drops up to 3 times daily. Take no more than 10 ml a week.

OIL: Fresh roots (1:4). Caution: Wear rubber gloves while chopping and handling roots. Macerate for 6 weeks.

POLYGALA

Latin name: *Polygala tenuifolia*

Polygala is an underutilized traditional Chinese medicine remedy for anxiety and fear. Its effects are stronger than those of many commonly used anxiolytics, and it's a valuable addition to nerve sedative formulas. It is beneficial for stress-induced memory loss, and initial studies show promising benefits in age-related cognitive decline and Alzheimer's disease.

WARNINGS: Large doses can cause nausea and vomiting. Not for use by people who have gastritis or ulcers. Not for use during pregnancy.

ENERGETICS: Warming and drying

DOSAGE FORMS

TINCTURE: Dried root (1:5, 50% alcohol); 1–2 ml (0.2–0.4 tsp.) 3 times daily

PRICKLY ASH

Latin name: *Zanthoxylum americanum*

Prickly ash increases peripheral circulation and is indicated for people with cold extremities or Raynaud's disease. It is used for peripheral neuropathies or sciatica with damaged, numb, tingling, or extremely painful nerves that cause a person to writhe in agony.

WARNINGS: Not recommended during pregnancy

ENERGETICS: Warming and drying

PROPERTIES: Alterative (blood purifier), analgesic (anodyne), carminative, diaphoretic, and circulatory stimulant

SPECIFIC INDICATIONS: Felter: Relaxation of mucosa with hypersecretion. Atony of nervous system. Tympanites, gastrointestinal torpor, with deficient secretion; dryness of mouth and fauces.

SOURCES: Mountain Rose Herbs, Starwest Botanicals, Stony Mountain Botanicals

STANDARD DECOCTION: 1–3 ounces 3 times daily

TINCTURE: Dried bark (1:5, 65% alcohol); 5 drops to 1 ml (0.2 tsp.) 3 times daily before meals

PROPOLIS

Propolis is not an herb; it is a plant resin collected by bees. It is warming and stimulating. It has powerful antibiotic and immune-enhancing effects. Its antimicrobial activity is due largely to its richness in phenolic aglycones.

WARNINGS: Avoid propolis if you have bee allergies.

ENERGETICS: Warming and drying

PROPERTIES: Antibacterial, antifungal, expectorant, and immune amphoteric

DOSAGE FORMS

TINCTURE: Propolis gum (1:5, 95% alcohol); 5 drops to 2 ml (0.4 tsp.) up to 5 times daily. Spray directly onto tonsils or wound to create a resinous covering like a liquid Band-Aid. Give in a little honey for internal use. Don't give in water.

POWDER OR CAPSULES: 1,000–2,000 mg up to 3 times daily

PSYLLIUM

Latin name: *Plantago spp.*

Psyllium is a mucilaginous herb used as a bulk laxative, as an antidiarrhea remedy, or to soothe intestinal irritation. It is best taken first thing in the morning or right before going to bed. Take before meals to help regulate appetite and blood sugar. It also helps to lower cholesterol. Always take psyllium with plenty of water or other liquids.

WARNINGS: Psyllium is a mild laxative, suitable for use by children, by the elderly, and during pregnancy, but should be avoided in cases of bowel obstruction or perforations. It can cause constipation when a person is dehydrated.

ENERGETICS: Cooling and moistening

PROPERTIES: Absorbent, antidiarrheal, demulcent (mucilant), and bulk laxative

SOURCES: Bulk Herb Store, Frontier Herbs, Mountain Rose Herbs, San Francisco Herb Company, Starwest Botanicals, Stony Mountain Botanicals

DOSAGE FORMS

POWDER OR CAPSULES: 1,000–5,000 mg up to 3 times daily mixed with water or juice. Drink a large glass of water after consuming.

PULSATILLA

Latin name: *Pulsatilla vulgaris*

Pulsatilla helps promote restful sleep and counteract feeling overwrought, over-emotional, high strung, and nervous. It helps with shock, despondency, imagined fears of impending danger, depression, PMS, spontaneous crying, and related emotional states. It's also helpful for stress-induced headaches and headaches associated with menstruation.

WARNINGS: Pulsatilla is a strong gastric irritant, and overdoses cause violent gastroenteritis, vomiting, and diarrhea. Overdoses can also cause elevated heart rate, anxiety, and convulsions. This herb is recommended for use by professionals only. Not for use during pregnancy or lactation.

ENERGETICS: Cooling and drying

PROPERTIES: Antidepressant, antirheumatic, and nervine

SPECIFIC INDICATIONS: Felter: Nervousness with despondency, sadness, and disposition to weep, without being able to tell why, or to weep while asleep; unnatural fear; fear of impending danger or death; insomnia, with nervous exhaustion; pain, with debility; headache, with nervousness, not dependent on determination of blood to the head; amenorrhea with chilliness and mental depression; dysmenorrhea, with gloomy mentality and chilliness; pasty, creamy, or white coating upon the tongue, with greasy taste; thick, bland, and inoffensive mucus discharges; alternating constipation and diarrhea, with venous congestion.

DOSAGE FORMS

TINCTURE: Freshly dried herb (1:5, 50% alcohol); 1–3 drops 3 times daily diluted in water, or as a small part of a formula

PYGEUM BARK

Latin name: *Pygeum africanum, P. gardneri*

Pygeum is a urinary remedy from Africa that has been found to be helpful for prostate swelling. It is most often used in combination with other herbs.

WARNINGS: No known warnings

ENERGETICS: Cooling

PROPERTIES: Anti-inflammatory and diuretic

DOSAGE FORMS

TINCTURE: Dried bark (1:5, 50% alcohol); 1–2 ml (0.2–0.4 tsp.) 3 times daily

POWDER OR CAPSULES: 1,000–2,000 mg up to 3 times daily

QUASSIA

Latin name: *Picrasma excelsa*

Quassia is traditionally used for parasites, anorexia, and dyspepsia. It helps suppress pathogenic gut bacteria and stimulates the entire digestive process. It is often used in combination with other gastric antimicrobial herbs like andrographis and barberry.

WARNINGS: Excessive doses of the bark may cause irritation of the digestive tract and vomiting. Quassia should not be used during pregnancy.

ENERGETICS: Cooling and drying

PROPERTIES: Antibacterial, antispasmodic, and antiviral

SOURCES: San Francisco Herb Company, Starwest Botanicals

DOSAGE FORMS

COLD INFUSION: 2–4 ounces 3 times daily

TINCTURE: Dried bark (1:5, 50% alcohol); 1–3 ml (0.2–0.6 tsp.) 3 times daily

RED CLOVER

Latin name: *Trifolium pratense*

Red clover is a pleasant-tasting blood purifier that is used in combination with other blood purifiers for skin conditions, cancer, swollen lymph glands, and liver detoxification. Red clover contains phytoestrogens that block estrogen receptor sites, possibly inhibiting estrogen-dependent cancers.

WARNINGS: Due to its phytoestrogen content, some herbalists recommend avoiding red clover during pregnancy.

ENERGETICS: Cooling and balancing

PROPERTIES: Alterative (blood purifier), lymphatic, and phytoestrogen

SPECIFIC INDICATIONS: Rolla Thomas: An infusion of red clover has a specific influence in spasmodic cough, whooping cough, and the cough of measles.

SOURCES: Bulk Herb Store, Frontier Herbs, Mountain Rose Herbs, San Francisco Herb Company, Starwest Botanicals, Stony Mountain Botanicals

DOSAGE FORMS

STANDARD INFUSION: 4–8 ounces 3 times daily

TINCTURE: Recently dried flower (1:5, 40% alcohol); 1–5 ml (0.2–1 tsp.) 3 times daily

GLYCERITE: Dried flowers (1:8); 5–10 ml (1–2 tsp.) up to 3 times daily

RED RASPBERRY

Latin name: *Rubus idaeus*

Red raspberry leaves are rich in manganese, an essential element for oxygenation of the cells. It is used as a tonic to strengthen the uterine muscles in preparation for childbirth. It also helps to relieve and prevent morning sickness.

The berries contain anthocyanin, a compound found to contribute to heart health, protect the eyes, guard against cancer, and help protect against diabetes.

WARNINGS: No known warnings

ENERGETICS: Cooling, slightly drying, and slightly constricting

PROPERTIES: Antacid, anti-emetic (antinauseous), antidiarrheal, and uterine tonic

SOURCES: Bulk Herb Store, Stony Mountain Botanicals

DOSAGE FORMS

STANDARD INFUSION: 4–8 ounces 3 times daily

GLYCERITE: Dried leaves (1:8); 10–30 ml (1–3 tsp.) 3 times daily

CAPSULES: 1,000–2,000 mg, 3 times daily

RED ROOT

Latin name: *Ceanothus americanus*

A powerful lymphatic cleanser, red root helps to shrink swollen lymph nodes and reduce an enlarged spleen. Combined with echinacea, it works well for tonsillitis, cysts, and infections in the lymph glands. It is very good for AIDS patients with a low platelet count, enlarged spleen, or swollen lymph nodes.

WARNINGS: Not for use during acute inflammation of the spleen

ENERGETICS: Drying and constricting

PROPERTIES: Astringent and lymphatic

SPECIFIC INDICATIONS: Felter: Gastric and hepatic disorders with splenic hypertrophy, expressionless countenance; sallow, doughy skin. Catarrhal conditions with profuse mucus flow. Antihemorrhagic.

SOURCES: Mountain Rose Herbs, Starwest Botanicals

DOSAGE FORMS

STANDARD DECOCTION: 2–4 ounces 3 times daily

TINCTURE: Dried bark (1:5, 50% alcohol); 1–3 ml (0.2–0.6 tsp.) 3 times daily

REHMANNIA

Latin name: *Rehmannia glutinosa*

This Chinese herb is used to cool the blood, reduce fever, and rebuild the blood from blood loss. It is also a liver and kidney tonic.

WARNINGS: Contraindicated with loss of appetite and diarrhea.

ENERGETICS: Cooling and nourishing

PROPERTIES: Antibacterial, blood building, and immune amphoteric

SOURCES: Mountain Rose Herbs, Starwest Botanicals

DOSAGE FORMS

TINCTURE: Dried root (1:5, 50% alcohol); 1–3 ml (0.2–0.6 tsp.) up to 3 times daily

REISHI (GANODERMA)

Latin name: *Ganoderma lucidum*

Reishi is a medicinal mushroom that has been shown to have immune-enhancing effects as well as acting as a general health tonic. Research suggests that reishi relaxes muscles, improves sleep, eases chronic pain, aids heart function, reduces cholesterol, and has antioxidant effects. Alcohol is the preferred menstruum for extraction of the relaxing and anxiolytic properties. Decoction is preferred for immune support. Dual extracts can be used, but these do not work as well as using either alcohol or water extracts separately.

WARNINGS: This herb is generally regarded as safe and nontoxic. However, it may be contraindicated with fluid deficiency and dryness.

ENERGETICS: Balancing, slightly warming, and nourishing

PROPERTIES: Adaptogen, alterative (blood purifier), anti-allergenic, immune amphoteric, and nutritive

SOURCES: Mountain Rose Herbs, Starwest Botanicals

DOSAGE FORMS

STANDARD DECOCTION: 6–8 ounces 3 times daily

TINCTURE (AS DUAL EXTRACT): Dried mushroom (1:5, 75% alcohol); 2–8 ml (0.4–1.6 tsp.) 3 times daily

RHODIOLA

Latin name: *Rhodiola rosea*

An adaptogenic tonic, rhodiola aids mental clarity, memory, energy production, and stress reduction.

WARNINGS: No known warnings

ENERGETICS: Cooling, drying, and constricting

PROPERTIES: Adaptogen, antidepressant, and astringent

SOURCES: Mountain Rose Herbs, Starwest Botanicals

DOSAGE FORMS

TINCTURE: Dried herb (1:5, 50% alcohol); 1–3 ml (0.2–0.6 tsp.), 3 times daily

CAPSULE: 1,000–2,000 mg, 3 times daily

ROSE

Latin name: *Rosa spp.*

Rose hips (the fruits of the rose plant) strengthen capillaries and are rich in bioflavonoids and vitamin C. They are mildly astringent and can be helpful for acute illnesses like colds.

Rose petals are an uplifting addition to herbal teas. They reduce stress and help heal heartache.

WARNINGS: No known warnings

ENERGETICS: Cooling, drying, and slightly constricting

PROPERTIES: Anti-inflammatory, antibacterial, antidepressant, and astringent

SOURCES: Bulk Herb Store, Frontier Herbs, Mountain Rose Herbs, San Francisco Herb Company, Starwest Botanicals, Stony Mountain Botanicals

DOSAGE FORMS

WEAK INFUSION: Up to 3 cups daily as needed

TINCTURE: Dried petals (1:5, 40% alcohol); 5 drops to 2 ml (0.4 tsp.) 3 times daily

CAPSULE: 1,000–2,000 mg, 3 times daily

ROSEMARY

Latin name: *Rosmarinus officinalis*

This herb is considered a tonic for elderly people and may help improve circulation to the brain. In Germany, rosemary is approved by Commission E for use in treating indigestion, joint ailments, and stomach problems. Rosemary also has antioxidant properties that protect the brain and blood vessels.

WARNINGS: No known warnings

ENERGETICS: Warming, drying, and slightly constricting

PROPERTIES: Antidepressant, antioxidant, antirheumatic, antiseptic, carminative, cerebral tonic, and expectorant

SOURCES: Bulk Herb Store, Mountain Rose Herbs, San Francisco Herb Company, Stony Mountain Botanicals

DOSAGE FORMS

WEAK INFUSION: 1 cup up to 3 times daily

TINCTURE: Dried leaves (1:5, 65% alcohol, 10% glycerin); 10 drops to 3 ml (0.6 tsp.) up to 3 times daily

GLYCERITE: Fresh leaves (1:6, 80% glycerin sealed simmer method); dried leaves (1:6); 1–5 ml (0.2–1 tsp.) 1–3 times daily

CAPSULE: 500–1,500 mg up to 3 times daily

TOPICAL USE: Prepare a salve from oil (1:4) and apply as needed. The essential oil can be applied neat, or added to salves, oils, and ointments.

SAFFLOWER

Latin name: *Carthamus tinctorius*

Safflower aids digestion and helps increase the excretion of lactic acid. A tea of safflowers is a very dependable remedy for relieving muscle soreness from overexertion. It reduces swelling in the breasts, brings on delayed menses, helps move stagnant blood (such as bruises and blood clots), and heals injuries.

WARNINGS: No known warnings

ENERGETICS: Cooling

PROPERTIES: Anti-inflammatory, carminative, stomachic, and vulnerary

SOURCES: Frontier Herbs, Mountain Rose Herbs, San Francisco Herb Company, Starwest Botanicals

DOSAGE FORMS

STANDARD INFUSION: 2–8 ounces up to 3 times daily

CAPSULE: 1,000–2,000 mg, 3 times daily

SAFFRON

Latin name: *Crocus sativus*

Saffron is one of the strongest anti-inflammatories in the herbal materia medica. It works particularly well at reducing the inflammatory cytokines associated with depression. Its current popularity is limited by its cost; however, small doses are all that's needed, so the per-dose cost isn't as high as is commonly thought.

WARNINGS: Not for use during pregnancy

ENERGETICS: Warming and drying

PROPERTIES: Anti-inflammatory

SOURCES: Mountain Rose Herbs

DOSAGE FORMS

TINCTURE: Dried herb (1:10, 40% alcohol); best made by percolation; 5–20 drops 3 times daily

SAGE

Latin name: *Salvia officinalis*

Sage can be helpful for colds and fever, especially those involving intermittent chills and fever, hoarseness, or sweating at night. It is best taken as a cool tea for night sweats and as a hot tea to induce perspiration. The tea may be used for sore or hoarse throat and laryngitis and as a mouthwash or gargle for irritation of the throat or mouth. The tea is a nerve tonic, increasing the capacity to handle stress. Sage is antiseptic, used topically to prevent infection and inflammation in wounds.

WARNINGS: Not recommended as a medicinal herb during pregnancy. Sage will dry up breast milk, so it should be avoided by nursing mothers.

ENERGETICS: Warming, drying, and slightly constricting

PROPERTIES: Antigalactagogue, antiseptic, antidiaphoretic, aromatic, carminative, diaphoretic, emmenagogue, and nervine

SPECIFIC INDICATIONS: Rolla Thomas: Profuse sweating, continued inaction of the skin, feet sweat, and cold night sweats.

SOURCES: Bulk Herb Store, Frontier Herbs, Mountain Rose Herbs, San Francisco Herb Company, Starwest Botanicals, Stony Mountain Botanicals

DOSAGE FORMS

STANDARD INFUSION: 4–8 ounces 3 times daily

TINCTURE: Dried herb (1:5, 70% alcohol, 10% glycerin); 1–2 ml (0.2–0.4 tsp.) 2–4 times daily

GLYCERITE: Dried herb (1:6); 2–5 ml (0.4–1 tsp.); 2–4 times daily

CAPSULE: 500–1,000 mg, 2–3 times daily; 1,000–2,000 mg at bedtime for night sweats

SARSAPARILLA

Latin name: *Smilax spp.*

Sarsaparilla is the major flavoring found in old-fashioned root beer. It is a mild bittersweet herb used for strengthening the liver, purifying the blood, and balancing the glands. It helps relieve arthritic pains and clear skin conditions. It has a hormonal balancing action, possibly due to its action on gut bacteria.

WARNINGS: No known warnings

ENERGETICS: Warming and moistening

PROPERTIES: Alterative (blood purifier) and diuretic

SOURCES: Frontier Herbs, Mountain Rose Herbs, San Francisco Herb Company, Starwest Botanicals

DOSAGE FORMS

STANDARD DECOCTION: 6–8 ounces 1–3 times daily

TINCTURE: Dried root (1:5, 40% alcohol); 1–3 ml (0.2–0.6 tsp.) 2–3 times daily

GLYCERITE: Dried root (1:5); 5–10 ml (1–2 tsp.) 2–3 times daily

CAPSULES: 1,000–2,000 mg, 3 times daily

SAW PALMETTO

Latin name: *Sabal serrulata, syn. Serenoa serrulata*

Widely used for prostate enlargement and urinary problems in men, saw palmetto is a general tonic for elderly men and may be helpful with other problems associated with aging. It aids digestion and weight gain in wasting conditions and has a slight effect in stimulating breast tissue in women.

WARNINGS: Women who are breastfeeding should avoid this herb, as it inhibits prolactin and may interfere with lactation.

ENERGETICS: Moistening and nourishing

PROPERTIES: Antigalactagogue, digestive tonic, and expectorant

SPECIFIC INDICATIONS: Rolla Thomas: Has a special action on the glands of the reproductive system, as mammae, ovaries, prostate, testes, etc., tending to increase their functional activity; best effect produced upon enlarged prostate. Especially useful in atrophy of testes or uterus, and in all prostatic troubles.

SOURCES: Bulk Herb Store, Frontier Herbs, Mountain Rose Herbs, San Francisco Herb Company, Starwest Botanicals

DOSAGE FORMS

DECOCTION: 1 teaspoon in 8 ounces, decoct for 15 minutes, steep for 30 minutes; 2–3 cups daily

TINCTURE: Dried berries (1:5, 50% alcohol); 2–5 ml (0.4–1 tsp.) 3 times daily

GLYCERITE: Dried berries (1:8); 0.1–10 ml (0.5–2 tsp.) 2–4 times daily

CAPSULE: 1,000–2,000 mg, 3 times daily; standardized extracts (85%–95% fatty acids and sterols); 1–2 times daily for a total dose of 320 mg

SCHISANDRA (SCHIZANDRA)

Latin name: *Schisandra chinensis*

Schisandra is a stimulating adaptogen and general tonic. It improves circulation, strengthens the heart, aids digestion, and increases bile secretion. In traditional Chinese medicine it is thought to harmonize the body and help retain energy. It helps to keep the nervous system balanced, increasing both excitatory and inhibitory action. The seeds have a hepatoprotective effect similar to that of milk thistle.

WARNINGS: Contraindicated with acute ailments like colds, flu, and fevers. Overuse can lead to insomnia and anxiety.

ENERGETICS: Cooling and moistening

PROPERTIES: Adaptogen, antitussive, hepatoprotective, immune amphoteric, lung tonic, and moistening

SOURCES: Frontier Herbs, Mountain Rose Herbs, Starwest Botanicals, Stony Mountain Botanicals

DOSAGE FORMS

DRIED BERRIES: 10 berries once daily

STANDARD INFUSION: 4–8 ounces 3 times daily

TINCTURE: Dried berries (1:3, 40% alcohol); 1–3 ml (0.2–0.6 tsp.) 3 times daily

CAPSULE: 500–1,500 mg, 1–2 times daily

SCULLCAP (SKULLCAP)

Latin name: *Scutellaria lateriflora*

A relaxing nervine, scullcap helps to calm brain function and is helpful for insomnia and chronic stress. It is also a good remedy for vasoconstrictive (or tension) headaches and migraines. It was used by nineteenth-century herbalists for hysteria, epilepsy, convulsions, and schizophrenia. The person who needs scullcap often has an inability to pay attention or a dull headache in the front or base of the skull. Symptoms are worse with noise, odors, and light, but improve with rest. Scullcap also seems to work well when people feel as if every sound, touch, and ray of light is personally attacking them. These people are oversensitive to any stimulation, and are twitchy even during sleep. Scullcap seems to works best as a tonic when tinctured fresh. Dried scullcap has a more sedative action.

WARNINGS: No known warnings

ENERGETICS: Cooling and relaxing

PROPERTIES: Analgesic (anodyne), antispasmodic, nervine, sedative, and soporific (hypnotic)

SPECIFIC INDICATIONS: Rolla Thomas: Hysteria with inability to control the voluntary muscles; nervousness manifesting itself in muscular action.

SOURCES: Frontier Herbs, Mountain Rose Herbs, Starwest Botanicals, Stony Mountain Botanicals

DOSAGE FORMS

STANDARD INFUSION: 4–8 ounces 3 times daily

TINCTURE: Fresh aerial parts (1:2, 95% alcohol); recently dried leaf and flower (1:5, 60% alcohol); 10 drops to 5 ml (1 tsp.) 2–4 times daily

GLYCERITE: Dried herb (1:6); 2–5 ml (0.4–1 tsp.) 2–4 times daily

SENNA LEAVES

Latin name: *Cassia senna, syn. Senna alexandrina*

Senna is a very strong stimulant laxative, best used in combination with other herbs.

WARNINGS: Can cause cramping and be habit forming. Use short-term only.

ENERGETICS: Drying and cooling

PROPERTIES: Purgative (cathartic) and stimulant laxative

SOURCES: Frontier Herbs, Mountain Rose Herbs, San Francisco Herb Company, Starwest Botanicals

DOSAGE FORMS

STANDARD INFUSION: ½–1 cup daily

TINCTURE: Dried leaf (1:5, 50% alcohol); 10 drops to 2 ml (0.4 tsp.) 1–2 times daily

CAPSULE: 100–500 mg, 1–2 times daily

SHATAVARI

Latin name: *Asparagus racemosus*

Shatavari is the root of a species of asparagus. It is a reproductive tonic that comes to us from Ayurvedic medicine. It is used as a restorative in people suffering from nervous exhaustion and has been used in a wide range of other ailments.

WARNINGS: Shatavari should be avoided by pregnant women.

ENERGETICS: Cooling and nourishing

PROPERTIES: Adaptogen and diuretic

SOURCES: Mountain Rose Herbs, Starwest Botanicals

DOSAGE FORMS

STANDARD DECOCTION: 2–4 ounces 3 times daily

CAPSULE: 1,000–2,000 mg, 3 times daily

SHEEP SORREL

Latin name: *Rumex acetosella*

Sheep sorrel is an ingredient in the famous anticancer formula Essiac. It is a detoxifying herb, rich in iron like other members of the dock genus. It has a mild laxative and intestinal tonic effect like yellow dock. It is also used as a salad green.

WARNINGS: Contains oxalic acid; don't use if you have a history of kidney stones.

ENERGETICS: Cooling and slightly drying

PROPERTIES: Anticancer, antiseptic, and hepatic

SOURCES: Frontier Herbs, Mountain Rose Herbs

DOSAGE FORMS

STANDARD INFUSION: 2–4 ounces 3 times daily. Don't take longer than 3 weeks out of a year.

TINCTURE: Recently dried aerial parts (1:5, 50% alcohol); 10 drops to 2 ml (0.4 tsp.) up to 3 times daily

SHEPHERD'S PURSE

Latin name: *Capsella bursa-pastoris*

Shepherd's purse is one of the best herbs to use for heavy bleeding during menstruation. It is an important herb in midwifery: It helps deliver the placenta after childbirth and cuts down on postpartum bleeding. It helps to constrict blood vessels, and it is one of the few remedies that will increase blood pressure. It can also be used to soothe the bladder and treat blood in the urine.

WARNINGS: Not for use during pregnancy

ENERGETICS: Warming, drying, and constricting

PROPERTIES: Astringent, hypertensive, styptic, and vasoconstrictor

SOURCES: Frontier Herbs, Mountain Rose Herbs, San Francisco Herb Company, Starwest Botanicals

DOSAGE FORMS

STANDARD INFUSION: 2–3 cups daily

TINCTURE: Fresh plant (1:2, 95% alcohol); dried plant (1:5, 60% alcohol); 1–2 ml (0.2–0.4 tsp.) 2–4 times daily

SHIITAKE

Latin name: *Lentinula edodes*

Shiitake mushroom is finding increasing use as a medicinal treatment for cancer and other health problems. It can be helpful in lowering cholesterol and fighting various types of cancer. It stimulates the immune system to increase the body's ability to fight infections.

WARNINGS: No known warnings

ENERGETICS: Balancing and nourishing

PROPERTIES: Adaptogen, alterative (blood purifier), anti-allergenic, immune amphoteric, and restorative

SOURCES: Mountain Rose Herbs, Starwest Botanicals; fresh shiitake can be found in many grocery stores.

DOSAGE FORMS

FRESH MUSHROOMS: Often available in supermarkets; can be cooked and eaten in a variety of ways

STANDARD DECOCTION: 4–8 ounces 3 times daily

SKUNK CABBAGE

Latin name: *Symplocarpus foetidus*

Skunk cabbage is a powerful antispasmodic, useful for cramps and muscle spasms of all kinds. It is a specific for severe bronchial asthmatic spasms associated with emotional distress, and coughing to the point of vomiting. It may also be helpful for fluid retention, headache, irritability, nervousness, tightness in the chest, and whooping cough.

WARNINGS: The fresh root can be irritating to mucous membranes. It should be used cautiously by people with a history of kidney stones.

ENERGETICS: Relaxing and slightly warming

PROPERTIES: Acrid, antispasmodic, emetic, and expectorant

TINCTURE: Fresh flowering plant (1:2, 95% alcohol); dried flowering plant (1:5, 50% alcohol); 5 drops to 1 ml (0.2 tsp.) 3 times daily in water

SLIPPERY ELM

Latin name: *Ulmus rubra*

Slippery elm is a soothing and nourishing mucilaginous herb that helps absorb acid and irritants in the stomach. It is used internally for irritation of the stomach and intestines, for diarrhea (especially in children), and as a mild, nourishing food for weak and debilitated persons.

Slippery elm is overharvested and at-risk. Unless you happen to have a slippery elm tree fall in your yard, use marshmallow instead. Marshmallow root will do everything slippery elm will do, and is sustainable and usually cheaper.

WARNINGS: A mild and very safe remedy

ENERGETICS: Cooling, moistening, and nourishing

PROPERTIES: Absorbent, demulcent (mucilant), emollient, nutritive, soothing, and vulnerary

SOURCES: Bulk Herb Store, Frontier Herbs, Mountain Rose Herbs, San Francisco Herb Company, Starwest Botanicals, Stony Mountain Botanicals

DOSAGE FORMS

BULK HERB: Can be made into a gruel, mixed with juice or applesauce

COLD INFUSION: 4–8 ounces 1–4 times daily. If it doesn't have a slimy texture, you probably didn't make it right.

CAPSULES: 1,000–2,000 mg, 3 times daily

TOPICAL USE: Mix the powdered herb with enough water to form a paste, and apply as a poultice.

SOLOMON'S SEAL

Latin name: *Polygonatum multiflorum*

Solomon's seal helps adjust tension on ligaments and tendons. It is an amazing anti-inflammatory, both topically and internally. It is specific for healing and repairing any connective tissue. It is the most reliable remedy for osteoarthritis and rheumatoid arthritis in the herbal materia medica.

WARNINGS: No known warnings

ENERGETICS: Cooling and balancing

PROPERTIES: Demulcent (mucilant) and emollient

SOURCES: Mountain Rose Herbs

DOSAGE FORMS

STANDARD DECOCTION: 2–4 ounces up to 3 times daily

TINCTURE: Fresh root (1:3, 95% alcohol); dried root (1:5, 50% alcohol); 5 drops to 3 ml (0.6 tsp.) 3 times daily

TOPICAL USE: A salve made from the oil extract (1:4) works amazingly well. You can apply the tincture or decoction as a compress, or use the decoction as a soak or in a bath. Try combining kava-kava and Solomon's seal decoction in a bath together.

SPIKENARD

Latin name: *Aralia racemosa*

Spikenard's expectorant properties make it an excellent lung tonic, helpful for colds, chronic coughs, bronchitis, and asthma. Use for chronic weak lungs with cough or after quitting smoking. Spikenard is also used as an alterative for arthritis and in the treatment of skin diseases (like sarsaparilla).

ENERGETICS: Warming and drying

PROPERTIES: Anti-inflammatory and expectorant

SOURCES: Mountain Rose Herbs

DOSAGE FORMS

STANDARD INFUSION: 1–2 tsp. powdered root per cup; ½–1 cup daily in small doses throughout the day

TINCTURE: Dried root (1:5, 50% alcohol); 20–40 drops (1–2 ml) daily as a tonic; for acute respiratory problems, 60–80 drops (3–4 ml) 2–3 times daily or as part of a formula

SPILANTHES

Latin name: *Spilanthes acmella*

Spilanthes is an antibacterial and antifungal herb that stimulates mucous membrane secretions and the immune system to fight respiratory infections. It acts as a local anesthetic to ease pain while reducing inflammation. One of its common names is toothache plant: it can be applied on an infected tooth to ease pain and help fight the infection.

WARNINGS: No known warnings

ENERGETICS: Warming and constricting

PROPERTIES: Analgesic (anodyne), antibacterial, antifungal, and astringent

DOSAGE FORMS

FRESH HERB: Chew the flower heads or leaves to relieve toothaches.

STANDARD INFUSION: 1–4 ounces 1–4 times daily

TINCTURE: Fresh plant (1:2, 95% alcohol); dried plant (1:5, 50% alcohol); 5 drops to 1 ml (0.2 tsp.) 3 times daily

ST. JOHN'S WORT

Latin name: *Hypericum perforatum*

St. John's wort became a popular herb when research suggested it could be helpful for mild to moderate depression. It is indeed helpful for some cases of depression, especially those accompanied by anxiety, but the herb has many other valuable properties. It is a nervine herb that helps to regulate the solar plexus, which are the nerves that regulate digestion. It can be helpful for insomnia, fear, nerve pain, and nerve damage. It stimulates nerve regeneration and repair and helps heal wounds. St. John's wort is antiviral and is used for infections such as shingles, herpes, mononucleosis, and flu.

WARNINGS: The fresh plant is phototoxic. It contains a chemical that changes to a toxin in the body after exposure to sunlight. This does not appear to be a problem when taking St. John's wort internally. Avoid when taking SSRI antidepressants.

ENERGETICS: Slightly warming

PROPERTIES: Antidepressant, antiseptic, antiviral, digestive tonic, nervine, and vulnerary

SPECIFIC INDICATIONS: Rolla Thomas: It is claimed that it exerts a marked influence in relieving irritation in injuries of the spine, and in punctured or lacerated wounds of the extremities, preventing tetanus. Relieves the excruciating pain of such injuries.

SOURCES: Bulk Herb Store, Mountain Rose Herbs, San Francisco Herb Company, Starwest Botanicals

DOSAGE FORMS

STANDARD INFUSION: 4–8 ounces 1–4 times daily

TINCTURE: Fresh plant (1:2, 95% alcohol); 5 drops to 3 ml (0.6 tsp.) 3 times daily

NOTE: Both tincture and infusion will turn a deep red when you're using a good-quality herb. If it doesn't turn red, you probably have old plant material or the wrong species.

OIL: Fresh flowers (1:4); apply topically.

CAPSULE: 500–1,500 mg, 3–4 times daily; standardized capsules to 0.3% hypericin, take 300 mg, 3–4 times daily.

STILLINGIA

Latin name: *Stillingia spp.*

Stillingia, also known as queen's root, is an herb in the Hoxsey anticancer formula. It is used primarily to improve lymphatic drainage and stimulate the immune system in chronic infections.

WARNINGS: No known warnings

ENERGETICS: Warming and balancing

SPECIFIC INDICATIONS: Rolla Thomas: Irritation of superior pharynx, and just behind the fauces, causing cough; hoarse croupal cough, paroxysmal, as if from great laryngeal irritation; skin disease, showing marked irritation, with ichorous discharge.

SOURCES: Starwest Botanicals

DOSAGE FORMS

TINCTURE: Fresh root (1:2, 95% alcohol); dried root (1:5, 50% alcohol); 5 drops to 1 ml (0.2 tsp.) 6 times daily

STONE BREAKER

Latin name: *Phyllanthus niruri*

Stone breaker has been shown to inhibit the growth of calcium oxalate crystals, stopping the formation or development of kidney stones. It stimulates bile flow and aids in digesting fats. It has hepatoprotective properties, and its action on the kidneys may be helpful in hypertension.

WARNINGS: No known warnings

ENERGETICS: Cooling and drying

PROPERTIES: Cholagogue, diuretic, and lipotropic

DOSAGE FORMS

STANDARD DECOCTION: 2–4 ounces 3 times daily

CAPSULE: 1,000–2,000 mg, 1–2 times daily with food

SWEET ANNIE (CHING-HAO)

Latin name: *Artemisia annua*

Sweet annie is a close relative of wormwood and is used for malaria and a number of bacterial infections. It is also a good remedy for intestinal parasites.

WARNINGS: Not for use when pregnant or nursing. All artemisia species can be toxic in large doses.

ENERGETICS: Cooling and drying

PROPERTIES: Anthelminthic, antibacterial, antiparasitic, and antiseptic

DOSAGE FORMS

TINCTURE: Fresh leaf (1:2, 95% alcohol); dried leaf (1:5, 60% alcohol); 10 drops to 2 ml (0.4 tsp.) 3 times daily

CAPSULE: 500–1,000 mg, 1–2 times daily with food. Do not exceed 3 grams daily.

STANDARDIZED EXTRACT: Artemisinin extract; 1–2 mg per 2 pounds of body weight 2 times daily with fatty food

TEASEL

Latin name: *Dipsacus asper*

Teasel root has been used for muscle and joint pain and as a tonic to aid repair of damaged tissues. It is also employed in the treatment of Lyme disease. It does not seem to cure Lyme disease but is helpful in pain management and relief of symptoms.

SOURCES: Mountain Rose Herbs

ENERGETICS: Cooling and drying

PROPERTIES: Kidney tonic and vulnerary

DOSAGE FORMS

STANDARD INFUSION: 4-8 ounces 1–3 times daily

TINCTURE: Dried root (1:5, 40% alcohol); 5–50 drops 1–3 times daily

THUJA

Latin name: *Thuja occidentalis*

The leaves of thuja are a strong antifungal remedy, useful for candida, athlete's foot, and jock itch. They also have antiparasitic effects against ringworm, amoebic dysentery, and giardia. The leaves are antiviral.

WARNINGS: In the 1930s thuja was used as an abortifacient in Europe and North America. It is not recommended for use during pregnancy. Not recommended for long-term use, as the herb may irritate the kidneys. There is a risk of toxicity with the tincture, but not with the infusion.

ENERGETICS: Warming and drying

PROPERTIES: Anthelminthic, antifungal, antiparasitic, aromatic, emmenagogue, and expectorant

SPECIFIC INDICATIONS: Rolla Thomas: Syphilitic or other diseases of bad blood, with warty excrescences, or ulceration, showing prominence of papillae.

DOSAGE FORMS

STANDARD INFUSION: 4–8 ounces 3 times daily

TINCTURE: Fresh needles (1:2, 95% alcohol); 0.5–1 ml (0.1–0.2 tsp.) 3 times daily

TOPICAL USE: The essential oil can be diluted 1:5 and applied to venereal warts (HPV), common warts, skin tags, and itchy skin conditions.

THYME

Latin name: *Thymus vulgaris*

Thyme is a very powerful remedy for infections of all kinds, especially in the lungs and digestive tract. It is indicated for spasmodic conditions of the respiratory and urinary tracts with infectious symptoms. It is a good antifungal and can be used to treat gut dysbiosis. The combination of fenugreek and thyme is excellent for clearing sinus congestion. Applied topically, it helps with insect bites, stings, and minor pain.

WARNINGS: Avoid large doses in pregnancy (culinary use and standard dosages in products are perfectly safe).

ENERGETICS: Warming and drying

PROPERTIES: Antibacterial, antifungal, antiviral, aromatic, carminative, decongestant, emmenagogue, and circulatory stimulant

SOURCES: Bulk Herb Store, Mountain Rose Herbs, San Francisco Herb Company, Stony Mountain Botanicals

STANDARD INFUSION: 2–4 ounces 3 times daily

TINCTURE: Dried leaf (1:5, 50% alcohol, 10% glycerin); 10 drops to 4 ml (0.8 tsp.) 3 times daily

GLYCERITE: Fresh leaves (1:8, 80% glycerin sealed simmer method); dried leaves (1:6, 80% glycerin sealed simmer method); 1–3 ml (0.2–0.6 tsp.) 3 times daily

TOPICAL USE: The essential oil, diluted to 1% or less, can be used in mouth-washes or vaginal douches for yeast infections.

TIENCHI GINSENG

Latin name: *Panax notoginseng*

Tienchi ginseng is used to control bleeding and hemorrhaging of all kinds. It is the main ingredient in Yunnan Bai Yao, a famous formula given to Vietcong soldiers to stop bleeding from bullet wounds. It is a mild circulatory stimulant and may be helpful for angina.

WARNINGS: No known warnings

ENERGETICS: Warming and constricting

PROPERTIES: Circulatory stimulant and styptic

DOSAGE FORMS

STANDARD DECOCTION: 2–4 ounces 3 times daily

TINCTURE: Dried herb (1:3, 60% alcohol); 1–2 ml (0.2–0.4 tsp.) 3 times daily

TRIBULUS

Latin name: *Tribulus terrestris*

Tribulus has long been used as a sexual tonic and as a means of restoring vigor to the body. Modern herbalists use tribulus as a restorative tonic to assist the male reproductive system and bring about an increase in health and stamina. It is used to support testosterone metabolism and hormone function, especially in aging men. The fruit of tribulus is used to treat urinary tract infections and kidney stones that make urination painful.

WARNINGS: No known warnings

ENERGETICS: Drying, slightly warming, and slightly relaxing

PROPERTIES: Aphrodisiac, hypotensive, and testosterone-enhancing

SOURCES: Mountain Rose Herbs, Starwest Botanicals, Stony Mountain Botanicals

DOSAGE FORMS

TINCTURE: Dried seed (1:5, 60% alcohol); 1–2 ml (0.2–0.4 tsp.) 3 times daily

CAPSULE: 500–1,000 mg, 1–2 daily with food

TRIPHALA

Latin name: *Emblica officinalis, Terminalia bellirica, and Terminalia chebula*

Triphala is not an herb, but a blend of three fruits used in Ayurvedic medicine as a gentle laxative, bowel tonic, and blood purifier. The first fruit in this blend is haritaki (Terminalia chebula). It has a balanced energy, containing five flavors (bitter, sour, astringent, salty, and sweet). It is a mild laxative that also tones the intestinal membranes. It lubricates tissues and relaxes muscle spasms.

The second fruit in this blend is bibhitaki (Terminalia bellirica), an antispasmodic herb that is pungent and warming. It is an expectorant and decongestant and is used to treat asthma, bronchial problems, and allergies.

The third and final fruit in triphala is amalaki or Indian gooseberry (Emblica officinalis), which also has a balanced energy, containing five flavors (sour, astringent, sweet, pungent, and bitter). It contains a small amount of anthraquinones, but is also astringent, so it has both a laxative action and a bowel toning action. This means it corrects both constipation and diarrhea. It is a cooling remedy and is also used to treat ulcers, intestinal inflammation, burning sensations, skin eruptions, and skin infections.

In various formulas these three fruits may also be referred to as belleric myrobalan fruit, chebulic myrobalan fruit, and Indian gooseberry fruit, or as harada fruit, amla fruit, and behada fruit. No matter what it is called, triphala is quite possibly the best formula for normalizing gastrointestinal function available.

Besides normalizing colon function, triphala improves liver function, protects the liver against environmental toxins, and improves digestion. It is antioxidant and anti-inflammatory, so it slows aging and protects the body from degenerative disease. It enhances circulation, lowers blood pressure, and protects the heart. It helps expel mucus from the respiratory passages and fights infection. In Ayurvedic medicine, triphala is used for constipation, indigestion, flatulence, poor appetite, digestive headaches, sinus congestion, joint pain, and general toxicity.

WARNINGS: None

ENERGETICS: Slightly cooling and slightly drying

PROPERTIES: Anti-inflammatory, antioxidant, aperient, decongestant, expectorant, and hepatoprotective

SOURCES: Mountain Rose Herbs, Starwest Botanicals

DOSAGE FORMS

CAPSULE OR POWDER: 1,000–2,000 mg, 1–2 times daily with food

TURKEY RHUBARB

Latin name: *Rheum palmatum*

A common ingredient in stimulant laxatives, this bitter is also used in small doses as a digestive tonic.

WARNINGS: Some people react with abdominal pain. Ginger or nervine herbs can help to counteract this.

ENERGETICS: Drying and cooling

PROPERTIES: Antacid and laxative (stimulant)

SOURCES: Frontier Herbs, Mountain Rose Herbs, Starwest Botanicals, Stony Mountain Botanicals

DOSAGE FORMS

TINCTURE: Dried leaf (1:5, 60% alcohol); 1–3 ml (0.2–0.6 tsp.) 1–2 times daily with food

CAPSULE: 500–1,000 mg, 1–2 times daily with food

TURMERIC

Latin name: *Curcuma longa, syn. C. domestica*

Turmeric stimulates digestion and aids assimilation. It is a very good liver and gallbladder remedy. It aids liver function and helps dissolve and prevent gallstones. Its potent ability to reduce inflammation and ease chronic pain makes it useful for treating arthritis and a number of chronic inflammatory disorders. It's one of the few anti-inflammatories that cross the blood-brain barrier, and studies show it's effective for inflammation-induced depression.

WARNINGS: Overuse in constitutionally hot/dry individuals can cause nervous agitation.

ENERGETICS: Warming and slightly drying

PROPERTIES: Anti-inflammatory, antimutagenic, antioxidant, cholagogue, and hepatoprotective

SOURCES: Bulk Herb Store, Mountain Rose Herbs, San Francisco Herb Company, Stony Mountain Botanicals

DOSAGE FORMS

STANDARD DECOCTION: 2–4 ounces 3 times daily (Water is acceptable, but a better menstruum for the decoction is coconut milk.)

TINCTURE: Fresh root (juice, then decoct to 50% of its original volume and preserve with 25% alcohol); 1–5 ml (0.2–1 tsp.) 3 times daily

POWDER OR CAPSULE: 1,000–3,000 mg, 3 times daily

USNEA

Latin name: *Usnea spp*

Actually a lichen, or a symbiotic combination of algae and fungi, usnea has been used for thousands of years in Chinese, Greek, and Egyptian medicine to treat a variety of health conditions. Its antibiotic and antifungal properties may be helpful for treating gastrointestinal infections, sore throats, and urinary tract infections. It's also a useful antibacterial for the mouth to promote oral hygiene.

WARNINGS: No known warnings

ENERGETICS: Cooling and drying

PROPERTIES: Antibacterial and antifungal

SOURCES: Mountain Rose Herbs, Starwest Botanicals, Stony Mountain Botanicals

DOSAGE FORMS

TINCTURE: Dried herb (1:5, 50% alcohol made as a hot alcohol extract); 1–5 ml (0.2–1 tsp.) 3 times daily

UVA URSI

Latin name: *Arctostaphylos uva-ursi*

A reliable diuretic with strong disinfectant and infection fighting properties, uva ursi is useful for kidney and bladder infections, irritated female organs, and other urogenital problems.

WARNINGS: Not for use in cases involving fluid deficiency, wasting, or dryness. Not recommended for long-term use, because of strong astringency. Prolonged use may irritate the stomach and cause constipation. Not recommended during pregnancy.

ENERGETICS: Warming, drying, and constricting

PROPERTIES: Antiseptic and diuretic

SOURCES: Frontier Herbs, Mountain Rose Herbs, San Francisco Herb Company, Starwest Botanicals, Stony Mountain Botanicals

DOSAGE FORMS

STANDARD INFUSION: 4–8 ounces 3 times daily

TINCTURE: Dried leaf (1:5, 50% alcohol); 10 drops to 3 ml (0.6 tsp.) 1–4 times daily

GLYCERITE: Dried leaf (1:6); 1–6 ml (0.2–1 tsp.) 1–4 times daily

CAPSULE: 1,000–2,000 mg, 3 times daily

VALERIAN

Latin name: *Valeriana officinalis*

Valerian is a popular and potent nervine with strong tranquilizing effects on the central nervous system. It has been used to treat a wide variety of nervous system conditions, insomnia, and mild pain. Valerian seems to work most consistently on people with sympathetic excess, as seen by their enlarged pupil size. People with parasympathetic excess (with small pupils) are more prone to be stimulated by valerian.

WARNINGS: Not recommended for persons with "hot" disorders, i.e., high strung, nervous, and excitable. (Scullcap or passionflower are better for such individuals.) Not recommended for long-term use in large doses, although there is no risk of addiction. Does not generally cause drowsiness that could affect driving. Some people react "backward" to valerian and find it stimulating rather than sedating. Low thyroid and the dosage appear to be factors. Some persons using valerian may experience a "light" feeling, as if floating in air, and they may experience hallucinations at night.

ENERGETICS: Relaxing and slightly warming

PROPERTIES: Analgesic (anodyne), antispasmodic, nervine, sedative, and soporific (hypnotic)

SOURCES: Frontier Herbs, Mountain Rose Herbs, San Francisco Herb Company, Starwest Botanicals, Stony Mountain Botanicals

DOSAGE FORMS

STANDARD INFUSION: 4–8 ounces 30 minutes before bed

TINCTURE: Fresh root (1:2, 95% alcohol); dried root (1:5, 60% alcohol); 10 drops to 3 ml (0.6 tsp.) 30 minutes before bed for insomnia or up to 4 times daily for mild pain or stress

CAPSULE: 500–1,000 mg, 30 minutes before bed for insomnia or up to 4 times daily for mild pain or stress

VENUS FLY TRAP

Latin name: *Dionaea muscipula*

Venus fly trap is used in cases of malignant conditions such as tumors in advanced stages (mammary, bladder, prostate carcinomas, and osteosarcoma) and solid tumors. It is also used for Hodgkin's and non-Hodgkin's lymphoma and other related conditions. Limited research seems to indicate it's a strong immune stimulant.

WARNINGS: Not for use during pregnancy

ENERGETICS: Cooling

PROPERTIES: Analgesic (anodyne), antimutagenic, antiviral, cytotoxic, and immune stimulant

DOSAGE FORMS

TINCTURE: Fresh plant (1:2, 95% alcohol); 1–4 ml (0.2–0.8 tsp.) 3 times daily

VIOLET

Latin name: *Viola odorata and related species*

Violet is a good remedy for cooling heat and relieving congestion in the lymphatic and respiratory systems.

WARNINGS: No known warnings

ENERGETICS: Cooling and moistening

PROPERTIES: Demulcent (mucilant) and lymphatic

SOURCES: Mountain Rose Herbs, Stony Mountain Botanicals

DOSAGE FORMS

STANDARD INFUSION: 4–8 ounces 3 times daily

TINCTURE: Fresh leaf (1:2, 95% alcohol); dried leaf (1:5, 60% alcohol); 1–5 ml (0.2–1 tsp.) 3 times daily

WHITE OAK

Latin name: *Quercus alba and other species*

A powerful astringent, white oak bark is used internally for hemorrhoids and varicose veins. A decoction can be used as a rectal injection for hemorrhoids, as a douche to stop bleeding, or as a fomentation for swelling, varicose veins, and other injuries. Use as a gargle for sore throats, or use as a mouthwash for bleeding gums. Use white oak bark powder with black walnut powder as a tooth powder for bleeding gums and loose teeth.

WARNINGS: Can be constipating when taken internally. Can interfere with digestion (take between meals). Contains large amounts of tannin, which may be associated with mouth and stomach cancer with consistent, long-term use. Use only for short periods internally. No warnings for external use.

ENERGETICS: Drying and constricting

PROPERTIES: Antidiarrheal, antiseptic, antivenomous, astringent, hemostatic, and styptic

SOURCES: Mountain Rose Herbs, Starwest Botanicals, Stony Mountain Botanicals

DOSAGE FORMS

POWDERED BARK: Powdered oak bark may be sniffed to treat nasal polyps, or sprinkled on eczema to dry the affected area.

STANDARD DECOCTION: 2–4 ounces 3 times daily

TINCTURE: Dried bark (1:5, 30% alcohol, 10% glycerin); 1–4 ml (0.2–0.8 tsp.) 3 times daily

GLYCERITE: Dried bark (1:5); 1–4 ml (0.2–0.8 tsp.) 3 times daily

TOPICAL USES: Tincture can be applied to bites and stings. Decoction can be used as a compress or soak.

WHITE POND LILY

Latin name: *Nymphaea odorata*

A cooling and constricting remedy, white pond lily and white water lily (N. alba) have been used to reduce restlessness, inflammation, and irritation in tissues. They also have a calming effect on libido.

WARNINGS: No known warnings

ENERGETICS: Cooling and constricting

PROPERTIES: Anaphrodisiac, anti-inflammatory, astringent, and uterine tonic

DOSAGE FORMS

TINCTURE: Fresh root (1:2, 95% alcohol); 1–2 ml (0.2–0.4 tsp.) 3 times daily

STANDARD DECOCTION: 2–4 ounces 3 times daily

TOPICAL USE: The decoction can be used as a vaginal douche.

WILD CHERRY

Latin name: *Prunus serotina*

An aromatic and astringent, wild cherry has a long history of use in cough remedies (ever wondered why so many cough remedies are cherry-flavored?). It is a cooling remedy that expels phlegm and soothes and dries out mucous membranes, making it helpful for a variety of respiratory and digestive system problems. It may also help normalize histamine reactions in allergies. In traditional Chinese medicine, it is indicated when there is heart fire blazing, consisting of palpitations, mental restlessness, agitation, insomnia, rapid pulse, and a yellow-coated tongue with a red tip.

WARNINGS: There is a slight toxicity to wild cherry, so it should not be used in large amounts or for long periods of time. It contains hydrocyanic acid, which, in high doses, may cause spasms and difficulty breathing. Medicinal doses have never proved harmful. Not recommended for use by pregnant women.

ENERGETICS: Cooling and drying

PROPERTIES: Astringent and expectorant

SPECIFIC INDICATIONS: Fyfe: Irregular or intermittent heart action; convulsive action due to overstrain. Irritation of stomach with cough, bronchial irritation. Impaired appetite. Lack of muscular tone.

SOURCES: Bulk Herb Store, Frontier Herbs, Mountain Rose Herbs, Starwest Botanicals, Stony Mountain Botanicals

DOSAGE FORMS

Many authors insist that a dried bark tincture is the safest and best preparation. After much experimentation, we believe the fresh bark tincture to be superior.

COLD INFUSION (STRONG): 1–5 ounces 3–5 times daily

TINCTURE: Fresh bark (1:3, in 40% alcohol); 10–40 drops 1–4 times daily

INFUSED WINE: Dried bark (1:5 in sherry) 1–2 ounces 3–5 times daily

GLYCERITE: Fresh or dried bark (1:8, 60% glycerin, cold maceration for 3 weeks; do not use heat); 1–2 tsp. 3–5 times daily

SYRUP: Make a strong cold infusion and add 50% honey.

WILD INDIGO (BAPTISTA)

Latin name: *Baptisia tinctoria*

A very valuable remedy for serious infections causing toxicity and blood poisoning, wild indigo is specifically indicated in conditions where there is a foul discharge and an odor reminiscent of decaying meat. It works very well for many bacterial infections, especially when combined with echinacea and poke.

WARNINGS: This herb should be used with caution. It is potentially toxic and is a strong purgative and emetic in larger doses.

ENERGETICS: Cooling and drying

PROPERTIES: Bitter, cathartic, emetic, and lymphatic

SPECIFIC INDICATIONS: Felter: Fullness of tissue, with dusky, leaden, purplish discoloration; tendency to ulceration and sloughing; face swollen and bluish, enfeebled circulation, fetid discharges.

SOURCES: Mountain Rose Herbs, Starwest Botanicals

DOSAGE FORMS

TINCTURE: Fresh plant (1:2, 95% alcohol); dried plant (1:5, 60% alcohol); 10 drops to 1 ml (0.2 tsp.) 3 times daily

WILD YAM

Latin name: *Dioscorea villosa*

Contrary to popular myth, wild yam is not a source of progesterone and is not a reliable herb for birth control. It contains compounds that are used in the synthetic production of hormones like progesterone, but these compounds are not converted to progesterone in the body, nor do they have a progesterone-like action.

Wild yam is, however, a valuable antispasmodic and anti-inflammatory remedy. It has been used to ease menstrual cramps and ovarian pain, and is also helpful for irritable bowel and intestinal cramps (gripping). It has also been used in conditions like arthritis and neuralgia.

WARNINGS: Overdose may cause nausea, vomiting, and diarrhea.

ENERGETICS: Cooling, slightly moistening, and relaxing

PROPERTIES: Analgesic (anodyne), anti-inflammatory, and antispasmodic

SPECIFIC INDICATIONS: Felter: Spasmodic abdominal colic, nausea, with skin and conjunctiva yellow. Twisting, boring distress centered at umbilicus.

SOURCES: Bulk Herb Store, Frontier Herbs, Mountain Rose Herbs, Starwest Botanicals, Stony Mountain Botanicals

DOSAGE FORMS

STANDARD DECOCTION: Simmer long enough for decoction to release soapy bubbles, turn red, and smell like Christmas; 3–6 ounces 3 times daily

TINCTURE: Fresh root (1:2, 95% alcohol); dried root (1:5, 60% alcohol); 10 drops to 3 ml (0.6 tsp.) 3 times daily

WILLOW

Latin name: *Salix alba, Salix lucida, and other species*

Willow bark has long been used for pain, fevers, and inflammation. Its active compound, salicin, is the original source of the synthetic derivative aspirin. The action of white willow is much slower than that of the synthetic drug, but is less likely to cause stomach problems. Willow takes about 8 hours to kick in. It generally works best at easing pain when combined with other analgesic herbs.

WARNINGS: Not recommended with ulcers or a weak digestive system. Also not recommended during pregnancy.

ENERGETICS: Cooling and slightly drying

PROPERTIES: Analgesic (anodyne), anti-inflammatory, antiseptic, and febrifuge

SOURCES: Bulk Herb Store, Frontier Herbs, Mountain Rose Herbs, San Francisco Herb Company, Starwest Botanicals, Stony Mountain Botanicals

DOSAGE FORMS

STANDARD DECOCTION: 4–8 ounces 3 times daily

CAPSULE: 500–2,000 mg up to 3 times daily

GLYCERITE: Dried bark (1:5); 10–30 ml (1–3 tsp.) up to 3 times daily

WINTERGREEN

Latin name: *Gaultheria procumbens*

Wintergreen contains salicylic acid (a natural aspirin), which can help to reduce inflammation and pain. It has been taken internally as a tea to ease pain, but it is seldom used internally today. The oil of wintergreen, however, is frequently used as a topical analgesic.

WARNINGS: The essential oil of wintergreen can trigger contact dermatitis in some people. The essential oil should never be taken internally. People who are sensitive to aspirin should avoid wintergreen.

ENERGETICS: Cooling

PROPERTIES: Analgesic (anodyne), anesthetic, and anti-inflammatory

SOURCES: Starwest Botanicals

DOSAGE FORMS

TOPICAL USE: Apply the essential oil of wintergreen, diluted to 10%, as needed for muscular pain.

WITCH HAZEL

Latin name: *Hamamelis virginiana*

Witch hazel is primarily used topically as an astringent. It can also be used as a suppository for hemorrhoids and anal fistulas.

WARNINGS: No known warnings

ENERGETICS: Drying and constricting

PROPERTIES: Anti-inflammatory, astringent, styptic, and vulnerary

SOURCES: Mountain Rose Herbs, Stony Mountain Botanicals

DOSAGE FORMS

TOPICAL USE: Apply decoction or tincture as a compress, as a fomentation, or in lotion as needed.

TINCTURE: Dried bark (1:5, 40% alcohol); for topical use only

WOOD BETONY

Latin name: *Betonica officinalis, syn. Stachys officinalis*

Wood betony is an analgesic nervine that relaxes tension in the muscles. It is frequently used in formulas for headaches and is used to relieve middle back pain and tension, facial pain, and muscle tension. It is helpful for people whose minds are overactive and stressed, and helps ease tension in one's thoughts and emotions.

WARNINGS: No known warnings

ENERGETICS: Cooling and relaxing

PROPERTIES: Analgesic (anodyne), nervine, and sedative

SOURCES: Mountain Rose Herbs, Starwest Botanicals

DOSAGE FORMS

STANDARD INFUSION: 4–8 ounces 3 times daily

TINCTURE: Dried leaf (1:5, 50% alcohol); 10 drops to 3 ml (0.6 tsp.) 3 times daily

WORMWOOD

Latin name: *Artemisia absinthium*

As its name implies, wormwood is a powerful antiparasitic herb, used for expelling tapeworms and other internal worms and parasites. It is also used to stimulate digestion and appetite.

WARNINGS: A very strong and potentially toxic herb, wormwood should not be used by pregnant women, nursing mothers, or weak persons. It should be used only for short periods of time and preferably as part of a formula. Take for no longer than 4–5 weeks at a time.

ENERGETICS: Cooling and drying

PROPERTIES: Antiparasitic, bitter, stomachic, and vermifuge

SOURCES: Bulk Herb Store, Frontier Herbs, Mountain Rose Herbs, San Francisco Herb Company, Starwest Botanicals, Stony Mountain Botanicals

DOSAGE FORMS

STANDARD INFUSION: 2–4 ounces 3 times daily (extremely bitter)

TINCTURE: Dried herb (1:5, 70% alcohol); 5 drops to 2 ml (0.4 tsp.) as needed

YARROW

Latin name: *Achillea millefolium*

Yarrow's hemostatic properties (ability to stem bleeding) made it the medication of choice for treating war injuries in ancient times. Yarrow leaves were traditionally applied to wounds to stop bleeding. Its hemostatic effects are not as reliable as proper bandaging and pressure, so it's rarely used for bleeding now. However, yarrow can be taken internally to stop internal bleeding. Yarrow flowers are also a strong diaphoretic and are used to cool high fevers and help the body fight infection. A warm tea of yarrow is one of the best remedies for inducing a sweat and breaking a fever. Add a little peppermint to improve the flavor. The flowers are highest in the volatile oil during dry weather, so a fresh flower tincture or sealed simmer glycerite made from flowers gathered after a 3-week drought makes a very strong medicine.

WARNINGS: Yarrow is a safe remedy, but should be reserved for medicinal use and not taken regularly.

ENERGETICS: Cooling, drying, and constricting

PROPERTIES: Anti-inflammatory, antiviral, diaphoretic, febrifuge, hemostatic, and vulnerary

SPECIFIC INDICATIONS: Rolla Thomas: In irritative conditions of the urinary apparatus, strangury, and suppression of urine. The best results are obtained from the infusion.

SOURCES: Bulk Herb Store, Frontier Herbs, Mountain Rose Herbs, San Francisco Herb Company, Starwest Botanicals, Stony Mountain Botanicals

DOSAGE FORMS

FRESH LEAVES: Can be crushed and applied topically as a poultice for cuts and insect bites

STANDARD INFUSION: 4–8 ounces 3 times daily. The tea tastes better when mixed with equal parts peppermint.

TINCTURE: Fresh flower and leaf (1:2, 95% alcohol); dried flowers and leaf (1:5, 40% alcohol); 5 drops to 2 ml (0.4 tsp.) 3 times daily

GLYCERITE: Fresh flowers (1:6, 80% glycerin sealed simmer method), 0.25–1 ml (0.05–0.2 tsp.) 3 times daily; dried flowers (1:6), 1–3 ml (0.2–0.6 tsp.) 3 times daily; add full dose to a cup of hot water for an instant diaphoretic tea.

TOPICAL USE: An infusion can be used as a soak or as a compress. The tincture can be applied to bites and stings, or used as a wound wash (it burns).

YELLOW DOCK

Latin name: *Rumex crispus*

Yellow dock is high in organic iron compounds and seems to free iron stored in the liver. This makes it useful for anemia, especially when combined with alfalfa, beets, and other iron-rich herbs. It is also used as a blood purifier for skin disorders (acne, boils, etc.) and general liver problems. It stimulates the flow of bile and acts as a mild laxative while reducing heat and irritation in the digestive tract. It is especially indicated when a person has a geographic tongue (a tongue with heavily coated patches and bare, bright-red areas) and intestinal inflammation with constipation.

WARNINGS: No known warnings

ENERGETICS: Cooling and slightly drying

PROPERTIES: Alterative (blood purifier), aperient, cholagogue, and hepatic

SPECIFIC INDICATIONS: Felter: Vitiated blood, with skin disorders; low glandular and cellular deposits, with tendency to ulceration. Dyspnea, with epigastric fullness and pectoral distress. Anorexia, with disturbed nutrition.

SOURCES: Bulk Herb Store, Mountain Rose Herbs, San Francisco Herb Company, Starwest Botanicals, Stony Mountain Botanicals

DOSAGE FORMS

STANDARD DECOCTION: 2–4 ounces 2 times daily

TINCTURE: Fresh root (1:2, 95% alcohol); dried root (1:5, 60% alcohol); 10 drops to 2 ml (0.4 tsp.) 3 times daily

POWDER OR CAPSULE: 100 mg, 3 times daily; the looser the stool, the smaller the dose

YERBA MANSA

Latin name: *Anemopsis californica*

Yerba mansa is a strong anti-inflammatory and antimicrobial. It is helpful for mouth, throat, sinus, and gastric infections. It can be used topically for boils and abscesses.

ENERGETICS: Warming and drying

PROPERTIES: Antibacterial, anti-inflammatory, and antifungal

SOURCES: Starwest Botanicals

DOSAGE FORMS

TINCTURE: Freshly dried (1:4, 75% alcohol); fresh root (1:2, 95% alcohol, 10% glycerin); 10 drops to 2 ml (0.4 tsp.) 3 times daily

YERBA SANTA

Latin name: *Eriodictyon californicum*

A warming and stimulating expectorant, yerba santa clears phlegm from the chest and opens air passages. It is a reliable herb for most respiratory problems, but is especially helpful for asthma, profuse expectoration, and respiratory complaints with obscure symptoms. It is also an effective diuretic and urinary antiseptic. It can be applied topically to insect bites and stings, poison oak and ivy, bruises, sprains, and cuts.

WARNINGS: No known warnings

ENERGETICS: Warming and drying

PROPERTIES: Decongestant and expectorant

SPECIFIC INDICATIONS: Rolla Thomas: Cough with abundant and easy expectoration.

SOURCES: Mountain Rose Herbs, Starwest Botanicals

DOSAGE FORMS

STANDARD INFUSION: 2–4 ounces 3 times daily

TINCTURE: Fresh leaf (1:2, 95% alcohol); dried leaf (1:5, 60% alcohol); 1–2 ml (0.2–0.4 tsp.) 2–4 times daily

CAPSULE: 500–1,000 mg up to 4 times daily

YOHIMBE

Latin name: *Pausinystalia johimbe*

Yohimbe causes dilation of blood vessels, including those in the genitalia, thus helping men to achieve an erection. Unfortunately it's also likely to cause elevated blood pressure and heart rate, agitation, and even mania. In short, yohimbe has some nasty side effects, and we feel that the benefits don't outweigh the cost. We don't recommend using it.

WARNINGS: Avoid long-term use, as it can irritate the urinary tract. Contraindicated in cases of emaciation or inflammation.

ENERGETICS: Warming

PROPERTIES: Vasodilator

YUCCA

Latin name: *Yucca glauca*

A blood purifier with anti-inflammatory and detergent properties, yucca leaf has antioxidant, anti-inflammatory, and antifungal properties. It is helpful as an analgesic and anti-inflammatory in arthritis, neuralgia, and other inflammatory conditions.

WARNINGS: Excessive consumption may cause diarrhea, nausea, upset stomach, and vomiting. Use only under professional supervision during pregnancy.

ENERGETICS: Cooling and moistening

PROPERTIES: Alterative (blood purifier), anti-inflammatory, and antiseptic

SOURCES: Frontier Herbs, Mountain Rose Herbs, San Francisco Herb Company, Starwest Botanicals, Stony Mountain Botanicals

DOSAGE FORMS

STANDARD DECOCTION: 2–4 ounces 3 times daily

TINCTURE: Fresh root (1:2, 95% alcohol); dried root (1:5, 60% alcohol); 1–3 ml (0.2–0.6 tsp.) 3 times daily

GLYCERITE: Dried root (1:5); 2.5–5 ml (0.5–1 tsp.) 3 times daily

CAPSULE: 500–1,000 mg, 3 times daily

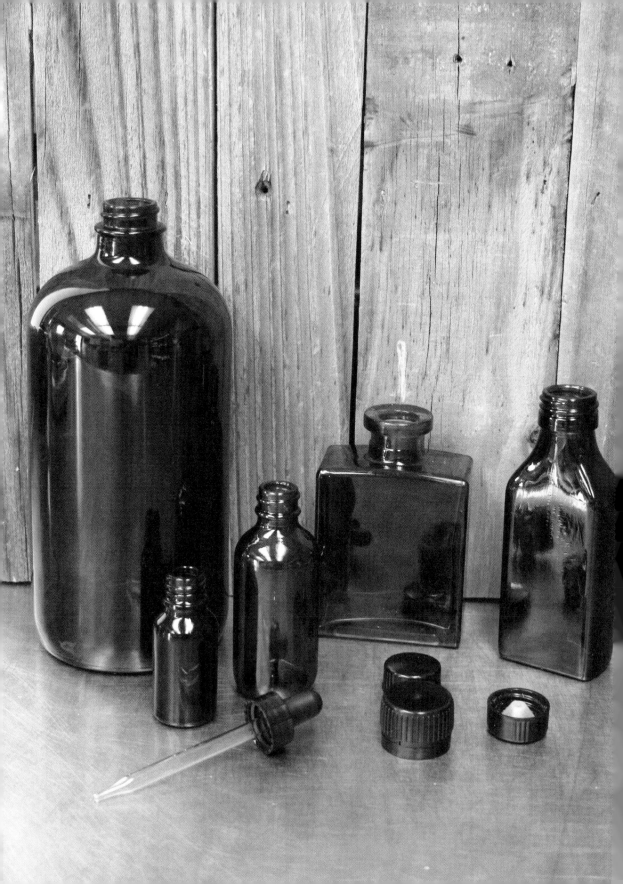

Herbal Hydrotherapy

COMBINING HERBS AND WATER FOR HEALING

Hydrotherapy is a term that means water therapy, which is the use of water for therapeutic purposes. Water can be used as ice, hot or cold water, or steam to help ease pain, improve circulation, reduce inflammation, detoxify the body, or stimulate healing. Hydrotherapy treatments include enemas and douches, baths, foot soaks, and steams.

Herbal hydrotherapy combines these water therapies with herbs. Herbs and water are powerful allies in healing a wide variety of ailments. This appendix covers the various ways of combining hydrotherapy and herbs for healing.

ENEMAS

Enemas can be an important therapeutic aid for healing the colon. They can be used to hydrate the bowel and cleanse the body. They are even more effective when herbs are added to the water used in the enema.

Herbal enemas can be used to:

- Cleanse the colon by removing large intestinal impactions
- Soothe colon irritation and inflammation
- Promote healing of colon tissues
- Relax bowel spasms and ease severe gas and bloating
- Reduce fevers (the majority of all fevers in children will come down once the colon is cleared)
- Relieve respiratory and lymphatic congestion

- Restore healthy intestinal flora (when probiotics or healthy fecal material are used in the enema)
- Get rid of intestinal parasites

HERBAL ENEMA SOLUTIONS

Herbal enemas have been used extensively in Ayurveda (basti) and traditional Chinese medicine, with many of the most popular herbs either being nutritive or having strong antimicrobial and anti-inflammatory properties.

Start by making the herbal enema solution using either 2 cups of a very strong tea or decoction per quart of water used in the enema, or add ½–2 teaspoons of tinctures or glycerites per quart of water. The water may be warm or cool, depending on the situation.

Some good herbs for enemas include catnip (for fevers), pau d'arco (for fungal infections), lobelia or lavender (for spasms), aloe vera (for inflammation and tissue healing), Oregon grape (for infection), and anise (for gas and bloating). Several of the formulas in Chapter Twelve work very well as an enema. These include: Herbal Composition, Children's Composition, and Herbal Crisis. These formulas are helpful for enemas for colds, fever, and congestion. The Herbal Crisis formula is particularly useful for clearing out sticky fecal matter as it loosens mucus.

You can make an enema for infections using raw garlic. Place 1 clove raw garlic per quart of water in a blender. Blend thoroughly, then strain the solution, and use small amounts as a rectal injection. This works well for respiratory infections and fevers.

HOW TO TAKE THE ENEMA

Always test the enema solution to make sure it is warm, not hot or cold. If you place a couple of drops on your wrist (like testing a baby bottle), it should feel neutral, slightly warm, or slightly cool in temperature. Add cool or warm water to adjust the temperature if necessary, then put the enema solution into the enema bag or bucket. Release the catch on the tube and allow the solution to flow through the tube to clear all the air out of the tube, then close the catch.

Lubricate the end of the enema tip and the rectal area with a petroleum jelly (Vaseline®), herbal salve, or other lubricant. Lie down on your left side and gently insert the tip into the rectum. Release the catch, and allow the solution to flow into the colon.

During this process, anytime you feel pain or discomfort, stop the flow of enema solution. Wait a minute or two and perhaps even lightly massage the area where you feel the pain and discomfort. If it does not go away, then use the toilet, expelling the liquid and waste material. Then start again.

Once the fluid flows freely into the colon while you are lying on your left side, you can move to your back and continue the procedure. Finish the procedure by lying on your right side.

To do what is called a "high enema," when you clear the entire colon from ascending to descending, you may need to fill the bag or enema bucket several times. In fact, the first few times you try this, you may not be able to do this at all. You may encounter spasms or other obstructions that won't want to move. Don't worry about this; just cleanse the colon as far as it wants to go.

Don't be discouraged; it took me several months of doing an enema once per week before I was able to get fluid past the halfway point in my colon due to a muscle spasm in my transverse colon. I finally learned to use lobelia or lavender oil (mentioned above) to relax that spasm and clean out the entire length of the colon.

GIVING AN ENEMA TO A CHILD

When giving a child or an infant an enema, you use a syringe. There are special syringes made just for giving enemas, but a regular bulb syringe can also be used. Prepare the enema solution and test the temperature as before.

Place a towel on the floor and lay the child on his or her back or left side on the towel. When doing this with a baby, place a diaper on top of the towel. Explain to the child that this procedure will be uncomfortable, but it will help him or her feel better. Be gentle and patient. If you were taking the child to the doctor, the child might have to get a shot or have blood drawn, which would hurt far more, but you'd probably make the child hold still for that anyway, so think of it in this same manner. An enema is nowhere near as painful as a shot, and you can explain this to a child.

Lubricate the anal opening and the tip of the syringe. Fill the syringe with the enema solution by squeezing the syringe and then sucking up the solution. Turn the syringe upright and squeeze any remaining air out of it. Fill it the rest of the way, so that the syringe is completely full. Gently insert the tip of the syringe into the anus. Then give a gentle squeeze. If you encounter strong resistance, or the child seems to be in pain, stop squeezing and withdraw the syringe. Make sure you don't "suck" with the syringe as you withdraw.

If nothing comes out, repeat the process. It may take several tries before anything passes, but don't be concerned; just be patient. Putting in a small amount of fluid every 5 minutes will not hurt the bowel. In fact, often small children get dehydrated from not drinking enough fluids when they are feverish or sick, so the body could be absorbing all of the liquid that you have put into the bowel.

Tell an older child they can go "potty" if they feel that they need to. If they don't, repeat the process. Then wait a minute or two and put a little more fluid in.

With a baby, on the other hand, put a diaper on the baby's bottom after putting one syringe-full into the rectum, and then wrap the diaper in a towel. (Enemas can make the stool "runny," and you don't want it to leak onto you.) Then cuddle and hold the baby for a few minutes. If nothing comes out after about 10–20 minutes, repeat the procedure.

The stool should be soft. If only a small amount of hard stool is passed, you may still need to repeat the process until a soft stool passes. The trick is to get the bowel to move freely.

RECTAL INJECTIONS

Rectal injections are similar to enemas, but they are not used to try to clear the colon. Instead, a small amount of herbal fluid is injected into the rectum, and it is left there to be absorbed rather than being expelled.

Rectal injections can be used to:

- Shrink hemorrhoids or anal fistulas (using liquid preparations of astringent herbs)

- Administer an herbal remedy to a child or elderly person who is having trouble swallowing an herb they need
- Hydrate a person or child who is severely dehydrated but can't or won't drink fluids (using solutions of mineral-rich herbs like alfalfa or oat straw to provide electrolytes)

DOUCHES

Douches can be helpful for vaginal infections, vaginal irritation, and excessive bleeding. For a douche, you will need an enema bag with a vaginal tip. Mix the douche solution the same way that you would mix an enema solution. Hold the liquid in the vagina for 5–15 minutes, using pillows to prop the hips up, before expelling it.

Here are some suggestions for herbs to use in douches. For vaginal yeast infections, consider using calendula flowers, pau d'arco bark, or barberry root. Tea tree oil can also be used cautiously (some women find it highly irritating), following the same directions for making an enema solution with essential oils described in the previous section. Use only 1 drop per quart.

For bacterial vaginosis, mix 10% povidone iodine and 90% distilled water for a douche solution. For excessive bleeding, use styptic herbs like bayberry root bark, calendula, yarrow, or white oak bark.

Regular douching is not recommended and can cause an imbalance of beneficial vaginal microbes.

BATHS AND SOAKS

Baths and soaks invigorate and stimulate circulation, or relax and soothe sore muscles. They can help to ease itching and skin eruptions and to hasten recovery from colds and fevers.

Add herbs to a bath by hanging 3–4 tea bags from the tap, or put a tea infuser in the water. A large gauze bag or a cotton sock will hold larger amounts of herbs. You can also make a strong decoction, strain it, and add the liquid to the bath.

Essential oils may be added to a bath as well; mix in a few drops of soap to disperse the oil in the bath water. Use caution: essential oils can burn the skin if not well diluted.

A sitz bath is useful for hemorrhoids and for prostate, vaginal, and uterine problems. It is also used to relax the pelvic floor in preparation for labor. Fill a large basin as above, and sit down in the water.

Foot soaks can help restore circulation to the legs, reduce swelling in the ankles or feet, and heal injuries. Fill a wash basin with hot water and herbs and soak the feet.

HERBS FOR BATHS AND SOAKS

The following are useful herbs for herbal baths and soaks:

Itching (Hives, Chicken Pox, etc.) Yellow dock, burdock, Oregon grape, barberry, comfrey, chickweed, lavender, vinegar (hot bath only), clay

Swelling and Inflammation Comfrey, plantain, white oak bark, calendula, witch hazel, chamomile

Cleansing Skin Pores Ginger, chamomile, vinegar (hot bath only)

Relaxing Nerves Kava-kava (seriously, try this as a whole-body soak), lavender, chamomile, rose, catnip, Epsom salts

SWEAT BATHS

Many people in temperate climates the world over have used sweating to both prevent and treat disease. Scandinavians built saunas; Native Americans built sweat lodges. The pioneer herbalist Samuel Thomson would wrap a person sitting in a chair in blankets and place a hot stone in a pail at his feet. By pouring water into the pail, the steam would come up under the blankets until the patient started to perspire.

A sweat bath can be used to:

- Help break a fever
- Speed recovery from colds, flu, or other acute infections

- General detoxification of the blood and lymph
- Stimulate the immune system

This therapy is contraindicated if you have a weak heart or high blood pressure or if you are weak, pale, and feeble. It is also not good for small children or very elderly people.

Mildly overheating the body simulates a slight fever and can be a powerful natural healing tool against serious disease. Fever is a natural defense and healing response of the immune system, created and sustained by the body to rid itself of harmful pathogens and to restore health. The high body temperature speeds up metabolism and inhibits the replication of the harmful virus or bacteria.

Here's how to take a sweat bath:

Step one: Drink plenty of water, and do not eat for 2 hours prior to the sweat bath.

Step two: Prepare an infusion with herbs that enhance perspiration. Drink some of the tea before entering the bath, and sip the tea frequently while in the bath. Examples of sweat-enhancing teas include:

- Herbal Composition, Children's Composition, or Herbal Crisis (see Chapter Twelve)
- Yarrow and peppermint tea (equal parts)
- Fresh ginger juice tea

Step three: Fill the tub with water as hot as can be tolerated comfortably. Epsom salts, Redmond clay, ginger, or essential oils may be added to the bath. If adding essential oils, mix them with a tablespoon of natural salt or ½ cup Epsom salts before adding them to the bath. This helps the oils dissolve in the water. (See more about aromatherapy in Chapter Ten.)

Step four: Soak in the tub for at least 20 minutes. Keep the water as hot as you can tolerate comfortably. Keep as much of your body submerged in the water as possible. If you start to feel faint, sit up and drape a cool washcloth over your face. Drain the tub if you become too uncomfortable.

Step five: Gentle massage with a skin brush helps bring the blood to the surface of the skin.

Step six: Optional: After soaking in the bath, stand up and rinse off with a quick, cool shower. This will enhance the sweating effect. **Step seven:** Go to bed and pile on the covers. Drink plenty of fluids. Stay in bed for at least an hour. It's fine to fall asleep. When finished, take a shower to cleanse the skin and close your pores.

Don't put small children into a really hot bath. Use a warm bath and gently wash their body down with some natural soap and a washcloth to make certain their pores are open. Add 3–4 drops lavender oil or tea tree oil (diluted with a natural liquid soap) or a little bit of Dr. Bronner's peppermint, tea tree, or eucalyptus soap to the bath. The essential oils will help to stimulate the circulation and draw the blood to the extremities.

COLD-SHEET TREATMENT

A cold-sheet treatment is performed using the same basic procedures as for the sweat bath, but is much more effective in inducing perspiration. It is a powerful way to detoxify the body.

Here's how to do the cold-sheet treatment:

Step one: Follow steps 1–5 for the sweat bath.

Step two: Cover the bed with a piece of plastic.

Step three: Soak a sheet in water (warm for a milder effect; cold for a stronger effect). As the person gets out of the bath, immediately wrap them in the damp sheet and have them lie down on the plastic sheet. Wrap the plastic around the damp sheet, and cover the person with blankets to warm up the body and induce perspiration.

Step four: After about 1 hour, have the person get up and shower to clean off the skin.

DRAWING BATHS

Sweat baths open the sweat glands to cause perspiration, whereas drawing baths target the sebaceous glands (or oil ducts) in the skin. Drawing baths are useful for skin eruptive diseases, rashes, hives, pox, acne, and so forth. They can also be helpful for detoxification from heavy metals, especially the clay baths.

A variety of herbs may be used in a drawing bath. You can also use Epsom salts and/or clay. Herbs that are good for drawing baths include mucilaginous herbs like comfrey leaf, plantain, and various seaweeds and alterative herbs like Oregon grape, goldenseal, burdock, yellow dock, and red clover. Oregon grape, goldenseal, and yellow dock all contain a yellow dye that can color the skin. It wears off rather quickly, but be warned.

To make an herbal drawing bath, make a decoction of any of these herbs in a large pot containing 1–2 gallons of water. Use about ¼–½ cup herbs per gallon. Simmer the herbs for at least 20–30 minutes, add this to the bath, then fill the tub with more water, adjusting the temperature to make the bath comfortable.

You can also use commercially prepared liquid herbal extracts in a bath, but you need about 2–4 ounces of extract per bath, which can be expensive.

Two other agents that are really effective for drawing baths are Epsom salts and fine clays. Epsom salts are available at any supermarket or drugstore. Use about 2 cups Epsom salts per bath. Epsom salts are also helpful for sweat baths. They relax the skin pores and encourage elimination through the skin.

Fine clay is even more effective than Epsom salts as a drawing agent. You have probably heard of or maybe even used a clay mask for drawing oil out of skin pores. Clay can be used in a similar manner in a bath, to absorb both fat- and water-soluble toxins from the body. Redmond clay, which is mined in Utah, is a good brand to use, and you can buy it in large boxes; but any fine clay will do.

HERBAL STEAM BATHS

Herbs rich in essential oils, such as basil, eucalyptus, and lavender, will release their properties into steam. Set a hot plate on the floor, and warm a pot of herbs and water on it. Sit on a cushioned metal chair over the hot plate and pot, and wrap a large blanket from your neck down to the floor. Be sure that the blanket doesn't get too close to the hot plate and catch on fire! This leaves your head out of the steam and keeps it cool, but heats up the rest of your body nicely.

Pelvic Steams

Pelvic steams are used for vaginal problems and hemorrhoids. Vaginal steams are less invasive than douching, and hemorrhoid steams are a nice pain reliever. Boil 1 gallon of water, add 100 grams of herbs, and let steep for 10 minutes. Place the entire pot of water in your toilet. Test the temperature by holding your inner arm over the steam at toilet-seat level. If it's too hot, let it cool for a few minutes and retest. When you feel comfortable with the temperature, sit on the toilet. Our favorite herbs for vaginal steams are yarrow, oregano, basil, calendula, and rosemary. Don't put essential oils into a vaginal steam; they are too irritating to the mucous membranes. For hemorrhoids, a steam of yarrow, calendula, and arnica works well.

CONTRAST THERAPY (ALTERNATING HOT AND COLD SOAKS)

Hot water has a relaxing, opening effect, whereas cold water causes constriction and a reduction in blood flow. Alternating hot and cold hydrotherapy stimulates blood circulation, lymphatic drainage, and nerve energy. It can ease spasmodic pain and cramping, improve circulation, enhance muscle tone, and improve mood.

One form of this method is to alternate hot and cold showers. Start with a comfortable hot shower for 3 minutes. Follow with a sudden change to cold water for 2 minutes. Repeat this cycle 3 times, ending with cold. After the shower, have a full or partial massage, or a brisk towel rub.

Another form of this therapy is to alternate hot and cold soaks for a body part, such as the feet. This therapy has proved helpful for gangrene or other illnesses involving poor circulation to the extremities. Alternate the hot and cold soaks in the same manner as the hot and cold showers. To further enhance the effect, stimulating herbs (like capsicum, garlic, and ginger) may be added to the hot soak, and soothing herbs (like comfrey or plantain) to the cold soak.

SITZ BATHS

Alternating hot and cold sitz baths may provide symptom relief and help speed recovery from a variety of ailments. It may be used as a healing technique for a patient who cannot take a full shower. It is especially beneficial for increasing circulation in the pelvic and urethral area, and is commonly recommended for vaginal yeast infections, hemorrhoids, and the like.

Step one: Fill a washtub with warm water so that you can soak your bottom in the water. As an alternative, fill the bathtub with water up to about ½ inch above your navel when seated.

Step two: Soak in the bath for 20–30 minutes. Cover the upper body with a towel, and place a cool, wet washcloth on the forehead.

Step three: Take a quick, cool rinse in the shower, or splash the body with cool water, before drying off, to further stimulate circulation.

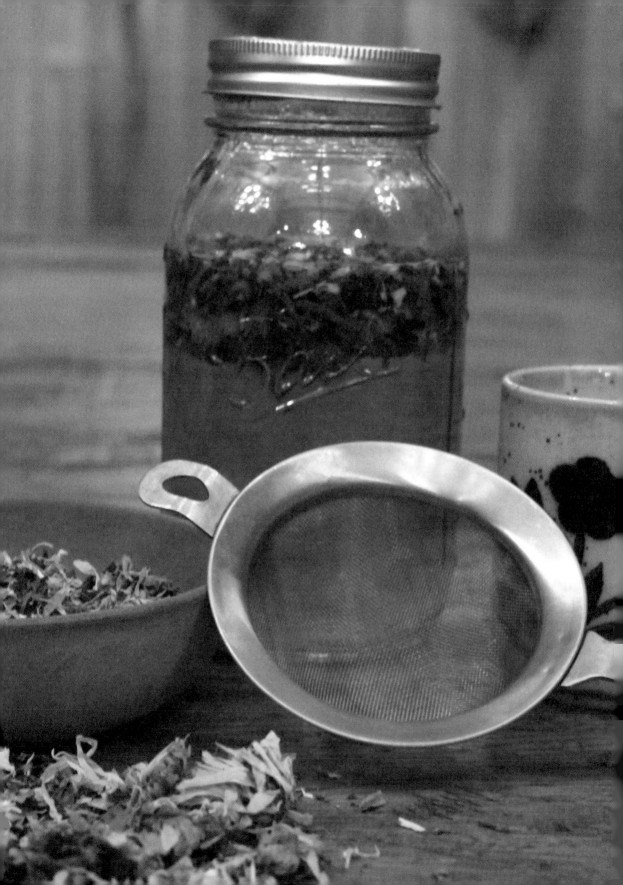

Recommended Suppliers

SOURCES FOR HERB PLANTS AND SEEDS, BULK HERBS, BOTTLES, GLYCERIN, AND OTHER SUPPLIES

The quality of the plants you use to make your herbal medicines is important. Growing or gathering your own herbs can be a very rewarding experience. Therefore, we encourage you to grow your own medicinal plants if possible. Sources for herb plants and seeds are listed below.

You can also learn how to sustainably harvest medicinal herbs growing in your area. To learn to identify local herbs, take a field botany class or plant walks with local herbalists and get to know the plants around you. To look for herbalists who do plant walks, visit http://findanherbalist.com.

If you can't harvest your own plants, purchase them from ethical suppliers. It's a good thing to know who is picking the herbs you purchase. Are they harvesting these plants with reverence and respect for nature? Are they harvesting them ethically and sustainably? Are the herbs correctly identified and free from contaminants?

This appendix contains a list of small companies that grow and collect herbs themselves. Small suppliers don't have the variety of plants that large suppliers do, but purchasing from them supports small scale family growers and local economies. You're also supporting people who are passionate about the quality of herbs they provide.

Larger bulk herb companies offer a better selection, and sometimes better prices. You may also be able to save on shipping if you're ordering a wide variety of herbs. Our favorite company in this category is Mountain Rose Herbs. Their commitment to quality herbs, and the time and money they spend supporting multiple free herbal clinics, great educational experiences, herb conferences, and the herbal community as a whole, is amazing.

In Chapter Thirteen we've listed larger bulk herb companies that supplied each herb at the time this book was written. A more up-to-date database of herb companies and suppliers for individual herbs, herbal formulas, and supplements is found in the member area at http://herbiverse.com.

SOURCES FOR PLANTS AND SEEDS

Companion Plants
7247 N. Coolville Ridge Road
Athens, OH 45701
(740) 592-4643
www.companionplants.com

Goodwin Creek Gardens
Grants Pass, OR
(800) 846-7359
www.goodwincreekgardens.com

Mountain Valley Growers
38325 Pepperweed Road
Squaw Valley, CA 93675
(559) 338-2775
www.mountainvalleygrowers.com

Sandy Mush Herb Nursery

316 Surret Cove Road
Leicester, NC 28748
(828) 683-2014
www.sandymushherbs.com

Strictly Medicinal Seeds
PO Box 69
Williams, OR 97544
(541) 846-6704
www.strictlymedicinalseeds.com

The Thyme Garden
20546 Alsea Hwy.

Alsea, OR 97324
(541) 487-8671
www.thymegarden.com

SMALLER HERB SUPPLIERS

AncesTree Herbals
PO Box 641
Twisp, WA 98856
(509) 997-3365
www.ancestreeherbals.com

Flack Family Farm
3971 Pumpkin Village Road
Enosburg Falls, VT 05450
(802) 933-7752
www.flackfamilyfarm.com

Gentle Harmony Farm
3354 Friendship Church Road
Lexington, NC 27295
(336) 787-3223
www.gentleharmonyfarm.com

Healing Spirits Herb Farm
61247 Rt. 415
Avoca, NY 14809
(607) 566-2701
www.healingspiritsherbfarm.com

Heartsong Farm Healing Herbs
859 Lost Nation Road
Groveton, NH 03582
(603) 636-2286
www.herbsandapples.com

Maple Spring Gardens
9812 Allison Road
Cedar Grove, NC 27231
(336) 562-5719
www.maplespringgardens.com

Mountain Gardens
546 Shuford Creek Road
Burnsville, NC 28714
(828) 675-5664
http://mountaingardensherbs.com

Oregon's Wild Harvest
1601 NE Hemlock Avenue
Redmond, OR 97756
(541) 548-9400
www.oregonswildharvest.com

Pacific Botanicals
4840 Fish Hatchery Road
Grants Pass, OR 97527
(541) 479-7777
www.pacificbotanicals.com

Pharmacopia Herbals
PO Box 1791
Eugene, OR 97440
(877) 243-5373
www.pharmacopiaherbals.com

Zack Woods Herbs
278 Mead Road
Hyde Park, VT 05655
(802) 888-7278
www.zackwoodsherbs.com

LARGER HERB SUPPLIERS

The following are some suppliers who sell bulk herbs, glycerin, and other materials for making your own herbal preparations.

Bulk Herb Store
26 West 6th Avenue
Lobelville, TN 83097
(877) 278-4257
www.bulkherbstore.com

Frontier Herbs
PO Box 229
Norway, IA 52318
(800) 669-3275
www.frontiercoop.com

Mountain Rose Herbs
PO Box 50220
Eugene, OR 97405
(800) 879-3337
www.mountainroseherbs.com

San Francisco Herb Company
250 14th Street
San Francisco, CA 94103
(800) 227-4530
www.sfherb.com

Starwest Botanicals
11253 Trade Center Drive
Rancho Cordova, CA 95742
(888) 369-4372
www.starwest-botanicals.com

Stony Mountain Botanicals
PO Box 106
Loudonville, OH 44842
www.wildroots.com

BOTTLES AND OTHER SUPPLIES

Bulk Apothecary
125 Lena Drive
Aurora, OH 44202
(888) 728-7612
www.bulkapothecary.com

The Chemistry Store.com
1133 Walter Price Street
Cayce, SC 29033
(800) 224-1430
www.chemistrystore.com

Industrial Container and Supply Company
1845 South 5200 West
Salt Lake City, UT 84104
(801) 972-1561
www.industrialcontainer.com

Specialty Bottle
3434 4th Avenue S.
Seattle, WA 98134
(206) 382-1100
www.specialtybottle.com

Uline
12575 Uline Drive
Pleasant Prairie, WI 53158
(800) 295-5510
www.uline.com

Recommended Reading

Chevallier, Andrew. *Encyclopedia of Herbal Medicine*. A nice general reference for 550 common herbs.

Foster, Steven and Hobbs, Christopher; *Western Medicinal Plants and Herbs*. A nice field guide to herbal medicines.

Gladstar, Rosemary: *Herbal Recipes for Vibrant Health*. A great reference for making herbal products, with useful recipes.

Hall, Dorothy: *Creating Your Herbal Profile*. A good reference on personality profiles for medicinal herbs.

Kaminski, Patricia and Katz, Richard; *Flower Essence Repertory*. A great guide to flower essences, both Bach flower remedies and North American remedies.

Kuhn, Merrily A. and Winston, David; *Herbal Therapy and Supplements: A Scientific and Traditional Approach*. An excellent and reliable reference on scientific research, constituents and clinical use of many common herbs.

McGuffin, Michael; Hobbs, Christopher; Upton, Roy; Goldberg, Alicia; *Botanical Safety Handbook*. A reliable, well-recognized safety handbook from the American Herbal Products Association.

McIntyre, Anne; *Flower Power: Flower Remedies for Healing Body and Soul*. A great guide to emotional indications of herbs, flower essences and essential oils.

Mills, Simon and Bone, Kerry; *The Essential Guide to Herbal Safety*. Another good safety reference.

Moore, Micheal; *Medicinal Plants of the Desert and Canyon West*.

—— *Medicinal Plants of the Mountain West*.

—— Southwest School of Botanical Medicine Website (www.swsbm.com).

Michael Moore is a great resource for dependable herbal information. His website is loaded with valuable material.

PDR for Herbal Medicines. A good reference for scientific information on herbs, but not a good clinical resource.

Wardwell, Joyce A: *The Herbal Home Remedy Book*. A nice guide to medicine making.

Willard, Terry; *Edible and Medicinal Plants of the Rocky Mountains and Neighboring Territories*. A nice field guide to wild medicinal plants in the Western U.S.

Wood, Matthew; *The Book of Herbal Wisdom: Using Plants as Medicine*.

—— Wood, Matthew; *The Earthwise Herbal: A Complete Guide to New World Medicinal Plants*. An essential guide to eclectic materia medica.

—— Wood, Matthew; The Earthwise Herbal: A Complete Guide to Old World Medicinal Plants.

Matthew Wood is a great resource for detailed clinical indications for herbal remedies including emotional profiles.

Ellingwood, 1919: *The American Materia Medica*. A great example of the work of Eclectic Physicians. Ellingwood has great indications not found in other Eclectic books.

Culpeper, Nicholas. *English Physician and Complete Herbal*. A classic that still hold relevance for practitioners wanting a glimpse at herbalism 400 years ago.

Felter, Harvey Wickes, MD, and John Uri Lloyd, PhrM, PhD, 1898: *King's American Dispensatory*.

Scudder, John M, MD, 1898: *The American Eclectic Materia Medica*. Scudder added valuable contributions to the Eclectic Materia Medica and almost single handedly changed their practice.

Fyfe, William, MD, 1935: *The Essentials of Modern Materia Medica*. The last great Eclectic materia medica.

Remington, Wood, 1918: *The Dispensatory of the United States of America*. An allopathic materia medica from when doctors still used botanical medicine.

Shook, Edward. *Advanced Treatise in Herbology*. A semi-modern classic in the Neo-Thomsonianism style and a key book in the Mormon herbal revival.

Grieve, Maude; *A Modern Herbal*. A classic guide to early 20th century herbal medicine.

Alexander, Leslie M., and Linda A. Straub-Bruce. *Dental Herbalism: Natural Therapies for the Mouth*. The only comprehensive book on taking care of your mouth naturally! Includes great recipes for tooth powders, tooth paste and more.

Hoffmann, David. *Medical Herbalism: The Science and Practice of Herbal Medicine*. A wonderful guide through the body systems from a great herbalist. David's formulas are lovely!

Plant Healer Magazine. Each year the magazine is printed and bound in 2 volumes. These are a wonderful resource for contemporary herbalist and feature great articles from both well-known and up and coming herbalists.

Menzies-Trull, Christopher. *Herbal Medicine: Keys to Physiomedicalism including Pharmacopoeia*. A valuable addition to the modern Physiomedical revival from England.

Ganora, Lisa. *Herbal Constituents: Foundations of Phytochemistry*. The best introduction to phytochemistry for herbalists out there!

Romm, Aviva Jill. *Botanical Medicine for Women's Health*. An integrative approach to women's health from a great herbalist and M.D.

Masé, Guido. *The Wild Medicine Solution: Healing with Aromatic, Bitter, and Tonic Plants*. An inspiring guide every herbalist should read.

Rogers, Robert Dale. *The Fungal Pharmacy: The Complete Guide to Medicinal Mushrooms and Lichens of North America*. The authoritative reference work to medicinal mushrooms from a great practitioner.

Coffman, Sam; *The Herbal Medic*. A unique guide to emergency medicine using plants. A must read!

Index

Athlete's foot, 187, 310
Atractylodes (*Actractylodes ovata, A. macrocephala*), 179–80
Atrophy, 9, 10, 11
Avena sativa. See Oat
Azadirachta indica. See Neem

B

Bach, Edward, 131–32
Back pain, 185, 219, 251, 257, 270, 324
Bacopa (*Bacopa monnieri*), 180
 David Winston's Anxiety Formula, 152
Bacterial infections, 173, 179, 209, 225, 234, 236, 270, 307, 309, 315, 321
Baking, 121
Balanced Bitters, 150
Balancing herbs, 140
Balms, 107
Baptisia tinctoria. See Wild indigo
Barberry (*Berberis vulgaris, B. aristata*), 180–81
 for baths and soaks, 336
 for douches, 335
 fluid extract of, 94
 GI Infection and Parasite Formula, 154
 for mouthwashes and gargles, 112
Barks
 harvesting, 36–37, 42–43
 outer vs. inner, 42
Barosma betulina. See Buchu
Basic Blood Purifier, 150
Basic Healing Salve, 162–63
Basic Poultice Formula, 163
Basil, 339, 340
Baths, 130, 335–41
Bayberry (*Myrica cerifera*), 181–82
 for douches, 335
 Herbal Composition, 155
 Herbal Crisis, 156–57
 Herbal Sinus Snuff, 165
 for mouthwashes and gargles, 112
 for sinus snuffs, 112
Bedstraw. *See* Cleavers
Bee pollen, 182
Beers, herbal, 76
Bee stings, 44, 157, 163, 184
Berberine, 180, 240
Berberis aristata. See Barberry
Berberis vulgaris. See Barberry
Berry syrup, fresh, 74
Betonica officinalis. See Wood betony

Bian Que, 75
Bibhitaki (*Terminalia bellirica*), 313
Bilberry (*Vaccinium myrtillus*), 183
Bitter melon (*Momordica charantia*), 183–84
Bitters, 152–53
 alkaloidal, 4–5
 Balanced Bitters, 150
 fragrant, 5
 simple (nonalkaloidal), 4
Blackberry (*Rubus fruticosus*), 187–88
Black cohosh (*Cimicifuga racemosa, Actaea racemosa*), 184–85
Black haw (*Viburnum prunifolium*), 185–86
Black pepper (*Piper nigrum*), 186
Black walnut (*Juglans nigra*), 187
 fluid extract of, 94
 GI Infection and Parasite Formula, 154
 for tooth powders, 112
Bladder infections, 316
Bladderwrack (*Fucus vesiculosus*), 188
Bleeding
 capillary, 228
 excessive, 257, 303, 312, 325, 335
 gums, 319
 internal, 284, 325
Blessed thistle (*Cnicus benedictus*), 189
Bloating, 186, 233, 331, 332
Blood clots, 199, 297
Blood pressure
 high, 176, 184, 185, 234, 246, 257, 265, 268, 275, 279, 283, 309, 314
 low, 261, 272, 303
Blood purifiers, 209, 298, 313, 326, 329
 Basic Blood Purifier, 150
Bloodroot (*Sanguinaria canadensis*), 189–90
Blood sugar, regulating, 223, 231, 238, 240, 244, 246, 254, 260, 289
Blue cohosh (*Caulophyllum thalictroides*), 190–91
Blue flag (*Iris versicolor*), 191
Blue vervain (*Verbena hastata, V. officinalis*), 101, 192
Boils, 187, 277, 326, 327
Boluses, 111
Bone fractures, 267
Boneset (*Eupatorium perfoliatum*), 193
Borage (*Borago officinalis*), 193–94
Boswellia (*Boswellia serrata*), 194–95
Bottles, 346
BPH (benign prostatic hypertrophy), 272
Breast cancer, 287
Brigham tea (*Ephedra viridis*), 195

Clove (*Eugenia caryophyllata, Syzygium aromaticum*), 112, 213–14

Clover. *See* Red clover

Cnicus benedictus. See Blessed thistle

Codonopsis (*Codonopsis pilosula*), 214–15

Coffee grinders, 58

Coffey, Aeneas, 77

Coffman, Sam, ix

Colds, 149, 151, 153–54, 155, 157, 173, 174, 179, 192, 193, 206, 208, 225, 230, 236, 250, 259, 270, 278, 283, 295, 298, 306, 335, 336

Cold-sheet treatment, 338

Cold sores, 259

Colic, 174, 175, 184, 206, 208, 231

Colitis, 194, 201

Collinsonia (*Collinsonia canadensis*), 215

Colon cleansing, 204, 221

Coltsfoot (*Tussilago farfara*), 216

Comfrey (*Symphytum officinale*), 216–17
  Basic Healing Salve, 162–63
  for baths and soaks, 336, 339
  dry-roasting, 120
  for plasters and poultices, 110
  for suppositories and boluses, 111

Commiphora molmol. See Myrrh

Commiphora mukul. See Guggul

Commiphora myrrha. See Myrrh

Compound Wine of Solomon's Seal, 152

Compresses, 103–4, 109–10

Concentrates, powdered, 115–17

Congestive heart failure, 176

Conjunctivitis, 164

Constipation, 184, 196, 204, 233, 314, 327

Constriction, 9, 11, 12

Contrast therapy, 340

Convallaria majalis. See Lily of the valley

COPD, 229, 270

Cordyceps (*Cordyceps sinensis, C. militaris*), 217–18

Coriander (*Coriandrum sativum*). *See* Cilantro

Corns, 207

Corn silk (*Zea mays*), 218

Corydalis (*Corydalis yanhusuo*), 218–19
  fluid extract of, 94
  Pain Formula, 160

Cotton root (*Gossypium herbaceum*), 219

Cough drops, 118–19

Coughs, 151, 153, 229, 248, 260, 265, 270, 284, 285, 304, 306, 320

Cough syrups
  Herbal Cough Syrup (Drying), 156

Herbal Cough Syrup (Moistening), 156
  Horehound Cough Syrup, 158

Cramp bark (*Viburnum opulus*), 219–20

Cramps, 199, 219, 269, 304, 340
  abdominal, 282
  intestinal, 174, 322
  menstrual, 190, 219, 269, 282, 322

Cranberry (*Vaccinium macrocarpon*), 220

Cranesbill, 111

Crataegus monogyna. See Hawthorn

Crataegus oxyacantha. See Hawthorn

Crocus sativus. See Saffron

Crohn's disease, 194, 201, 205

Culpeper, Nicholas, 39

Culver's root (*Leptandra virginica*), 221

Curcuma domestica. See Turmeric

Curcuma longa. See Turmeric

Cuts, 44, 252, 263, 328

Cynara scolymus. See Artichoke

Cynarin, 177

Cystitis, 162, 170, 207, 255, 285

D

Damiana (*Turnera diffusa*), 221–22

Dandelion (*Taraxacum officinale*), x, 222
  Balanced Bitters, 150
  David Winston's DOPAA Bitters, 152–53
  dry-roasting, 120
  fluid extract of, 94
  in green drinks, 44
  harvesting root of, 40
  Liver Formula, 159

Datura, 166

David Winston's Anxiety Formula, 152

David Winston's DOPAA Bitters, 152–53

David Winston's SAD Formula, 153

Decanting, 57

Decoctions, 22–23, 71–72

Dehydrated herb juice, 45

Dehydration, 335

Dehydrators, 61

Dementia, 283

Depression, 9, 10, 125, 137, 155, 174, 178, 184, 194, 221, 258, 259, 267, 269, 290, 297, 307, 315

Devil's claw (*Harpagophytum procumbens*), 222–23

Devil's club (*Oplopanax horridus*), 223

Diabetes, 183, 188, 212, 231, 237, 242, 244, 254, 260, 265, 273, 293

Eyebright (*Euphrasia officinalis*), 229–30
    Antiallergy Formula, 148
    for eyewashes, 113
    Herbal Eyewash, 164
Eyes
    infections, 164, 229
    irritated, 183, 210
    red and itchy, 148
Eyewashes, 113
    Herbal Eyewash, 164

F

False unicorn (*Chamaelirium luteum, Helonias dioica*), 230–31
Fatigue, 238, 248
Feet, swollen, 336
Fennel (*Foeniculum vulgare*), 112, 231
Fenugreek (*Trigonella foenum-graecum*), 231–32
Fever, 151, 174, 193, 208, 232, 253, 282, 283, 294, 298, 322, 325, 331, 332, 335, 336, 337
Feverfew (*Tanacetum parthenium*), 232–33
Fiber Blend, Gentle, 154
Filipendula ulmaria. See Meadowsweet
Filters, 59
Fire Cider, 153–54
Flavonoids, 6
Flaxseed (*Linum usitatissimum*), 233
    Gentle Fiber Blend, 154
    for plasters and poultices, 110
Fleabane. *See* Erigeron
Flower essences, 131–33
Flowers
    drying, 38–39
    harvesting, 37, 38
Flu, 149, 151, 153–54, 155, 157, 173, 174, 192, 193, 208, 225, 226, 236, 250, 259, 278, 282, 308, 336
Fluid extracts, 92–93
Foeniculum vulgare. See Fennel
Fomentations, 110
Foot soaks, 331, 336, 340
Formulas
    designing, 135–36, 137–41
    reading, 147
    sample, 147–67
    singles vs., 136–37
Fo-ti. *See* He shou wu
Fouquieria splendens. See Ocotillo
Frankincense. *See* Boswellia
Fried's Rule, 144

Fringe tree (*Chionanthus virginicus*), 233–34
Fruits
    drying, 42
    harvesting, 42
Fucoidan, 188
Fucus vesiculosus. See Bladderwrack
Fungal infections, 148, 179, 189, 234, 258, 271, 281, 307, 310, 311, 315, 329, 332
Funnels, 61

G

Galium aparine. See Cleavers
Gallbladder problems, 191, 233, 254, 315
Gallstones, 233, 259, 275, 315
Gambier. *See* Cat's claw
Ganoderma lucidum. See Reishi
Garbling, 55
Gargles, 112
    Antiseptic Gargle, 148–49
Garlic (*Allium sativum*), 234
    for ear drops, 113
    for enemas, 332
    Fire Cider, 153–54
    Garlic Lemon Aid, 154
    Garlic-Mullein Ear Oil, 164
    oil extract of, 104
    raw, 45
Gas, 175, 186, 208, 233, 283, 314, 331, 332
Gastritis, 201, 205, 232
Gastroenteritis, 236
Gattefossé, René-Maurice, 124
Gaultheria procumbens. See Wintergreen
Gentian (*Gentiana lutea*), 235
Gentle Fiber Blend, 154
Ghost pipe (*Monotropa uniflora*), 235–36
Giardia, 240, 310
GI Infection and Parasite Formula, 154
Ginger (*Zingiber officinale*), 236–37
    baking herbs with, 121
    for baths and soaks, 336
    Fire Cider, 153–54
    Ginger Magic, 155
    for mouthwashes and gargles, 112
Ginkgo (*Ginkgo biloba*), 237–38
Ginseng, American (*Panax quinquefolius*), 238
Ginseng, Asian or Korean (*Panax ginseng*), 238–39
Gladstar, Rosemary, 51, 153
Glycerin extractions (glycerites), 24–25, 78–81
Glycyrrhiza glabra. See Licorice

Goldenrod (*Solidago virgaurea, S. canadensis*), 239–40

Goldenseal (*Hydrastis canadensis*), 240–41
    for baths, 339
        Herbal Sinus Snuff, 165
        for plasters and poultices, 110
        for sinus snuffs, 112
        Suppository for Vaginal Infections, 167

Gossypium herbaceum. See Cotton root

Gotu kola (*Centella asiatica, Hydrocotyle asiatica*), 241–42

Gout, 207, 242, 272

Gravel root (*Eupatorium purpureum*), 242

Graves' disease, 197

Green drinks, 44

Grifola frondosa. See Maitake

Grindelia (*Grindelia spp.*), 44, 242–43

Guarana (*Paullinia cupana, P. sorbilis*), 243–44

Guggul (*Commiphora mukul*), 244

Gums, bleeding, 319

Gumweed. *See* Grindelia

Gymnema (*Gymnema sylvestre*), 244–45

H

Hamamelis virginiana. See Witch hazel

Hangover, 257

Happy Formula, 155

Haritaki (*Terminalia chebula*), 313

Harmonizing herbs, 140

Harpagophytum procumbens. See Devil's claw

Hawthorn (*Crataegus oxyacantha, C. monogyna*), 245–46

Hay fever, 148, 199, 239, 246, 250

Headaches, 192, 199, 232, 253, 258, 268, 283, 290, 301, 304, 314, 324

Healing Salve, Basic, 162–63

Hearing loss, 283

Heartache, 267, 273, 295

Heartbeat
    irregular, 197
    rapid, 197, 268, 273, 279
    strengthening, 203

Heart disease, 176, 179, 245, 268, 269, 273, 286

Heavy metal toxicity, 209, 211

Helicobacter pylori, 183, 220

Helonias dioica. See False unicorn

Hemorrhoids, 199, 200, 215, 249, 319, 324, 334, 336, 340, 341
    Hemorrhoid Suppository, 164

Hepatitis, 173, 254

Herbal Composition, 155, 332, 337

Herbal Cough Syrup (Drying), 156

Herbal Cough Syrup (Moistening), 156

Herbal Crisis, 156–57, 332, 337

Herbal Eyewash, 164

Herbalists, finding, 14

Herbal Mineral Tonic, 157–58

Herbal Nut Butter Balls, 51

Herbal Sinus Snuff, 112, 165

Herbal Tooth Powder, 165

Herb presses, 59–60

Herbs. *See also* Extractions/extracts;
   individual herbs
    assessment and, 12–14
    best dosage forms for, 30–31
    categories of, 3–8
    dosages of, 142–45
    dried, 18–21, 47–52
    energetics of, 1–2
    fresh, 17–18, 33–45
    growing, 34, 343
    harvesting, 35–43, 343
    identifying, x, 34–35, 343
    liquid, 21–26
    purchasing, 47–48
    quality of, 48
    remedy selection and, 14–15
    safety and, 34–35, 37
    sources for, 343–46
    topical use of, 51
    traditional Chinese processing methods for, 119–21

Herpes, 308

He shou wu (*Polygonum multiflorum*), 246

Holy basil (*Ocimum sanctum*), 246–47

Honey, 73

Hops (*Humulus lupulus*), 247–48

Horehound (*Marrubium vulgare*), 248
    Horehound Cough Syrup, 158

Horny goat weed (*Epimedium grandiflorum*), 248–49

Horse chestnut (*Aesculus hippocastanum*), 249

Horseradish (*Armoracia rusticana*), 250
    Fire Cider, 153–54

Horsetail (*Equisetum arvense*), 112, 250–51

Ho shou wu. *See* He shou wu

Hot alcohol extract, 119

Hot flashes, 269, 282

Humulus lupulus. See Hops

Hyaluronidase, 225

Hydrangea (*Hydrangea arborescens*), 251

Hydrastis canadensis. See Goldenseal
Hydrocotyle asiatica. See Gotu kola
Hydrotherapy
    baths and soaks, 335–41
    definition of, 331
    douches, 335
    enemas, 331–34
    rectal injections, 334–35
Hyperactivity, 208
Hypericum perforatum. See St. John's wort
Hypoglycemia, 191, 260
Hypothyroidism, 187
Hyssop (*Hyssopus officinalis*), 251–52

I

Ibn Sīnā, 76
Icariin, 248
Immune system
    Immune Boosting Formula, 158
    Immune Syrup, 158–59
    stimulating, 173, 278, 287, 304, 308, 337
    strengthening, 172, 205, 214, 228, 236,
       264–65, 289, 294
Incontinence, 170
Indian gooseberry. *See* Amalaki
Indian pipe. *See* Ghost pipe
Indigestion, 206, 231, 296, 314
Indigo. *See* Wild indigo
Inflammation Formula, 159
Infusions, 22, 23, 70–71
Insect bites, 44, 157, 163, 242, 252, 262, 285,
    311, 328
Insomnia, 201, 206, 218, 247, 253, 255, 267, 280,
    290, 301, 307, 317
Intestinal flora, restoring, 332
Inula helenium. See Elecampane
Iodine, 188, 197, 224, 252, 256
Irish moss (*Chondrus crispus*), 252
Iris versicolor. See Blue flag
Irritable bowel syndrome, 205, 206
Irritation, 9–10
Isatis (*Isatis tinctoria*), 253
Itching, 198, 210, 277, 335, 336

J

Jābir ibn Hayyān, 76
Jamaican dogwood (*Piscidia erythrina, P. piscipula*), 94, 253–54
Jambul (*Syzygium cumini*), 254

Jars, 57
Jewel weed, 44
Jock itch, 310
Joints
    inflammation, 184
    pain, 174, 310, 314
Juglans cinerea. See Butternut bark
Juglans nigra. See Black walnut
Juicing, 44–45
Juniper berry (*Juniper spp.*), 254–55
    Stimulating Diuretic, 161–62
    UTI Formula, 162

K

Kava-kava (*Piper methysticum*), 255–56
    for baths and soaks, 336
    fluid extract of, 94
Kelp (*Laminaria spp.*), 256
Key herbs, 139–40
Khella (*Ammi visnaga*), 256–57
Kidney infections, 242, 316
Kidney stones, 239, 251, 259, 265, 309, 312
Kudzu (*Pueraria lobata, P. thunbergiana*), 257

L

Labor
    inducing, 190, 219
    preparing for, 336
Lactation, 175, 189, 231, 265
Lady's mantle (*Alchemilla vulgaris*), 257–58
Laminaria spp. See Kelp
Larrea tridentata. See Chaparral
Laryngitis, 215, 298
Lavender (*Lavandula officinalis, L. angustifolia*), 258
    for baths and soaks, 336, 338, 339
    for ear drops, 113
    for enemas, 332
Laxatives, 52, 154, 196, 200, 226, 233, 274, 289,
    301, 303, 313, 314
Leaky gut, 232, 257
Leaves
    drying, 39–40
    harvesting, 39
Lemon (*Citrus limon*), 113, 259
Lemon balm (*Melissa officinalis*), 259–60
    David Winston's SAD Formula, 153
    Soxhlet extract of, 101
Lentinula edodes. See Shiitake
Leonurus cardiaca. See Motherwort

Mountain Rose Herbs, 344, 346
Mouthwashes, 112
    Antiseptic Mouthwash, 149
Mucilage, 52
Mucilants, 7–8
Muira puama (*Ptychopetalum olacoides*), 269
Mullein (*Verbascum spp.*), 270
    for ear drops, 113
    Garlic-Mullein Ear Oil, 164
    Herbal Cough Syrup (Moistening), 156
    oil extract of, 104
Muscles
    pain, 174, 257, 310
    sore, 239, 297, 335
Myrica cerifera. See Bayberry
Myrrh (*Commiphora molmol, C. myrrha*), 270–71
    Antiseptic Gargle, 148–49
    Antiseptic Mouthwash, 149
    for mouthwashes and gargles, 112
    for tooth powders, 112

N

Nausea, 236
Neck pain, 257
Neem (*Azadirachta indica*), 271
Nepeta cataria. See Catnip
Nerve Formula, 160
Nettle (*Urtica dioica*), 272–73
    Antiallergy Formula, 148
    Herbal Mineral Tonic, 157–58
    Soothing Diuretic, 161
Neuralgia, 192, 253, 322, 329
Night blooming cereus (*Selenicereus grandiflorus*), 273
Night sweats, 282, 298
Night vision, 183
Nopal. *See* Prickly pear cactus
Nut Butter Balls, Herbal, 51
Nymphaea odorata. See White pond lily

O

Oak. *See* White oak
Oat (*Avena sativa*), 274–75
Ocimum sanctum. See Holy basil
Ocotillo (*Fouquieria splendens*), 275
Oil extractions, 26, 103–6
Ointments, 44, 106–7
Olive (*Olea europaea*), 275–76
Omura, Yoshiaki, 211

Oplopanax horridus. See Devil's club
Opuntia ficus-indica. See Prickly pear cactus
Opuntia streptacantha. See Prickly pear cactus
Orange peel (*Citrus sinensis*), 276
    Balanced Bitters, 150
Oregano (*Origanum vulgare*), 276–77, 340
Oregon grape (*Berberis repens, B. aquifolium*), 277–78
    for baths and soaks, 336, 339
    for enemas, 332
    for suppositories and boluses, 111
Origanum vulgare. See Oregano
Osha (*Ligusticum porteri*), 278
Osteoarthritis, 194, 306
Ovarian pain, 190, 322

P

Paeonia lactiflora. See Peony
Pain, 201, 218, 235, 253, 266, 294, 307, 315, 317, 322–23, 331
    Pain Formula, 160
    Pain-Relieving Liniment, 165–66
Palmaria palmata. See Dulse
Palsy, 192
Panax ginseng. See Ginseng, Asian or Korean
Panax notoginseng. See Tienchi ginseng
Panax quinquefolius. See Ginseng, American
Panic attacks, 235
Papaya (*Carica papaya*), 278–79
Paracelsus, 77
Paralysis, 269
Parasites, 154, 173, 184, 209, 213, 291, 309, 310, 325, 332
Parsley (*Petroselinum crispum*), 44, 279
Partridge berry (*Mitchella repens*), 279–80
Passionflower (*Passiflora incarnata, P. quadrangularis*), 94, 280–81
Pastes, 44
Pau d'arco (*Tabebuia spp., Tecoma ochracea*), 281
    Antifungal Formula, 148
    for douches, 335
    for enemas, 332
Paullinia cupana. See Guarana
Paullinia sorbilis. See Guarana
Pausinystalia johimbe. See Yohimbe
Pelvic inflammatory disease, 242
Pelvic steams, 340
Pennyroyal (*Mentha pulegium*), 282
Peony (*Paeonia lactiflora*), 282–83
Peppermint (*Mentha × piperita*), 112, 283

Roots
 drying, 41
 harvesting, 37, 40–41
Rose (*Rosa spp.*), 295–96
 for baths and soaks, 336
 Rose Water Lotion, 166
Rosemary (*Rosmarinus officinalis*), 296, 340
Rubus fruticosus. See Blackberry
Rumex acetosella. See Sheep sorrel
Rumex crispus. See Yellow dock
Ruscus aculeatus. See Butcher's broom

S

Sabal serrulata. See Saw palmetto
Safflower (*Carthamus tinctorius*), 297
Saffron (*Crocus sativus*), 297
Sage (*Salvia officinalis*), 112, 298
St. John's wort (*Hypericum perforatum*), 307–8
 David Winston's SAD Formula, 153
 for ear drops, 113
 oil extract of, 104
Salicin, 266, 322
Salix spp. See Willow
Salt, processing with, 120
Salves, 106–7
 Basic Healing Salve, 162–63
Sand heating, 121
Sanguinaria canadensis. See Bloodroot
Sap, harvesting, 41–42
Sarsaparilla (*Smilax spp.*), 298–99
Saw palmetto (*Sabal serrulata, Serenoa serrulata*),
 299–300
Scabies, 189
Scales, 60
Scar prevention, 241
Schisandra (*Schisandra chinensis*), 300
Sciatica, 288
Scullcap (*Scutellaria lateriflora*), 301
 Happy Formula, 155
 Nerve Formula, 160
Seasonal affective disorder (SAD), 153
Seeds
 drying, 40
 harvesting, 40
Seizures, 180, 268
Selenicereus grandiflorus. See Night blooming
 cereus
Senna (*Cassia senna, Senna alexandrina*), 301–2
Serenoa serrulata. See Saw palmetto
Sexual dysfunction, 248, 264, 269, 312

Shatavari (*Asparagus racemosus*), 302
Sheep sorrel (*Rumex acetosella*), 302–3
Shepherd's purse (*Capsella bursa-pastoris*), 303
Shiitake (*Lentinula edodes*), 304
Shingles, 259, 308
Shock, 203, 290
Shook, Edward, 79
Silk tree. *See* Mimosa
Silybum marianum. See Milk thistle
Silymarin, 177
Sima Qian, 75
Sinus congestion, 148, 311, 314
 Herbal Sinus Snuff, 165
Sinus infections, 165, 173
Sitz baths, 336, 341
Skin. *See also individual skin conditions*
 cancer, 189
 dry, 165, 200
 eruptions, 272, 335
 irritations, 172, 210
 pores, cleansing, 336
Skullcap. *See* Scullcap
Skunk cabbage (*Symplocarpus foetidus*), 304–5
Slippery elm (*Ulmus rubra*), 52, 305
 for mouthwashes and gargles, 112
 for plasters and poultices, 110
Smilax spp. See Sarsaparilla
Smoking, 176
Snake bites, 44
Snuffs, 112
 Herbal Sinus Snuff, 165
Soaks, 130, 335–36, 340
Solidago canadensis. See Goldenrod
Solidago virgaurea. See Goldenrod
Solomon's seal (*Polygonatum multiflorum*), 306
 Compound Wine of Solomon's Seal, 152
 Inflammation Formula, 159
Solubility, 56
Solvents
 choosing, 61–62, 63
 definition of, 22, 56
 weights of, 64
Soothing Diuretic, 161
Soxhlet extraction, 94–101
Spasms, 149, 332, 340
Spatulas, rubber, 57
Spearmint, 101, 112
Spikenard (*Aralia racemosa*), 306–7
Spilanthes (*Spilanthes acmella*), 307
Sprains, 174, 263, 328
Squaw vine. *See* Partridge berry

About the Authors

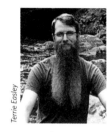

Terrie Easley

Thomas Easley is founder of the Eclectic School of Herbal Medicine. He is a clinical herbalist and professional member of the American Herbalists Guild. Easley integrates modern science and the deep and rich tradition of Western herbalism into a unified and systematic approach to health and healing. Easley emphasizes foods as primary medicine and uses intensive diets as well as stress reduction techniques, nutritional supplements, exercise and herbs to help people achieve their health goals. His approach draws on Traditional Western Herbalism, Clinical Nutrition, Functional Medicine, and his extensive clinical experience, which spans fifteen years of full-time practice and over 15,000 clients.

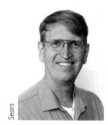

Sears

Steven Horne is a professional member and former president of the American Herbalists Guild and a professional member of the International Iridology Practioner's Association, having also served on the board of directors of both organizations. He has spoken at numerous conventions and conferences and has helped to start four different herbal companies, giving him extensive practical experience in formulating and manufacturing herbal extracts. Horne maintains a part-time consulting practice, working one-on-one with clients to help them resolve their health problems.

About North Atlantic Books

North Atlantic Books (NAB) is an independent, nonprofit publisher committed to a bold exploration of the relationships between mind, body, spirit, and nature. Founded in 1974, NAB aims to nurture a holistic view of the arts, sciences, humanities, and healing. To make a donation or to learn more about our books, authors, events, and newsletter, please visit www.northatlanticbooks.com.